FACTS AND COMPARISONS

A Wolters Kluwer Company
St. Louis

ODF

OPHTHALMIC DRUG FACTS

2002

THE UPJOHN COMPANY

U08FN9

Ophthalmic Drug Facts®

© Facts and Comparisons, 2002

All rights reserved. No part of this publication may be reproduced or transmitted in any form or by any means, electronic or mechanical, including photocopy, recording, or any information storage data base or retrieval system, or be put into a computer, without prior permission in writing from Facts and Comparisons®, the publisher.

Adapted from *Drug Facts and Comparisons®* loose-leaf drug information service.

ISBN 1-57439-113-5

Printed in the United States of America

The information contained in this publication is intended to supplement the knowledge of health care professionals regarding ophthalmic drug information. This information is advisory only and is not intended to replace sound clinical judgment or individualized patient care in the delivery of healthcare services. Facts and Comparisons® disclaims all warranties, whether expressed or implied, including any warranty as to the quality, accuracy or suitability of this information for any particular purpose.

Published by
Facts and Comparisons®
A Wolters Kluwer Company
111 West Port Plaza, Suite 300
St. Louis, Missouri 63146-3098
www.factsandcomparisons.com
Phone: 314/216-2100 • 800/223-0554
Fax: 314/878-5563

Ophthalmic Drug Facts Editorial Panel:

Jimmy D. Bartlett, OD, DOS
Professor of Optometry,
School of Optometry
Professor of Pharmacology
School of Medicine
University of Alabama at Birmingham
Birmingham, Alabama

Richard G. Fiscella, RPh, MPH
Clinical Associate Professor
Department of Pharmacy Practice
University of Illinois at Chicago
Chicago, Illinois

Dr. Edward Bennett
Associate Professor
Co-Chief, Contact Lens Service
School of Optometry
University of Missouri – St. Louis
St. Louis, Missouri

Siret D. Jaanus, PhD
Professor of Pharmacology
Southern California College of Optometry
Fullerton, California

J. James Rowsey, MD
Saint Luke's Cataract and Laser Institute
Tarpon Springs, Florida

Thom J. Zimmerman, MD, PhD
Chairman of Department of
  Ophthalmology and Visual Sciences
Professor of Pharmacology & Toxicology
University of Louisville
Louisville, Kentucky

Facts and Comparisons Editorial Advisory Panel:

Dennis J. Cada, PharmD, FASHP
Executive Editor, The Formulary, Hospital Pharmacy

Timothy R. Covington, PharmD, MS
Anthony and Marianne Bruno Professor of Pharmacy
Director, Managed Care Institute
School of Pharmacy, Samford University

Daniel A. Hussar, PhD
Remington Professor of Pharmacy
University of the Sciences in Philadelphia

Louis Lasagna, MD
Chairman and Adjunct Scholar
Tufts Center for the Study of Drug Development

James R. Selevan, BSEE, MD
Executive Vice President and
Chief Technology Officer
Monarch Healthcare

Richard W. Sloan, MD, RPh
Chairman and Residency Program Director
Department of Family Practice
York Hospital
Clinical Associate Professor
Pennsylvania State University

David S. Tatro, PharmD
Drug Information Analyst
San Carlos, California

Thomas L. Whitsett, MD
Professor of Medicine and Pharmacology
Director, Clinical Pharmacology Program
University of Oklahoma Health Sciences Center

Facts and Comparisons Staff:

Steven K. Hebel, RPh
president and CEO

Kenneth H. Killion
publisher

Bernie R. Olin, PharmD
director, drug information

Teri Hines Burnham
senior managing editor

Shephali A. Graf
managing editor

Jill A. Snitker
associate editor

Juanito R. Baladad, Jr.
Angela J. Schwalm
assistant editors

Beverly A. Donnell
senior composition specialist

Susan L. Polcyn
production and manufacturing manager

Robert E. Brown
director, sales and marketing

TABLE OF CONTENTS

Preface ix

Introduction xi

Chapter

1. **Dosage Forms and Routes of Administration** 1

2. **Ophthalmic Dyes** 13

3. **Local Anesthetics** 25

4. **Mydriatics and Cycloplegics** 39

5. **Antiallergy and Decongestant Agents** 57

6. **Anti-inflammatory Agents** 85

7. **Artificial Tear Solutions and Ocular Lubricants** 99

8. **Anti-infective Agents** 111

9. **Agents for Glaucoma** 179

10. **Hyperosmotic Agents** 251

11. **Surgical Adjuncts** 263

12.	Nonsurgical Adjuncts	289
13.	Contact Lens Care	299
14.	Extemporaneous Preparations	323
15.	Systemic Drugs Affecting the Eye	331
16.	Systemic Medications Used for Ocular Conditions	339
17.	Drugs with Off-labeled Ophthalmic Uses	347
18.	Orphan and Investigational Drugs	353

American Optometric Association Clinical Practice Guidelines ... 363

Excipient Glossary ... 367

Manufacturer Index ... 371

Chapter Summary Tables ... 377

Index ... 421

Editor's Preface

The mission of *Ophthalmic Drug Facts* is to provide reliable and objective ophthalmic drug information and facilitate therapeutic decision making. This book is intended to promote efficient, quality eye health care. Although general information is available for ophthalmic drugs, there are very few sources that provide comparative drug and drug product information in a concise format; none is as comprehensive.

Ophthalmic Drug Facts was conceived and developed through a team approach and will be of value to both the student and eyecare practitioner. Ophthalmologists, optometrists, and opticians should find this text particularly valuable in their daily practices.

Ophthalmic Drug Facts provides a broad range of information including pharmacologic and pharmacokinetic information on drug entities, commercial product information, and specific formulation availability. The text is arranged in a pharmacotherapeutic format, with emphasis on drug action and current product availability rather than on pathophysiology of disease states.

Ophthalmic Drug Facts is a comprehensive ophthalmic drug information resource. Detailed information on specific entities is included as well as many drug combinations. There is also a comprehensive section of contact lens products and extemporaneous preparations. Selected bibliographies are provided for all chapters. In addition, *Ophthalmic Drug Facts* includes valuable information on:

- Systemic medications for ocular conditions
- Systemic drugs affecting the eye
- Off-labeled uses for FDA-approved drugs
- Orphan ophthalmic agents and investigational drugs
- Selected Clinical Practice Guidelines of the American Optometric Association
- Excipient glossary
- Ophthalmic product manufacturer index
- Extemporaneous preparations

New information of importance in the *2002 Edition* includes: Three glaucoma agents, Brimonidine Tartrate (*Alphagan P*), bimatoprost (*Lumigan*), and Travoprost (*Travatan*).

We hope the reader finds this a valuable guide in ophthalmic drug product selection and use. As any practitioner is aware, ophthalmic practice is constantly adapting to incorporate the latest information. We intend to continue the effort with future editions; therefore, your comments, criticisms, and suggestions are always welcome.

Jimmy D. Bartlett, OD, DOS
Richard G. Fiscella, RPh, MPH
Edward S. Bennett, OD, MSEd
Siret D. Jaanus, PhD
J. James Rowsey, MD
Thom J. Zimmerman, MD, PhD

INTRODUCTION

Ophthalmic Drug Facts is a comprehensive ophthalmic drug information compendium. The unique format is designed to facilitate comparisons between drugs. To enable the reader to quickly locate needed information, it has been organized by:

- Therapeutic drug class
- Table of contents
- Chapter summary tables
- Comprehensive alphabetical index
- Extensive cross-referencing

The following pages explain the organization and contents of *Ophthalmic Drug Facts* in detail. All readers are urged to review this information to ensure efficient and effective use of *Ophthalmic Drug Facts*.

◆ Editorial Policy

Accurate, unbiased information; concise, standardized presentation; comparative, objective format; and timely delivery are the principal editorial guidelines governing *Ophthalmic Drug Facts*. Review of FDA-approved product labeling, hundreds of journal articles, textbooks, policies, and recommendations from many authoritative and official groups form the base of evaluation of information for *Ophthalmic Drug Facts*. FDA-approved indications and dosage recommendations are included. In addition, other established or potential uses are discussed and are designated as *"Off-labeled Uses."*

Most of the products listed are protected by letters of patent and their names are trademarked and registered by the firm whose name appears with the product. Identification of the product distributor is given in parentheses next to the brand name. The distributor may or may not be the actual manufacturer or fabricator of the final dosage form. Listing of specific products is an indication only of availability on the market and does not constitute an endorsement or recommendation.

Products that contain identical amounts of active ingredients are listed together for comparison as an aid in product selection. Drug product interchange is regulated by state laws; listing of products together does not imply that they are therapeutically equivalent or legally interchangeable. Caution is particularly advised when comparing sustained release, timed release, or repeat action dosage forms.

◆ Editorial Panel

The Editorial Panel for *Ophthalmic Drug Facts* is an interdisciplinary group of established, respected, and renowned clinicians and researchers. The panel includes recognized experts in the fields of ocular pharmacology, therapeutics, and drug information. These experts contribute the introductory material, review monographs, and provide direction for *Ophthalmic Drug Facts.*

The *Drug Facts and Comparisons* Editorial Advisory Panel consists of a very distinguished group of physicians, pharmacologists, and pharmacists. This panel reviews monographs and provides editorial direction for the entire Facts and Comparisons database.

◆ Organization

Information in *Ophthalmic Drug Facts* is organized by therapeutic use. Twelve chapters are divided into groups and subgroups to facilitate comparisons of drugs and drug products with similar uses. The remaining chapters provide information on chapter summary tables, ophthalmic dosage forms and routes of administration, nonsurgical adjuncts, contact lens care, systemic drugs affecting the eye, extemporaneous preparations, systemic medications used for ocular conditions, drugs with unlabeled ophthalmic uses, investigational and orphan drugs, and selected American Optometric Association Clinical Practice Guidelines.

Products most similar in content or use are listed together. This format of presenting the facts makes it easy to make comparisons of identical, similar, or related products. Because drugs are listed by use, some drugs may be listed in more than one section of the book.

◆ Index

The alphabetical index includes page references for drugs by their generic name, brand or trade name (in italics), and therapeutic group names. Additionally, many synonyms, pharmacological actions, and therapeutic uses for agents are included.

◆ Chapter Introductions

The chapter introductions provide information about the drugs in each therapeutic class, including general treatment guidelines. A selected bibliography located at the end of each chapter introduction provides additional sources of information.

◆ Drug Monographs

Prescribing information is presented in comprehensive drug monographs. General information on a group of closely related drugs may be presented in a group monograph. Specific information relating to a particular drug is presented in an individual monograph under the generic name of the drug. All monographs are divided into sections identified with bold titles for ease in locating the desired information.

Actions: Provides a brief summary of the known pharmacologic and pharmacokinetic properties.

Indications: All FDA-approved indications or uses are listed. When available, drug monographs also include "Off-labeled Uses." These include investigational uses for drugs and uses not yet approved by the FDA.

Contraindications: Specifies those conditions in which the drug should NOT be used.

Warnings and Precautions: Lists conditions in which use of the drug may be hazardous, precautions to observe, and parameters to monitor during therapy.

Drug Interactions: A brief summary of documented, clinically significant drug-drug, drug-food, and drug-lab test interactions is provided.

Adverse Reactions: Reported adverse reactions are presented. Incidence data on adverse effects are included when available.

Overdosage: Clinical manifestations of toxicity and treatment of overdosage are given for most agents.

Patient Information: Provides the essential information to be communicated to the patient by the health professional to allow the patient to safely and effectively administer the medication.

Administration and Dosage: Dosage ranges and administration methods are presented.

◆ Charts and Tables

Charts and tables are included in many monographs to make drug-drug comparisons easier. Examples of tables include: Pharmacokinetics (onset, peak and duration of action), routes of administration, dosage ranges, and adverse reactions.

◆ Special Features

Contact Lens Care: Chapter 13 provides guidelines and product information for soft and rigid gas permeable contact lens care.

Extemporaneous Preparations: Chapter 14 provides guidelines for the use and preparation of extemporaneous compounding of ophthalmic solutions.

Systemic Drugs Affecting the Eye: Chapter 15 discusses the effects systemic drugs have on ocular structures and functions.

Systemic Medications Used for Ocular Conditions: Chapter 16 discusses systemic medications and their uses and dosing in ocular conditions.

Drugs with Off-labeled Ophthalmic Uses: Chapter 17 discusses FDA-approved drugs that are being used for off-labeled ophthalmic purposes.

Orphan Drugs: Chapter 18 briefly describes Orphan Drug legislation and includes a table that provides generic name, trade name, indication, and manufacturer information on Orphan Drugs for ophthalmic conditions.

Investigational New Drugs: Chapter 18 also outlines the FDA drug approval process and includes a table that provides generic name, trade name (if available), therapeutic class or use, and manufacturer information for ophthalmic drugs on the horizon.

American Optometric Association Clinical Practice Guidelines: Three of the most relevant guidelines for the practicing eye care professional and student are reprinted in this appendix.

Excipient Glossary: This glossary lists pharmaceutical excipients found in ophthalmic products. The functions and strengths of these adjuncts are briefly described.

Manufacturer Index: This index provides the unique manufacturer/labeler codes found in the National Drug Code (NDC) numbers, as well as the addresses and phone numbers of the manufacturers and distributors of ophthalmic products listed in *Ophthalmic Drug Facts.*

♦ Product Listings

Individual products are listed following each monograph. The format and components of the product listings are discussed below and illustrated on the following page.

1. **Chapter title** is located at the top of the right-hand page.

2. **Generic titles** appear at the beginning of general drug monographs and individual drug monographs.

3. **Cross references** to the appropriate drug monograph appear for complete prescribing information.

4. **Distribution status** of products is indicated as *Rx* or *otc*.

5. **Identical brand name products** are listed in alphabetical order. Combination products are listed in tables to facilitate comparisons. Products most similar in formulation are listed next to each other.

6. **Products are grouped** by dosage form or strength.

7. **Package sizes** are given for all dosage forms and strengths of each product.

8. **Products available by their generic name** from multiple sources are indicated as available from (Various) distributors. Selected multiple-source distributors and manufacturers are provided. The list of distributors and manufacturers is intended to provide an example and is not an attempt to be comprehensive.

9. **Distributor's name** is given in parentheses next to the product name.

MYDRIATICS AND CYCLOPLEGICS 53

ATROPINE SULFATE

For complete prescribing information, refer to the Cycloplegic Mydriatrics group monograph.

Indications:

Mydriasis/Cycloplegia: For cycloplegic refraction or pupil dilation in acute inflammatory conditions of iris and uveal tract.

Administration and Dosage:

Solution:

　Adults - Uveitis – Instill 1 or 2 drops into the eye(s) up to 4 times daily.

　Children - Uveitis – Instill 1 or 2 drops of 0.5% solution into the eye(s) up to 3 times daily.

　Refraction – Instill 1 or 2 drops of 0.5% solution into the eye(s) twice daily for 1 to 3 days before examination.

Ointment: Apply a small amount in the conjunctival sac up to 3 times daily.

Compress the lacrimal sac by digital pressure during and for 2 to 3 minutes after instillation.

Individuals with heavily pigmented irides may require larger doses.

Storage: Keep away from heat.

Rx	**Atropine Sulfate Ophthalmic** (Various, eg, Bausch & Lomb, Fougera)	Ointment: 1%	In 3.5 and UD 1 g.
Rx	**Isopto Atropine** (Alcon)	Solution: 0.5%	In 5 mL Drop-Tainers.[1]
Rx	**Atropine Sulfate** (Various, eg, Alcon, Bausch & Lomb, Fougera, Ivax)	Solution: 1%	In 2, 5 and 15 mL and UD 1 mL.
Rx	**Atropine Care** (Akorn)		In 2, 5 and 15 mL.[2]
Rx	**Atropisol** (Novartis)		In 1 mL Dropperettes.[3]
Rx	**Isopto Atropine** (Alcon)		In 5 and 15 mL Drop-Tainers.[1]

[1] With 0.01% benzalkonium chloride, 0.5% hydroxypropyl methylcellulose, boric acid.
[2] With 0.01% benzalkonium chloride, hydroxypropyl methylcellulose, boric acid.
[3] With benzalkonium chloride, EDTA, boric acid.

Dosage Forms and Routes Of Administration

For ophthalmic drugs to be effective, they must reach ocular tissues in relatively high concentrations. Depending on the specific diagnostic or therapeutic objective, ophthalmic drugs may be delivered to the eye through various routes of administration, including the following:

- Topical
- Oral
- Parenteral
- Periocular
- Intracameral
- Intravitreal

TOPICAL ADMINISTRATION

Topical application is the most common route of administration for ophthalmic drugs. Advantages of topical application are convenience, simplicity, noninvasive nature, and the ability of the patient to self-administer. Because of blood and aqueous losses of drug, topical medications do not typically penetrate in useful concentrations to posterior ocular structures and usually are of no therapeutic benefit for diseases of the retina, optic nerve, and other posterior segment structures.

Inactive Ingredients

The following inactive agents may be present in ophthalmic products:

Preservatives: Destroy or inhibit multiplication of microorganisms introduced into the product by accident. Each preservative can cause epithelial toxicity, especially with more than 12 drops instilled per day.

benzalkonium chloride
benzethonium chloride
cetylpyridinium chloride
chlorobutanol
EDTA

mercurial preservatives
 (eg, phenylmercuric
 nitrate, phenylmercuric
 acetate, thimerosal)
methyl/propylparabens

phenylethyl alcohol
sodium benzoate
sodium propionate
sorbic acid

OPHTHALMIC DRUG FACTS

Viscosity-Increasing Agents: Slow drainage of the product from the eye, increasing retention time of the active drug. Increased bioavailability may result.

carboxymethylcellulose sodium
dextran 70
gelatin
glycerin
hydroxyethyl cellulose

hydroxypropyl methylcellulose
methylcellulose
PEG
poloxamer 407

polysorbate 80
propylene glycol
polyvinyl alcohol
polyvinylpyrrolidone (povidone)

Antioxidants: Prevent or delay deterioration of products by oxygen in the air.

EDTA
sodium bisulfite

sodium metabisulfite
sodium thiosulfate

thiourea

Wetting Agents: Reduce surface tension, allowing the drug solution to spread.

polysorbate 20 and 80

poloxamer 282

tyloxapol

Buffers: Help maintain ophthalmic products in the range of pH 6 to 8, which is the comfortable range for ophthalmic instillation.

acetic acid
boric acid
hydrochloric acid
phosphoric acid
potassium bicarbonate
potassium borate

potassium carbonate
potassium citrate
potassium phosphate
potassium tetraborate
sodium acetate
sodium bicarbonate

sodium biphosphate
sodium borate
sodium carbonate
sodium citrate
sodium hydroxide
sodium phosphate

Tonicity Agents: These agents help the ophthalmic product solutions to be isotonic with the preocular tear film. Products in the sodium chloride equivalence range of 0.9% ± 0.2% are considered isotonic and will help prevent ocular irritation and tissue damage. A range of 0.6% to 1.8% is usually comfortable for ophthalmic use.

buffers
dextran 40 and 70
dextrose

glycerin
potassium chloride

propylene glycol
sodium chloride

Packaging Standards

To help reduce confusion in labeling and identification of various topical ocular medications, drug packaging standards have been proposed. The standard colors for drug labels and bottle caps include the following:

Topical Ophthalmic Drug Packaging Standards	
Therapeutic class	Proposed color
Beta blockers	Yellow, blue, or both
Mydriatics and cycloplegics	Red
Miotics	Green
Nonsteroidal anti-inflammatory drugs	Grey
Anti-infectives	Brown, tan
Carbonic anhydrase inhibitors	Orange

Medications

Solutions and Suspensions: Most topical ocular preparations are commercially available as solutions or suspensions that are applied directly to the eye from the bottle, which serves as the eye dropper. Avoid touching the dropper tip to the eye because

DOSAGE FORMS AND ROUTES OF ADMINISTRATION

this can lead to contamination of the medication and may cause ocular injury. Resuspend suspensions (notably, many ocular steroids) by shaking to provide an accurate dosage of drug.

Betaxolol 0.25% (*Betoptic S*) and rimexolone (*Vexol*) are classified by the FDA as suspensions, but are much less viscous products suspended in carbonol gels than is pilocarpine (*Pilopine HS*). A drop can be administered with less concern for prolonged blurry vision. Although *Betoptic S* and *Vexol* are classified technically as suspensions, little shaking is required to suspend or resuspend these agents.

RECOMMENDED PROCEDURES FOR ADMINISTRATION OF SOLUTIONS AND SUSPENSIONS
1. Wash hands thoroughly before administration.
2. Tilt head backward or lie down and gaze upward.
3. Gently grasp lower eyelid below eyelashes and pull the eyelid away from the eye to form a pouch.
4. Place dropper directly over eye. Avoid contact of the dropper with the eye, finger, or any surface. Keep the tip 1 inch from the eye to avoid contact.
5. Look upward just before applying a drop.
6. Release the lid slowly and close eyes gently.
7. With eyes closed, apply gentle pressure with fingers to the inside corner of the eye for 2 to 3 minutes (see Figure 1). This retards drainage of the solution from the intended area.
8. Do not rinse the dropper.
9. Do not use eye drops that have changed color or contain a precipitate.
10. If > 1 type of ophthalmic drop is used, wait ≥ 5 minutes before administering the second agent.

Solutions and Suspensions - Drops

Nasolacrimal Occlusion

Ointments: The primary purpose for an ophthalmic ointment vehicle is to prolong drug contact time with the external ocular surface. This is particularly useful for treating children, who may "cry out" topically applied solutions, and for medicating ocular injuries, such as corneal abrasions, when the eye is to be patched. Administer solutions before ointments. Ointments may prevent entry of subsequent drops.

RECOMMENDED PROCEDURES FOR ADMINISTRATION OF OINTMENTS
1. Wash hands thoroughly before administration.
2. Tilt head backward or lie down and gaze upward.
3. Gently pull down the lower lid to form a pouch.
4. Place 0.25 to 0.5 inch of ointment with a sweeping motion inside the lower lid by squeezing the tube gently, and slowly release the eyelid.
5. Close the eye for 1 to 2 minutes.
6. Temporary blurring of vision may occur. Avoid activities requiring visual acuity until blurring clears.
7. Remove excessive ointment around the eye or ointment tube tip with a tissue.
8. If using > 1 kind of ointment, wait ≈ 10 minutes before applying the second agent.

DOSAGE FORMS AND ROUTES OF ADMINISTRATION

Ointments

- *Gels:* Ophthalmic gels are similar in viscosity and clinical usage to ophthalmic ointments. Pilocarpine (*Pilopine HS*) is formulated in carbopol gel. *Pilopine HS* is more viscous than a traditional gel and is applied at bedtime to avoid blurred vision. Timolol maleate (*Timoptic XE*) is a slightly viscous solution that forms a gel when it makes contact with the cations in the preocular tear fluid. This formulation provides a prolonged contact time for the timolol within the precorneal tear film. A limited number of gels are available as artificial tear products for treatment of dry eye. These products (eg, *GenTeal Gel*) make treatment more convenient by reducing required dosing frequency.

Sprays: Some practitioners use mydriatics or cycloplegics, alone or in combination, administered as a spray to the eye to dilate the pupil or for cycloplegic examination. This is most often used for pediatric patients, and the solution is administered using a sterile perfume atomizer or plastic spray bottle.

Lid Scrubs: Commercially available eyelid cleansers, antibiotic solutions, or ointments can be applied directly to the lid margin for the treatment of blepharitis. This is best accomplished by applying the medication to the end of a cotton-tipped applicator and then scrubbing the eyelid margin several times daily. The gauze pads supplied with commercially available eyelid cleansers are also convenient.

Lid Scrub - Cotton-Tipped Applicator

Lid Scrub - Gauze

DOSAGE FORMS AND ROUTES OF ADMINISTRATION

Devices

Contact Lenses: Soft contact lenses can absorb water-soluble drugs and release them to the eye over prolonged periods of time. This has the clinical advantage of promoting sustained-release of solutions or suspensions that would otherwise be removed quickly from the external ocular tissues. Soft contact lenses as drug delivery devices are most often used in the management of dry eye disorders, but the technique is occasionally used for the treatment of ocular infections, including corneal ulcers.

Corneal Shields: Non-cross-linked, homogenized, porcine, or bovine scleral collagen shields are available. These devices are placed as a bandage on the cornea following surgery or injury, protecting and lubricating the cornea. Topical antibiotics have been used in conjunction with the shield to promote healing of corneal ulcers.

Cotton Pledgets: Small pieces of cotton can be saturated with ophthalmic solutions and placed in the conjunctival sac. These devices allow a prolonged ocular contact time with solutions that are normally administered topically into the eye. The clinical use of pledgets is usually reserved for the administration of mydriatic solutions such as cocaine or phenylephrine. This drug delivery method promotes maximum mydriasis in an attempt to break posterior synechiae or to dilate sluggish pupils.

Filter Paper Strips: Sodium fluorescein, lissamine green, and rose bengal dyes are commercially available as drug-impregnated filter paper strips. The strips help ensure sterility of sodium fluorescein which, when prepared in solution, can be easily contaminated with *Pseudomonas aeruginosa*. These dyes are used diagnostically to disclose corneal injuries, infections such as herpes simplex, and dry eye disorders.

Artificial Tear Inserts: A rod-shaped pellet of hydroxypropyl cellulose without preservative (*Lacrisert*) is inserted into the inferior conjunctival sac with a specially designed applicator. Following placement, the device absorbs fluid, swells, and then releases the nonmedicated polymer to the eye for up to 24 hours. The device is designed as a sustained-release artificial tear for the treatment of dry eye disorders.

Membrane-Bound Inserts: A membrane-controlled drug delivery system (*Ocusert*) delivers a constant quantity of pilocarpine to the eye for up to 1 week. Placed onto the bulbar conjunctiva under the upper or lower eyelid, it is a useful substitute for pilocarpine drops or gel in glaucoma patients who cannot comply with more frequent drug instillation or in patients with ocular or visual side effects from pilocarpine solutions.

GENERAL CONSIDERATIONS IN TOPICAL OPHTHALMIC DRUG THERAPY

Proper administration is essential to optimal therapeutic response. In many instances, health professionals may be too casual when instructing patients on proper use of ophthalmics. The administration technique used often determines drug safety and efficacy.

- ◆ The normal eye retains ≈ 10 mcL of fluid (adjusted for blinking). The average dropper delivers 25 to 50 mcL/drop. There is no value in instilling > 1 properly placed drop.
- ◆ Minimize systemic absorption of ophthalmic drops by compressing the canaliculus and lacrimal sacs for 3 to 5 minutes after instillation. This retards passage of drops via the nasolacrimal duct into areas of potential absorption, such as nasal and pharyngeal mucosa.
- ◆ Because of rapid lacrimal drainage and limited eye capacity, if multiple-drop therapy is indicated, the best interval between drops is 5 minutes. This ensures that the first drop is not flushed away by the second or that the second is not diluted by the first.
- ◆ Factors that may increase absorption from ophthalmic doseforms include lax eyelids of some patients, usually the elderly, which creates a greater reservoir for retention of drops, and hyperemic or diseased eyes.
- ◆ Eyecup use is discouraged because of risk of contamination and spreading disease.
- ◆ Ophthalmic suspensions mix with tears less rapidly and remain in the cul-de-sac longer than solutions.
- ◆ Ophthalmic ointments maintain contact between the drug and ocular tissues by slowing the clearance rate to as little as 0.5% per minute. Ophthalmic ointments provide maximum contact between drug and external ocular tissues.
- ◆ Ophthalmic ointments may impede delivery of other ophthalmic drugs to the affected side by serving as a barrier to contact.
- ◆ Ointments may blur vision during the waking hours. Use with caution in conditions where visual clarity is critical (eg, operating motor equipment, reading) or use at bedtime.
- ◆ Monitor expiration dates closely. Do not use outdated medication.
- ◆ Solutions and ointments are frequently misused. Do not assume that patients know how to maximize safe and effective use of these agents. Combine appropriate patient education and counseling with prescribing and dispensing of ophthalmics.

ORAL ADMINISTRATION

Although most ocular diseases respond to topical therapy, some disorders require systemic drug administration to achieve adequate therapeutic levels of the drug in ocular tissue. Oral administration of certain drugs may be the most effective route of drug delivery. Examples of commonly used oral medications include the following: Carbonic anhydrase inhibitors for the treatment of glaucoma, corticosteroids for Graves' ophthalmopathy, analgesics for the management of pain associated with ocular injury, antibiotic therapy of preseptal cellulitis, and antihistamine therapy for acute allergic angioneurotic edema of the eyelids.

PARENTERAL ADMINISTRATION

Intramuscular (IM) and intravenous (IV) injections are occasionally used for the treatment of ocular disorders. Hydroxocobalamin (vitamin B_{12}; [eg, *Hydro Cobex*]) and some antibiotics (eg, penicillin) may be administered through the IM route. The continuous IV infusion of various antibiotics may be required for the treatment of endophthalmitis and other severe ocular infections.

DOSAGE FORMS AND ROUTES OF ADMINISTRATION

PERIOCULAR/PERIBULBAR ADMINISTRATION

Drugs can be injected locally into the periocular tissues when higher concentrations of drugs are required than can be delivered to the eye by topical, oral, or parenteral administration. Periocular drug administration includes injections under the bulbar conjunctiva (subconjunctival), under Tenon's capsule (sub-Tenon's), and behind the globe itself (retrobulbar). Drugs most often delivered in this manner include corticosteroids and antibiotics. Local anesthetics are commonly administered via retrobulbar or peribulbar injection prior to cataract extraction and other intraocular surgical procedures.

INTRACAMERAL ADMINISTRATION

Although the term "intracameral" technically denotes injection of drug into the globe, contemporary usage of the term implies administering the drug directly into the anterior chamber of the eye. This is most commonly associated with cataract extraction, during which a viscoelastic substance is injected into the anterior chamber to protect the corneal endothelium or lidocaine is administered for anesthesia. Antibiotics are not routinely injected into the anterior chamber. This procedure is associated with a significant risk of complications as well as drug toxicity.

INTRAVITREAL ADMINISTRATION

The intravitreal injection of drugs is primarily reserved as a heroic effort to rescue eyes with severe acute intraocular inflammation or eyes that have failed to respond to more conservative therapy. Intravitreal antibiotics may be the treatment of choice for endophthalmitis. Intravitreal liquid silicone is used for the treatment of complicated retinal detachment. Intravitreal ganciclovir has been used with some success in treating cytomegalovirus retinitis in patients with acquired immunodeficiency syndrome (AIDS). A ganciclovir implant (*Vitrasert*) is available that delivers the antiviral agent continuously to the vitreous and retina for periods of 4 to 6 months.

Jimmy D. Bartlett, OD, DOS
University of Alabama at Birmingham

DOSAGE FORMS AND ROUTES OF ADMINISTRATION

For More Information

Bartlett JD, Jaanus SD, eds. Clinical Ocular Pharmacology, ed. 4. Boston: Butterworth-Heinemann, 2001.

Bartlett JD, Wesson MD, et al. Efficacy of a pediatric cycloplegic administered as a spray. *J Am Optom Assoc* 1993;64:617.

Feibel RM. Current concepts in retrobulbar anesthesia. *Surv Ophthalmol* 1985;30:102.

Fraunfelder FT. Drug-packaging standards for eye drop medications. *Arch Ophthalmol* 1988;106:1029.

Fraunfelder FT. Extraocular fluid dynamics: How best to apply topical ocular medication. *Trans Am Ophthalmol Soc* 1976;74:457.

Fraunfelder FT, Hanna C. Ophthalmic drug delivery systems. *Surv Ophthalmol* 1974;18:292.

Jain MR. Drug delivery through soft contact lenses. *Br J Ophthalmol* 1988;72:150.

Lamberts DW. Solid delivery devices. *Int Ophthalmol Clin* 1980;20:63.

MacKeen DL. Aqueous formulations and ointments. *Int Ophthalmol Clin* 1980;20:79.

Martin DF, Parks DJ, Mellow SD, et al. Treatment of cytomegalovirus retinitis with intraocular sustained-release ganciclovir implant. A randomized controlled clinical trial. *Arch Opthalmol* 1994;112:1531.

Reynolds LA, Closson RG, eds. Extemporaneous Ophthalmic Preparations. Vancouver, WA: Applied Therapeutics, 1993.

Robin JS, Ellis PP. Ophthalmic ointments. *Surv Ophthalmol* 1978;22:335.

Sharp J, Hanna C. Use of a spray to deliver drugs to the eye. *J Arkansas Med Soc* 1977;73:462.

Silbiger J, Stern GA. Evaluation of corneal collagen shields as a drug delivery device for the treatment of experimental *Pseudomonas* keratitis. *Ophthalmology* 1992;99:889.

Wesson MD, Bartlett JD, Swiatocha J, et al. Efficacy of a cycloplegic administered as a spray. *J Am Optom Assoc* 1993;64:637.

Zimmerman TJ, et al. Improving the therapeutic index of topically applied ocular drugs. *Arch Ophthalmol* 1984;102:551.

Zimmerman TJ, Sharir M, et al. Therapeutic index of pilocarpine, carbachol and timolol with nasolacrimal occlusion. *Am J Ophthalmol* 1992;114:1.

OPHTHALMIC DYES

Dyes are used for a variety of diagnostic ocular procedures. Ophthalmic dyes in current use include sodium fluorescein, fluorexon, rose bengal, lissamine green, and indocyanine green. Topical sodium fluorescein and rose bengal have proven valuable for assessment of ocular surface integrity, while IV fluorescein has proven useful for evaluating retinal vascular function. More recently, indocyanine green has greatly enhanced observation of the choroidal circulation.

FLUORESCEIN SODIUM

Fluorescein sodium is a yellow water-soluble dibasic acid dye of the xanthine series that produces an intense green fluorescent color in alkaline (pH > 5) solution. Fluorescein is used to demonstrate defects of corneal epithelium. It does not actually stain tissues, but is useful as an indicator dye. The normal precorneal tear film appears yellow or orange with fluorescein. The intact corneal epithelium resists penetration of water-soluble fluorescein and is not colored by it. Any break in the epithelial barrier permits rapid fluorescein penetration. Whether resulting from trauma, infection, or other causes, epithelial defects of the cornea appear bright green and are easily visualized. If epithelial loss is extensive, topical fluorescein will penetrate into the aqueous and is readily visible biomicroscopically as a green flare.

Fluorescein sodium exhibits a high degree of ionization at physiologic pH. Therefore, it does not penetrate the intact corneal epithelium or form a firm bond with vital tissue. When exposed to light, fluorescein absorbs certain wavelengths and emits fluorescent light of longer wavelength. Factors that can affect its fluorescence include its concentration, the pH of the solution, the presence of other substances, and the intensity and wavelength of the absorbed light. At pH 8, fluorescein reaches its maximum intensity.

Ophthalmic uses of fluorescein include applanation tonometry, detection of foreign bodies, fitting of rigid contact lenses, determination of tear breakup time, Seidel's test, fluorescein angiography, and vitreous fluorophotometry.

For topical ocular use, fluorescein may be administered as a solution or by fluorescein-impregnated filter paper strips (eg, *Fluorets*). Since fluorescein in solution is susceptible to bacterial contamination, multidose formulations are dispensed with a preservative such as chlorobutanol. For diagnostic purposes such as applanation tonometry, a local anesthetic is included in the formulation.

Fluorescein-impregnated filter paper strips are useful for routine office procedures such as contact lens fitting and lacrimal system evaluation. Bacterial contamination is minimized when the strips are stored in a dry state. When wetted with saline or an irrigating solution, the dye is released from the strip and can be applied to the eye by gently touching the conjunctiva.

IV fluorescein (fluorescein angiography) is used for detection of vascular abnormalities of the fundus. Following injection into the antecubital vein, the dye appears in the central retinal artery. Integrity of the retina and choroid may be determined.

Oral fluorescein can be administered by mixing fluorescein powder or several vials of 10% injectable fluorescein in a citrus drink over ice (see the Unlabeled Ophthalmic Uses chapter). Time of onset of maximal fluorescence is 45 to 60 minutes compared with seconds via the injectable route. Fasting enhances the serum concentration of the dye. Oral fluorescein can be used to study disorders characterized by late leakage of dye, such as cystoid macular edema, to study retinal vascular abnormalities in young diabetic patients, and to document retinal pigment epithelial detachment, central serous choroidopathy, and optic disc edema.

Topical application of fluorescein has been associated with minimum adverse effects. The most common side effect of IV use is nausea. The oral route appears to have the clinical advantage of less frequent side effects.

FLUOREXON

With a molecular size nearly twice that of fluorescein, fluorexon penetrates hydrophilic contact lenses at a much slower rate. Upon ocular instillation, it yields a pale, yellow-brown color. These properties make it useful as an adjunct in the fitting of soft contact lenses. However, the dye can stain hydrophilic lenses if significant amounts become trapped between the lens and cornea or if the dye remains in contact with the soft lens for ≥ 10 minutes. Fluorexon is not recommended for use with high-water content soft lenses since the possibility of discoloration is much greater and more difficult to reverse than with lower-water content lenses.

Fluorexon has a lower fluorescent intensity than fluorescein. For optimum fluorescence, a special yellow filter is recommended. The dye generally causes little or no discomfort when instilled on the eye. Because of its larger molecular size, it is a less effective stain for epithelial defects, erosions, and contact lens-induced effects than fluorescein. Like rose bengal, it will stain degenerated cells and mucus threads.

INDOCYANINE GREEN

Indocyanine green is a tricarbocyanine dye, available commercially under the trade name of *Cardio-Green*, and has been advocated for visualization of choroidal vessels with infrared absorption angiography. Toxic effects have not been associated with IV use of the dye when manufacturer's recommended dosage regimens have been followed.

ROSE BENGAL

An iodine derivative of fluorescein, rose bengal stains cells of the cornea and conjunctiva (including the nuclei and cell walls) a red color. More recent evidence indicates that this dye stains both normal and degenerated or dead cells. Staining will occur whenever there is poor protection of the surface epithelium by the preocular tear film. It appears that rose bengal is not a vital dye and that stained cells actually lose vitality upon exposure to the dye and undergo morphologic changes. It also will stain the mucus of the precorneal tear film. When applied from a moistened filter paper strip, this dye can aid in the evaluation of keratoconjunctivitis sicca, corneal abrasions, and detection of foreign bodies.

OPHTHALMIC DYES

Rose bengal can cause pronounced irritation and discomfort following instillation, particularly in more severely diseased eyes and with use of higher concentrations of dye. Rose bengal can stain eyelids, cheeks, fingers, and clothing in a concentration-dependent manner. Keeping the amount of dye at a minimum and irrigating the eye can help circumvent this problem.

LISSAMINE GREEN

Lissamine green stains the same structures of the eye as rose bengal, specifically degenerate cells, dead cells, and precipitated mucus a bluish-green color. The dye has been reported useful for assessing dry eye conditions and can be helpful in detecting recurrent corneal erosions and dendritic ulcers. The staining effect is easier to see than rose bengal in red, inflamed, or hemorrhagic eyes, and the effect of dye appears to last longer.

Instillation of lissamine green into the conjunctival sac is nonirritating to most patients, and no adverse effects or contraindications for its topical ocular use have been observed.

Siret D. Jaanus, PhD
Southern California College of Optometry

For More Information

Bartlett JD, Jaanus SD, eds. Clinical Ocular Pharmacology, ed. 4. Boston: Butterworth-Heinemann, 2001.

Berkow JW, Flower RW, Orth D, et al. Fluorescein and Indocyanine Green Angiography Technique and Interpretation, 2nd ed. American Academy of Optometry, San Francisco, 1997.

Brooks SE, Kaza V, Nakanura T, et al. Photo inactivation of herpes simplex virus by rose bengal and fluorescein. *Cornea* 1994;13:43.

Chodosh J, Dix RD, Howell RC, et al. Staining characteristics and antiviral activity of sulforhodamine B and lissamine green B. *Invest Ophthalmol Vis Sci* 1994;35:1046.

Dakryon Pharmaceuticals. Lissamine green colored ophthalmic demulcent. Product information, 1997.

Feenstra RPG, Tseng SCG. Comparison of fluorescein and rose bengal staining. *Arch Ophthalmol* 1992;99:605.

Hayashi K, et al. Indocyanine green angiography of central serous chorioretinopathy. *Int Ophthalmol Clin* 1986;9:37.

Kelley JS, Kincaid M. Retinal fluorography using oral fluorescein. *Arch Ophthalmol* 1979;97:2331.

Khurana AK, Chaudhary R, Ahluwalia BK, et al. Tear film profile in dry eye. *Acta Ophthamol* 1991;69:79-86.

Norn MS. Lissamine green. Vital staining of the cornea and conjunctiva. *Acta Ophthalmol* 1973;51:483.

Romanchuk KG. Fluorescein: Physiochemical factors affecting its fluorescence. *Surv Ophthalmol* 1982;26:269.

Yannuzzi LA, Slakter JS, Sorenson JA, et al. Digital indocyanine green videoangiography and choroidal neovascularization. *Retina* 1992;12:191.

Yannuzzi LA, Sorenson JA, Guyer DR, et al. Indocyanine green videoangiography: current status. *Eur J Opthalmol* 1994;4:69.

FLUORESCEIN SODIUM

Actions:

Pharmacology: Sodium fluorescein, a yellow water-soluble dibasic acid xanthine dye, produces an intense green fluorescent color in alkaline (pH > 5) solution. Fluorescein demonstrates defects of corneal epithelium. It does not stain tissues, but is a useful indicator dye. Normal precorneal tear film will appear yellow or orange. The intact corneal epithelium resists fluorescein penetration and is not colored. Any break in the epithelial barrier permits rapid penetration. Whether resulting from trauma, infection, or other causes, epithelial corneal defects appear bright green and are easily seen. If epithelial loss is extensive, topical fluorescein penetrates into the aqueous humor and is readily visible biomicroscopically as a green flare.

Indications:

Topical: In fitting contact lenses; in applanation tonometry; diagnosis and detection of corneal stippling, abrasions, ulcerations, herpetic lesions, foreign bodies (not epithelialized), contact lens pressure points; making lacrimal drainage test; wound leakage tests (Seidel's Test).

Injection: Diagnostic aid in ophthalmic angiography, including examination of the fundus; evaluation of the iris vasculature; distinction between viable and nonviable tissue; observation of the aqueous flow; differential diagnosis of malignant and nonmalignant tumors; determination of circulation time and adequacy.

Off-labeled use(s): Oral fluorography for diagnosis of retinal vascular diseases.

Contraindications:

Hypersensitivity to fluorescein or any other component of the product; do not use with soft contact lenses (lenses may become discolored).

Topical: Not for injection. Do not use in intraocular surgery.

Warnings:

Topical (drops): Discontinue if sensitivity develops. May stain soft contact lenses. Do not touch dropper tip to any surface, as this may contaminate the solution.

Extravasation: Avoid extravasation during injection. The high pH can result in severe local tissue damage. Complications have occurred from extravasation: Sloughing of skin, superficial phlebitis, SC granuloma, and toxic neuritis along the median curve in the antecubital area. Extravasation can cause severe pain in the arm for several hours. When significant extravasation occurs, discontinue injection and use conservative measures to treat damaged tissue and relieve pain (see Warnings).

Hypersensitivity: Exercise caution when administering to patients with a history of hypersensitivity, allergies, or asthma. If signs of sensitivity develop, discontinue use.

Pregnancy: Category C. Avoid parenteral fluorescein angiography during pregnancy, especially in the first trimester. There are no reports of fetal complications during pregnancy.

OPHTHALMIC DYES

17

Lactation: Fluorescein is excreted in breast milk. Use caution when administering to a nursing woman.

Children: Safety and efficacy for use in children have not been established.

Adverse Reactions:

Miscellaneous:

Injection – Nausea; headache; GI distress; vomiting; syncope; hypotension and other symptoms and signs of hypersensitivity; cardiac arrest; basilar artery ischemia; thrombophlebitis at injection site; severe shock; convulsions; death (rare); temporary yellowish skin discoloration. Hives, itching, bronchospasm, anaphylaxis, pyrexia, transient dyspnea, angioneurotic edema and slight dizziness may occur. A strong taste may develop with use. Urine becomes bright yellow. Skin discoloration fades in 6 to 12 hours, urine fluorescence in 24 to 36 hours. Extravasation at injection site causes intense pain at the site and dull aching pain in the injected arm (see Warnings).

Patient Information:

May cause strong taste with use.

May cause temporary yellowish discoloration of the skin. Urine will turn bright yellow. Discoloration of skin fades in 6 to 12 hours; urine fluorescence fades in 24 to 36 hours.

Soft contact lenses may become stained. Do not wear lenses while fluorescein is being used. Whenever fluorescein is used, flush the eyes with sterile normal saline solution and wait ≥ 1 hour before replacing the lenses.

Administration and Dosage:

Topical: To detect foreign bodies and corneal abrasions, instill 1 or 2 drops of 2% solution; allow a few seconds for staining. Wash out the excess with sterile irrigating solution.

Strips: Moisten the strip with sterile water. Place the moistened strip at the fornix in the lower cul-de-sac close to the punctum. For best results, the patient should close their lid tightly over the strip until the desired amount of staining is obtained. The patient should blink several times after application.

Applanation tonometry strips – Anesthetize the eyes. Retract the upper lid and touch the tip of the strip moistened with saline or ocular irrigating solution (eg, *Blinx*) to the bulbar conjunctiva on the temporal side until an adequate amount of stain is available for a clearly defined endpoint reading.

Injection: Inject the contents of the ampule or prefilled syringe rapidly into the antecubital vein *after taking precautions to avoid extravasation.* A syringe filled with fluorescein is attached to transparent tubing and a 25-gauge scalp vein needle for injection. Insert the needle and draw blood to the hub of the syringe so that a *small* air bubble separates the blood in the tubing from the fluorescein. With the room lights on, slowly inject the blood back into the vein while watching the skin over the needle tip. If the needle has extravasated, the patient's blood will bulge the skin, and the injection should be stopped before any fluorescein is injected. When assured that extravasation has not occurred, the room light may be turned off and the fluorescein injection

OPHTHALMIC DRUG FACTS

completed. Luminescence appears in the retina and choroidal vessels in 9 to 15 seconds and can be observed by standard viewing equipment.

If potential allergy is suspected, an intradermal skin test may be performed prior to IV administration (ie, 0.05 mL injected intradermally to be evaluated 30 to 60 minutes following injection).

In patients with inaccessible veins where early phases of an angiogram are not necessary, such as cystoid macular edema, 1 g fluorescein has been given orally. Ten to 15 minutes are usually required before evidence of dye appears in the fundus.

Adults – 500 to 750 mg injected rapidly into the antecubital vein.

Children – 7.5 mg/kg (3.5 mg/lb) injected rapidly into the antecubital vein.

Have 0.1% epinephrine IM or IV, an antihistamine, soluble steroid, aminophylline IV, and oxygen available.

Storage: Store at 8° to 30°C (46° to 86°F). Do not use if the solution contains a precipitate. Discard any unused solution. Keep out of the reach of children.

Rx	**AK-Fluor** (Akorn)	**Injection:** 10%	In 5 mL amps and vials.
Rx	**Fluorescite** (Alcon)		In 5 mL amps with syringes.
Rx	**AK-Fluor** (Akorn)	**Injection:** 25%	In 2 mL amps and vials.
Rx	**Fluorescite** (Alcon)		In 2 mL amps.
Rx	**Fluorescein Sodium** (Various, eg, Alcon)	**Solution:** 2%	In 15 mL.
Rx	**Ful-Glo** (Akorn)	**Strips:** 0.6 mg	In 300s.
Rx	**Fluorets** (Akorn)	**Strips:** 1 mg	In 100s.

FLUOREXON

Actions:

Pharmacology: Fluorexon is a large-molecular weight fluorescent solution for use as a diagnostic and fitting aid for patients with hydrogel (soft) contact lenses. Used with or without lens in place when fluorescein is contraindicated to avoid staining lenses. It may be used in both soft and hard lenses.

Indications:

Contact lens fitting aid: Assessment of proper fitting characteristics of hydrogel lenses. For quickly and accurately locating the optic zone in aphakic or low-plus lenses.

Evaluation of corneal integrity of patients wearing hydrogel contact lenses. In many instances, arcuate staining will show definite correlation with the edge of the optic zone, indicating improper bearing surfaces.

For use in place of sodium fluorescein when conducting the tear breakup time (BUT) test.

For conducting the applanation tonometry procedure without removing the lens.

OPHTHALMIC DYES

For locating the lathe-cut index markings (toric lenses). Use as directed for fitting contact lenses.

Contraindications:

Hypersensitivity to fluorescein sodium.

Warnings:

Contact lenses: When used with lenses with > 55% hydration, some color may remain on lens. Remove by washing repeatedly with washing solution approved for the lens. Rinse with saline or water. Any residual coloring will wash out with the tear flow when the lens is reinserted in the eye. With highly hydrated lenses, the amount of coloring picked up will vary with exposure. Avoid unnecessary delays in the examination procedure.

Precautions:

Hydrogen peroxide: Do not use hydrogen peroxide solutions to clean or sterilize lenses until all traces of fluorexon are removed because fluorexon molecules may bind to the lens.

Administration and Dosage:

Place 1 drop on the concave surface of the lens and place the lens immediately on the eye. Alternately place 1 or 2 drops in the lower cul-de-sac and have the patient blink several times.

As the dye passes under the lens, observe a central dark zone of 6 to 9 mm in diameter (ie, a limbal fluorescent ring about 2 mm wide), which forms after each blink. If such staining pattern cannot be observed immediately, slide the lens upward by gently pushing it with a finger, causing the dye to penetrate under the lens as it slides back into normal position. Additional drops may be used if the fluorescence starts to dissipate after prolonged examination. When the examination is completed, rinse the eye and lens with saline. The lens may be reinserted immediately, as opposed to the long waiting period required after the use of fluorescein.

Begin the examination immediately after instillation of fluorexon drops. The material tends to dissipate readily with the tear flow, leading to a progressive reduction in fluorescence. Prolonged examination may require sequential application of drops.

Applanation tonometry (without removing lens): After seating the patient at the slit lamp and instilling a drop of fluorexon with a drop of proparacaine or similar topical anesthetic, the contact lens is displaced to one side onto the sclera with the finger and the procedure begun.

---

otc   **Fluoresoft** (Various, eg, Holles)   **Solution:** 0.35%   In 0.5 mL pipettes (12s).

INDOCYANINE GREEN

Actions:

Pharmacology: Sterile, water-soluble, tricarbocyanine dye with a peak spectral absorption at 800 to 810 nm in blood or blood plasma. Indocyanine green contains ≤ 5% sodium iodide.

Indocyanine green permits recording of indicator-dilution curves for both diagnostic and research purposes independent of fluctuations in oxygen saturation. In the performance of dye dilution curves, a known amount of dye is usually injected as a single bolus as rapidly as possible via a cardiac catheter into selected sites in the vascular system. A recording instrument (oximeter or densitometer) is attached to a needle or catheter for sampling of the blood-dye mixture from a systemic arterial sampling site.

The peak absorption and emission of indocyanine green lie in a region (800 to 850 nm) where transmission of energy by the pigment epithelium is more efficient than in the region of visible light energy. Because indocyanine green is also nearly 98% bound to blood protein, excessive dye extravasation does not take place in the highly fenestrated choroidal vasculature. Therefore, it is useful in both absorption and fluorescence infrared angiography of the choroidal vasculature when using appropriate filters and film in a fundus camera.

Pharmacokinetics: Following IV injection, indocyanine green is rapidly bound to plasma protein, of which albumin is the principle carrier (95%). Indocyanine green undergoes no significant extrahepatic or enterohepatic circulation; simultaneous arterial and venous blood estimations have shown negligible renal, peripheral, lung, or cerebrospinal uptake of the dye. Indocyanine green is taken up from the plasma almost exclusively by the hepatic parenchymal cells and is secreted entirely into the bile. After biliary obstruction, the dye appears in the hepatic lymph, independent of the bile, suggesting that the biliary mucosa is sufficiently intact to prevent diffusion of the dye, though allowing diffusion of bilirubin. These characteristics make indocyanine green a helpful index of hepatic function.

Indications:

Angiography: For ophthalmic angiography.

In vivo diagnostics: For determining cardiac output, hepatic function, and liver blood flow.

Warnings:

Pregnancy: Category C. It is not known whether indocyanine green can cause fetal harm when administered to a pregnant woman or can affect reproduction capacity. Give to a pregnant woman only if clearly indicated.

Lactation: It is not known whether this drug is excreted in breast milk. Exercise caution when indocyanine green is administered to a nursing woman.

OPHTHALMIC DYES

Precautions:

Plasma fractional disappearance: Plasma fractional disappearance rate at the recommended 0.5 mg/kg dose has been reported to be significantly greater in women than in men; however, there was no significant difference in the calculated value for clearance.

Radioactive iodine uptake studies: Do not perform for at least a week following the use of indocyanine green.

Iodide allergy: Contains sodium iodide. Use with caution in individuals who have a history of allergy to iodides.

Drug Interactions:

Drug/Lab test interactions: Heparin preparations containing sodium bisulfite reduce the absorption peak of indocyanine green in blood. Do not use heparin as an anticoagulant for the collection of samples for analysis.

Adverse Reactions:

Anaphylactic or urticarial reactions have also occurred in patients without history of allergy to iodides. If such reactions occur, treat with appropriate agents (eg, epinephrine, antihistamines, corticosteroids).

Administration and Dosage:

Use 40 mg dye in 2 mL of aqueous solvent. In some patients, half the volume has been found to produce angiograms of comparable resolution. Immediately follow the injected dye bolus with a 5 mL bolus of normal saline. This injection regimen is designed to provide delivery of a spatially limited dye bolus of optimal concentration to the choroidal vasculature following IV injection.

Compatibility: Use only the Aqueous Solvent (pH 5.5 to 6.5) provided, which is specially prepared Sterile Water for Injection, to dissolve indocyanine green because there have been reports of incompatibility with some commercially available Water for Injection products.

Storage/Stability: Indocyanine green is unstable in aqueous solution and must be used within 10 hours. However, the dye is stable in plasma and whole blood so that samples obtained in discontinuous sampling techniques may be read hours later. Use sterile techniques in handling the dye solution and in the performance of the dilution curves.

Indocyanine green powder may cling to the vial or lump together because it is freeze-dried in the vials. *This is not due to the presence of water.*

Rx	**Cardio-Green (CG)** (Becton-Dickinson)	**Powder for Injection:** 25 mg	In 10 mL amps of aqueous solvent (2s).

ROSE BENGAL

Actions:

Pharmacology: Stains dead or degenerated epithelial cells (corneal and conjunctival) and mucus.

Indications:

Suspected corneal/conjunctival damage: A diagnostic agent when superficial corneal or conjunctival tissue damage is suspected. Effective aid for diagnosis of keratitis, squamous cell carcinomas, keratoconjunctivitis sicca, corrosions, or abrasions, and for the detection of foreign bodies.

Contraindications:

Hypersensitivity to rose bengal or any component of the formulation.

Precautions:

Irritation: The solution may be irritating.

Contact lenses: Whenever rose bengal is used in patients with soft contact lenses, flush the eyes thoroughly with sterile normal saline solution and wait ≥ 1 hour before replacing the lens.

Administration and Dosage:

Strips: Thoroughly saturate tip of strip with sterile irrigating solution. Touch bulbar conjunctiva or lower fornix with moistened strip. The patient should blink several times after application.

Rx	**Rosets** (Akorn)	**Strips:** 1.3 mg/strip	In 100s.

LISSAMINE GREEN

Actions:

Pharmacology: Stains dead or degenerated corneal and conjunctival cells and precipitated mucus.

Indications:

For use as a diagnostic agent when superficial corneal or conjunctival tissue change is suspect.

Off-labeled Uses: Diagnostic aid for dry eye conditions and squamous cell metaplasia.

OPHTHALMIC DYES

Contraindications:

Hypersensitivity to lissamine green or any component of the formulation.

Warnings:

Not to be used with soft contact lenses. For external use only. Keep out of reach of children.

Administration and Dosage:

Moisten the lissamine green impregnated tip before application. One or 2 drops of sterile irrigating or saline solution should be used for this purpose. Touch conjunctiva or fornix as required with moistened tip. It is recommended that the patient blink several times after application.

otc	**Lissamine Green** (Cyanacon/Ocusoft)	**Strips:** 1.5 mg	100 sterile strips per carton.

LOCAL ANESTHETICS

Although the exact mechanism of action is unknown, local anesthetics prevent the generation and conduction of nerve impulses by reducing sodium permeability, increasing the electrical excitation threshold, slowing the nerve impulse propagation, and reducing the rate of rise of the action potential. Their action is reversible; complete recovery of nerve function occurs with no evidence of structural damage to nerve tissue.

With the exception of cocaine, local anesthetics are synthetic, aromatic, or heterocyclic compounds. Nearly all local anesthetics in current use are weakly basic tertiary amines. The structural components consist of an aromatic lipophilic portion, an intermediate alkyl chain, and a hydrophilic hydrocarbon chain containing nitrogen. The intermediate chain is linked to the aromatic group by either an ester or an amide, which determines certain pharmacologic properties of the molecule.

CLASSIFICATION

Local anesthetics are divided into 2 groups: *Esters*, which are derivatives of para-aminobenzoic acid, and *amides*, which are derivatives of aniline. The "ester" local anesthetics are metabolized by hydrolysis of the ester linkage by plasma esterase, probably plasma cholinesterase. The "amide" local anesthetics are metabolized in the liver, then excreted primarily in the urine as metabolites with a small fraction of unchanged drug. Biliary excretion may contribute to the disposition of lidocaine (eg, *Xylocaine*) and mepivacaine (eg, *Carbocaine*). Allergic reactions to local anesthetics occur almost exclusively to anesthetics with ester linkage (see Precautions). All commonly used topical anesthetics are of the ester type (see Table 1: Classification of Local Anesthetics).

Table 1: CLASSIFICATION OF LOCAL ANESTHETICS	
Ester Linkage	**Amide Linkage** (Amides of benzoic acid)
A.) Esters of benzoic acid: Cocaine	A. Lidocaine
B. Esters of meta-aminobenzoic acid: Proparacaine	B. Mepivacaine
	C. Bupivacaine
C. Esters of para-aminobenzoic acid:	D. Etidocaine
1. Procaine	
2. Chloroprocaine	
3. Tetracaine	
4. Benoxinate	

In the amine form, local anesthetics tend to be only slightly soluble in water and, therefore, are usually formulated in the form of their hydrochloride salt, which is water soluble. Because local anesthetics are weak bases, with a pK_a between 8 and 9, they ionize in solution, enhancing stability and shelf-life. Upon contact with more neutral or alkaline environments (eg, tears), the nonionized form is liberated. The nonionized drug can penetrate tissues, including the cornea.

PHARMACOKINETICS

Various pharmacokinetic parameters of the local anesthetics can be significantly altered by the presence of hepatic or renal disease, addition of epinephrine, factors affecting urinary pH, renal blood flow, route of administration, and patient age. Onset of local anesthesia is dependent on the dissociation constant (pK_a), lipid solubility, pH of the solution, protein binding, and molecular size. In general, local anesthetics with high lipid solubility or low pK_a have a faster onset. The duration of action of local anesthetics is proportional to the drug's contact time with nerve tissue. To prolong contact time of injectable local anesthetics, vasoconstrictors may be added, but such adjuncts are of no benefit when used with topical anesthetics. The use of vasoconstrictors (eg, epinephrine) in conjunction with local anesthetics promotes local hemostasis, decreases systemic absorption, and prolongs the duration of action.

Systemic absorption of local anesthetics affects the cardiovascular system and central nervous system. At blood concentrations achieved with normal therapeutic doses of injectable anesthetics, changes in cardiac conduction, excitability, refractoriness, contractility, and peripheral vascular resistance are minimal. However, toxic blood concentrations depress cardiac conduction and excitability, which may lead to atrioventricular block and, ultimately, to cardiac arrest. In addition, with toxic blood concentrations, myocardial contractility may be depressed and peripheral vasodilation may occur, leading to decreased cardiac output and arterial blood pressure.

Following systemic absorption, toxic blood concentrations of local anesthetics can produce CNS stimulation, depression, or both. Apparent central stimulation may be manifested as restlessness, tremors, and shivering, which may progress to convulsions. Depression and coma may occur, possibly progressing to respiratory arrest. Local anesthetics have a primary depressant effect on the medulla and on higher centers. The depressed stage may occur without a prior stage of CNS stimulation.

Rate of systemic absorption depends on total dose and concentration of drug, vascularity of administration site, and presence of vasoconstrictors. Depending on route of administration, local anesthetics are distributed to some extent to all body tissues. High concentrations are found in highly perfused organs (eg, liver, lungs, heart, brain). The rate and extent of placental diffusion is determined by plasma protein binding, ionization, and lipid solubility. It is the nonionized form of the drug that crosses cellular membranes to the site of action. Fetal:maternal ratios are inversely related to degree of protein binding. Only the free, unbound drug is available for placental transfer. Drugs with the highest protein binding capacity may have the lowest fetal:maternal ratios. Lipid-soluble, nonionized drugs readily enter the fetal blood from the maternal circulation.

OPHTHALMIC USES

Anesthetics in current clinical use have relatively low systemic and ocular toxicity. They have a sufficiently long duration of action, are stable in solution, and usually lack interference with the actions of other drugs. These advantages make local anesthetics useful for such ocular procedures as tonometry, foreign body and suture removal, gonioscopy, nasolacrimal irrigation and probing, and surgical procedures (see Table 2: Ophthalmic Uses of Local Anesthetics).

LOCAL ANESTHETICS

Table 2: OPHTHALMIC USES OF LOCAL ANESTHETICS	
Injectable	1. Facial nerve block 2. Retrobulbar or peribulbar anesthesia 3. Eyelid infiltration
Topical	1. Gonioscopy 2. Tonometry 3. Fundus contact lens biomicroscopy 4. Evaluation of corneal abrasions 5. Forced duction testing 6. Schirmer tear testing 7. Electroretinography 8. Lacrimal dilation and irrigation 9. Contact lens fitting 10. Superficial foreign body removal 11. Minor surgery of conjunctiva 12. Suture removal 13. Corneal epithelial debridement

Jimmy D. Bartlett, OD, DOS
University of Alabama at Birmingham

For More Information

Bartlett JD, Jaanus SD, eds. Clinical Ocular Pharmacology, ed. 4. Boston: Butterworth-Heinemann, 2001.

Burns RP, et al. Chronic toxicity of local anesthetics on the cornea. In: Leopold IH, Burns RP, eds. *Symposium on Ocular Therapy*. New York: Wiley, 1977.

Chandler MJ, et al. Provocative challenge with local anesthetics in patients with a prior history of reaction. *J Allergy Clin Immunol* 1987;79:883.

Gail H, Kaufman R, Kalveram CM. Adverse reactions to local anesthetics; analysis of 197 cases. *J Allergy Clin Immunol* 1996;97:933-37.

Greenbaum S. Anesthetics for eye surgery. In: Tasman W, Jaeger EA, eds. *Duane's Clinical Ophthalmology*. Philadelphia: JB Lippincott, 1998;6: Chapters 11–32.

Johnston RL, Whitfield LA, Giralt J, et al. Topical versus peribulbar anesthesic without sedation, for clear corneal phacoemulsification. *J Cataract Refract Surg* 1998;24:407-10.

Rosenwasser GOD. Complications of topical ocular anesthetics. *Int Ophthalmol Clin* 1989;29:153.

Smith RB, Everett WG. Physiology and pharmacology of local anesthetic agents. *Int Ophthalmol Clin* 1973;13: 35.

Sobol WM, McCrary JA. Ocular anesthetic properties and adverse reactions. *Int Ophthalmol Clin* 1989;29:195.

Vettesse T, Breslin CW. Retrobulbar anesthesia for cataract surgery: Comparison of bupivacaine and bupivacaine-lidocaine combinations. *Can J Ophthalmol* 1985;20:131.

OPHTHALMIC DRUG FACTS

LOCAL ANESTHETICS, INJECTABLE

Actions:

Pharmacology: These agents prevent generation and conduction of nerve impulses by inhibiting ionic fluxes, increasing electrical excitation threshold, slowing nerve impulse propagation, and reducing rate of rise of action potential. Progression of anesthesia is related to the diameter, myelination, and conduction velocity of affected nerve fibers.

The use of vasoconstrictors (eg, epinephrine) with local anesthetics promotes local hemostasis, decreases systemic absorption, and prolongs duration of action.

Pharmacokinetics: Various pharmacokinetic parameters can be significantly altered by presence of hepatic or renal disease, addition of epinephrine, factors affecting urinary pH, renal blood flow, administration route, and age of the patient.

Injectable Local Anesthetics Pharmacokinetics						
Anesthetic	Onset (minutes)	Duration (hours)	Equivalent anesthetic concentration (%)	pK$_a$	Partition coefficient[1]	Systemic protein binding (%)
ESTERS						
Procaine[2])	2-5	0.25-1	2	9.1	0.02	5.8[3]
(w/epinephrine)	nd	0.5-1.5				
Chloroprocaine[2]	6-12	0.5	2	9	0.14	nd
(w/epinephrine)	nd	0.5-1.5				
AMIDES						
Lidocaine[2]	h 2	0.5-1	1	7.9	2.9	64.3
(w/epinephrine)	h 2	2-6				
Mepivacaine[2]	3-5	0.75-1.5	1	7.8	0.8	77.5[4]
(w/epinephrine)	nd	2-6				
Bupivacaine[2]	5	2-4	0.25	8.2	27.5	95.6[4]
(w/epinephrine)	nd	3-7				
Etidocaine[2]	3-5	5-10	0.5	7.7	141	94[4]
(w/epinephrine)	nd	3-7				

[1] n-Heptane/Buffer, pH 7.4.   nd - No data.
[2] Values in this line are for infiltrative anesthesia.
[3] Nerve homogenate binding.
[4] Plasma protein binding.

Local anesthetics are divided into two groups: *Esters*, which are derivatives of para-aminobenzoic acid, and *amides*, which are derivatives of aniline. The "ester" local anesthetics are metabolized by hydrolysis of the ester linkage by plasma esterase, probably plasma cholinesterase. The "amide" local anesthetics are metabolized primarily in the liver, then excreted primarily in the urine as metabolites with a small fraction of unchanged drug. Hypersensitivity reactions may occur with local anesthetics of the ester type (see Warnings).

Indications:

Refer to individual product listings.

Ophthalmic Uses of Local Anesthetics	
Route	Use
Injectable	Facial nerve block Retrobulbar anesthesia Eyelid infiltration

LOCAL ANESTHETICS 29

Contraindications:

Hypersensitivity to local anesthetics, para-aminobenzoic acid (amides only), or parabens.

Warnings:

Head and neck area: Small doses of local anesthetics injected into the head and neck area, including retrobulbar, dental, and stellate ganglion blocks, may produce adverse reactions similar to systemic toxicity seen with unintentional intravascular injections of larger doses. The injection procedures require the utmost care. Confusion, convulsions, respiratory depression or arrest, and cardiovascular stimulation or depression have occurred. These reactions may be caused by intra-arterial injection of the local anesthetic with retrograde flow to cerebral circulation. They also may be caused by puncture of the dural sheath of the optic nerve during retrobulbar block with diffusion of any local anesthetic along the subdural space to the midbrain. Observe patient carefully. Monitor respiration and circulation. Do not exceed dosage recommendations.

Ophthalmic – When local anesthetic solutions are used for retrobulbar block, complete corneal anesthesia usually precedes onset of clinically acceptable external ocular muscle akinesia. Therefore, presence of akinesia rather than anesthesia alone should determine readiness of the patient for surgery.

Cardiovascular reactions – Cardiovascular reactions are depressants. They may be the result of direct drug effect, the result of vasovagal reaction, particularly if the patient is in the sitting position. Failure to recognize premonitory signs such as sweating, feeling of faintness, and changes in pulse or sensorium may result in progressive cerebral hypoxia and seizure or serious cardiovascular catastrophe. Place patient in recumbent position and administer oxygen. Vasoactive drugs such as ephedrine or methoxamine may be administered IV.

Hypersensitivity reactions: Hypersensitivity reactions, including anaphylaxis, may occur in a small segment of the population allergic to para-aminobenzoic acid derivatives (eg, procaine, tetracaine, benzocaine). The amide-type local anesthetics have not shown cross-sensitivity with the esters. Hypersensitivity reactions and anaphylaxis have occurred rarely with lidocaine. Administer ester-type local anesthetics cautiously to patients with abnormal or reduced levels of plasma esterases.

Renal function impairment: Use mepivacaine with caution in patients with renal disease.

Hepatic function impairment: Because amide-type local anesthetics are metabolized primarily in the liver, patients with hepatic disease, especially severe hepatic disease, may be more susceptible to potential toxicity. Use cautiously in such patients.

Elderly: Repeated doses may cause accumulation of the drug or its metabolites or slow metabolic degradation. Give reduced doses.

Pregnancy: Category B (etidocaine, lidocaine). *Category C* (bupivacaine, chloroprocaine, mepivacaine). Safety for use in pregnant women, other than those in labor, has not been established.

Lactation: Safety for use in the nursing mother has not been established. It is not known whether local anesthetic drugs are excreted in breast milk.

Children: Because of lack of clinical experience, the administration of bupivacaine to children < 12 years of age is not recommended. Dosages in children should be reduced to commensurate with age, body weight, and physical condition.

Precautions:

Dosage: Use the lowest dosage that results in effective anesthesia to avoid high plasma levels and serious adverse effects. Inject slowly with frequent aspirations before and during the injection to avoid intravascular injection. Perform syringe aspirations before and during each supplemental injection using continuous (intermittent) catheter techniques.

Inflammation or sepsis: Use local anesthetic procedures with caution when there is inflammation or sepsis in the region of proposed injection.

CNS toxicity: Monitor cardiovascular and respiratory vital signs and state of consciousness after each injection. Restlessness, anxiety, incoherent speech, lightheadedness, numbness and tingling of the mouth and lips, metallic taste, tinnitus, dizziness, blurred vision, tremors, twitching, depression, or drowsiness may be early signs of CNS toxicity.

Special risk patients: Debilitated patients, acutely ill patients, children, obstetric delivery patients, and patients with increased intra-abdominal pressure: Repeated doses may cause accumulation of the drug or its metabolites or slow metabolic degradation. Give reduced doses. Use anesthetics with caution in patients with severe disturbances of cardiac rhythm, hypotension, shock, or heart block. Local anesthetics should also be used with caution in patients with impaired cardiovascular function because they may be less able to compensate for functional changes associated with the prolongation of A-V conduction produced by these drugs.

Malignant hyperthermia: Many drugs used during anesthesia are considered potential triggering agents for familial malignant hyperthermia. It is not known whether amide-type local anesthetics trigger this reaction and the need for supplemental general anesthesia cannot be predicted in advance; therefore, have a standard protocol for management available.

Vasoconstrictors: Use solutions containing a vasoconstrictor with caution and in carefully circumscribed quantities in areas of the body supplied by end arteries or having otherwise compromised blood supply. Use with extreme caution in patients whose medical history and physical evaluation suggest the existence of hypertension, peripheral vascular disease, arteriosclerotic heart disease, cerebral vascular insufficiency, or heart block; these individuals may exhibit exaggerated vasoconstrictor response.

Sulfite sensitivity: Some of these products contain sulfites. Sulfites may cause allergic-type reactions (eg, hives, itching, wheezing, anaphylaxis) in certain susceptible persons. Although the overall prevalence of sulfite sensitivity in the general population is probably low, it is seen more frequently in asthmatics or in atopic nonasthmatic persons.

Drug Interactions:

Intercurrent use: Mixtures of local anesthetics are sometimes employed to compensate for the slower onset of one drug and the shorter duration of action of the second drug. Toxicity is probably additive with mixtures of local anesthetics, but some

LOCAL ANESTHETICS 31

experiments suggest synergisms. Exercise caution regarding toxic equivalence when mixtures of local anesthetics are employed.

Prior use of chloroprocaine may interfere with subsequent use of bupivacaine. For this reason, and because safety of intercurrent use of bupivacaine and chloroprocaine has not been established, such use is not recommended.

Some preparations contain vasoconstrictors. Keep this in mind when using concurrently with other drugs that may interact with vasoconstrictors.

Injectable Local Anesthetic Drug Interactions			
Precipitant drug	Object drug*		Description
Local anesthetics	Sulfonamides	↓	The para-aminobenzoic acid metabolite of procaine, chloroprocaine, and tetracaine inhibits the action of sulfonamides. Therefore, do not use procaine, chloroprocaine, or tetracaine in any condition in which a sulfonamide drug is employed.

* ↓ = Object drug decreased.

Adverse Reactions:

The most common acute adverse reactions are related to the CNS and cardiovascular systems. These are generally dose-related and may result from rapid absorption from the injection site, diminished tolerance, or unintentional intravascular injection.

Dermatologic: Cutaneous lesions, urticaria, pruritus, erythema, angioneurotic edema (including laryngeal edema), sneezing, syncope, excessive sweating, elevated temperature, and anaphylactoid symptoms (including severe hypotension). Skin testing is of limited value.

CNS: Restlessness, anxiety, dizziness, tinnitus, blurred vision, nausea, vomiting, chills, pupil constriction, or tremors may occur, possibly proceeding to convulsions ($\approx$ 0.1% of local anesthetic epidural administrations). Excitement may be transient or absent, with depression being the first manifestation. This may quickly be followed by drowsiness merging into unconsciousness and respiratory arrest.

Postspinal headache; meningismus; arachnoiditis; palsies; apprehension; double vision; euphoria; sensation of heat, cold, or numbness; and spinal nerve paralysis (spinal anesthesia) have also occurred.

Cardiovascular: Myocardial depression, hypotension (with spinal anesthesia because of vasomotor paralysis and pooling of blood in the venous bed), decreased cardiac output, heart block, syncope, bradycardia, ventricular arrhythmias (including tachycardia and fibrillation), cardiac arrest, and fetal bradycardia (see Warnings).

Overdosage:

Acute emergencies from local anesthetics are generally related to high plasma levels encountered during therapeutic use or because of unintended subarachnoid injection.

Management: The first consideration is prevention.

Convulsions – Convulsions, as well as underventilation or apnea, are caused by unintentional subarachnoid injection; maintain patent airway and assist or control ventilation with oxygen and a delivery system capable of permitting immediate positive airway pressure by mask. Evaluate circulation. If convulsions persist despite respiratory support, and if the status of the circulation permits, give small increments of an ultra short-acting barbiturate (eg, thiopental) or a benzodiazepine (eg, diazepam) IV. Circulatory depression may require administration of IV fluids and a vasopressor. If not treated immediately, convulsions and cardiovascular depression can result in hypoxia, acidosis, bradycardia, arrhythmias, and cardiac arrest. Underventilation or apnea may produce these same signs and also lead to cardiac arrest if ventilatory support is not instituted. If cardiac arrest occurs, institute standard cardiopulmonary resuscitative measures.

Endotracheal intubation may be indicated.

Administration and Dosage:

The dose of local anesthetic administered varies with the procedure, vascularity of the tissues, depth of anesthesia, degree of required muscle relaxation, duration of anesthesia desired, and the physical condition of the patient. Reduce dosages for children, elderly and debilitated patients, and patients with cardiac or liver disease.

Infiltration or regional block anesthesia: Always inject slowly, with frequent aspirations, to prevent intravascular injection.

For detailed administration and dosage, refer to specific manufacturers' labeling.

Individual drug monographs are on the following pages.

LOCAL ANESTHETICS 33

LIDOCAINE HCl and LIDOCAINE COMBINATIONS

For complete prescribing information, refer to the Injectable Local Anesthetics group monograph.

Indications:

Retrobulbar or transtracheal injection: 4% solution.

Rx	Xylocaine MPF (Astra)	Injection: 4%	In 5 mL amps and 5 mL disp. syringe with laryngotracheal cannula.
Rx	Xylocaine (Astra)	Injection: 0.5% with 1:200,000 epinephrine	In 50 mL multiple-dose vials.[1]
Rx	Xylocaine (Astra)	Injection: 1% with 1:100,000 epinephrine	In 10, 20, and 50 mL multiple-dose vials.[1]
Rx	Xylocaine MPF (Astra)	Injection: 1% with 1:200,000 epinephrine	In 30 mL ampules, and 5, 10, and 30 mL single-dose vials.[2]
Rx	Xylocaine MPF (Astra)	Injection: 1.5% with 1:200,000 epinephrine	In 5 and 30 mL ampules, and 5, 10, and 30 mL single-dose vials.[2]
Rx	Xylocaine (Astra)	Injection: 2% with 1:100,000 epinephrine	In 10, 20, and 50 mL multiple-dose vials.[1]
Rx	Xylocaine MPF (Astra)	Injection: 2% with 1:200,000 epinephrine	In 20 mL ampules, and 5, 10, and 20 mL single-dose vials.[2]

[1] With methylparaben.
[2] With sodium metabisulfite.

MEPIVACAINE HCl

For complete prescribing information, refer to the Injectable Local Anesthetics group monograph.

Indications:

Peripheral nerve block: 1% or 2% solution.

Infiltration: 0.5% (via dilution) or 1% solution

Rx	Polocaine (Astra)	Injection:1%	In 50 mL vials.
Rx	Polocaine MPF (Astra)		In 30 mL vials.
Rx	Polocaine MPF (Astra)	Injection:1.5%	In 30 mL vials.
Rx	Polocaine (Astra)	Injection: 2%	In 50 mL vials.
Rx	Polocaine MPF (Astra)		In 20 mL vials.

34 OPHTHALMIC DRUG FACTS

BUPIVACAINE HCl and BUPIVACAINE COMBINATIONS

For complete prescribing information, refer to the Injectable Local Anesthetics group monograph.

Indications:

Retrobulbar block: 0.75% solution.

Rx	**Bupivacaine HCl** (Abbott)	**Injection:** 0.75%	In 20 mL amps and 20 mL *Abboject.*
Rx	**Sensorcaine MPF** (Astra)		In 30 mL amps and 10 and 30 mL vials.
Rx	**Sensorcaine MPF** (Astra)	0.75% with 1:200,000 epinephrine	In 30 mL amps and 10 and 30 mL vials.[1]

[1] With sodium metabisulfite.

ETIDOCAINE HCl

For complete prescribing information, refer to the Injectable Local Anesthetics group monograph.

Indications:

Retrobulbar: 1% or 1.5% solution.

Rx	**Duranest** (Astra)	**Injection:** 1%	In 30 mL single-dose vials.
		1% with 1:200,000 epinephrine	In 30 mL single-dose vials.[1]
		1.5% with 1:200,000 epinephrine	In 20 mL amps.[1]

[1] With sodium metabisulfite.

LOCAL ANESTHETICS, TOPICAL

Actions:

Pharmacology: Local anesthetics stabilize the neuronal membrane so the neuron is less permeable to ions. This prevents the initiation and transmission of nerve impulses, thereby producing the local anesthetic action.

Studies indicate that local anesthetics influence permeability of the nerve cell membrane by limiting sodium ion permeability by closing the pores through which the ions migrate in the lipid layer of the nerve cell membrane. This limitation prevents the fundamental change necessary for the generation of the action potential.

Pharmacokinetics: Tetracaine and proparacaine are approximately equally potent. They have a rapid onset of anesthesia beginning within 13 to 30 seconds following instillation; the duration of action is 15 to 20 minutes.

LOCAL ANESTHETICS

Indications:

Corneal anesthesia of short duration (eg, tonometry, gonioscopy, removal of corneal foreign bodies and sutures); short corneal and conjunctival procedures; cataract surgery; conjunctival and corneal scraping for diagnostic purposes; paracentesis of the anterior chamber.

Ophthalmic Uses of Local Anesthetics	
Route	Use
Topical	Gonioscopy
	Tonometry
	Fundus contact lens biomicroscopy
	Evaluation of corneal abrasions
	Forced duction testing
	Schirmer tear testing
	Electroretinography
	Lacrimal dilation and irrigation
	Contact lens fitting
	Superficial foreign body removal
	Minor surgery of conjunctiva
	Suture removal
	Corneal epithelial debridement

Contraindications:

Hypersensitivity to similar drugs (ester-type local anesthetics), para-aminobenzoic acid or its derivatives, or to any other ingredient in these preparations; prolonged use, especially for self-medication (not recommended).

Warnings:

For topical ophthalmic use only: Prolonged use may diminish duration of anesthesia, retard wound healing, and cause corneal epithelial erosions (see Adverse Reactions).

Systemic toxicity: Systemic toxicity is rare with topical ophthalmic application of local anesthetics. It usually occurs as CNS stimulation followed by CNS and cardiovascular depression.

Protection of the eye: Protection of the eye from irritating chemicals, foreign bodies, and rubbing during the period of anesthesia is very important. Advise the patient to avoid touching the eye until anesthesia has worn off.

Pregnancy: Category C. Safety for use during pregnancy has not been established. Use only when clearly needed and when potential benefits outweigh potential hazards to the fetus.

Lactation: Safety for use during lactation has not been established. Use only when clearly needed and when potential benefits outweigh potential hazards to the infant.

Children: Safety and efficacy for use in children have been well established through clinical experience, although no studies exist.

Precautions:

Reduced plasma esterase: Use caution in patients with abnormal or reduced levels of plasma esterases.

36 OPHTHALMIC DRUG FACTS

Special risk patients: Use cautiously and sparingly in patients with known allergies, cardiac disease, or hyperthyroidism.

Adverse Reactions:

Prolonged ophthalmic use of topical anesthetics has been associated with corneal epithelial erosions, retardation, or prevention of healing of corneal erosions, and reports of severe keratitis and permanent corneal opacification with accompanying visual loss and scarring or corneal perforation. Inadvertent damage may be done to the anesthetized cornea and conjunctiva by rubbing an eye to which topical anesthetics have been applied.

Tetracaine:

Miscellaneous – Transient stinging, burning, and conjunctival redness may occur. A rare, severe, immediate-type allergic corneal reaction has been reported. It is characterized by acute diffuse epithelial keratitis with filament formation and sloughing of large areas of necrotic epithelium, diffuse stromal edema, descemetitis, and iritis.

Rarely, local reactions including lacrimation, photophobia, and chemosis have occurred.

Proparacaine:

Miscellaneous – Local or systemic sensitivity occurs occasionally. At recommended concentration and dosage, proparacaine usually produces little or no initial irritation, stinging, burning, conjunctival redness, lacrimation, or increased winking. However, some local irritation and stinging may occur several hours after instillation.

Rarely, a severe, immediate-type, hyperallergic corneal reaction may occur, which includes acute, intense, and diffuse epithelial keratitis, a gray, ground-glass appearance, sloughing of large areas of necrotic epithelium, corneal filaments, and, sometimes, iritis with descemetitis. Pupillary dilation or cycloplegic effects have been rarely observed.

Allergic contact dermatitis with drying and fissuring of the fingertips, softening and erosion of the corneal epithelium, and conjunctival congestion and hemorrhage have been reported.

Patient Information:

Avoid continuous or prolonged use.

Avoid touching or rubbing the eye until the anesthesia has worn off because inadvertent damage may be done to the anesthetized cornea and conjunctiva.

To avoid contamination, do not touch dropper tip to any surface. Replace cap after using.

Do not use if discolored, cloudy, or if it contains a precipitate. Protect from light.

Individual drug monographs are on the following pages.

LOCAL ANESTHETICS

TETRACAINE HCl

For complete prescribing information, refer to the Topical Local Anesthetics group monograph.

Administration and Dosage:

Solution: Instill 1 or 2 drops. Not for prolonged use.

Storage: Store at 8° to 27°C (46° to 80°F). Protect from light.

Rx	Tetracaine HCl (Various, eg, Alcon, Bausch & Lomb, Novartis, Schein)	Solution: 0.5%	In 1, 2, and 15 mL.
Rx	AK-T-Caine PF (Akorn)		Preservative free. In 15 mL.

[1] With 0.4% chlorobutanol and 0.75% sodium chloride.

PROPARACAINE HCl

For complete prescribing information, refer to the Topical Local Anesthetics group monograph.

Administration and Dosage:

Deep anesthesia as in cataract extraction: 1 drop every 5 to 10 minutes for 5 to 7 doses.

Removal of sutures: Instill 1 or 2 drops 2 or 3 minutes before removal of sutures.

Removal of foreign bodies: Instill 1 or 2 drops prior to operating.

Tonometry: Instill 1 or 2 drops immediately before measurement.

Storage: Store at 8° to 24°C (46° to 75°F). Protect from light.

Rx	Proparacaine HCl (Various, eg, Bausch & Lomb, Falcon)	Solution: 0.5%	In 15 mL.
Rx	AK-TAINE (Akorn)		In 15 mL.[1,2]
Rx	Alcaine (Alcon)		In 15 mL Drop-Tainers.[3,4]
Rx	Ophthetic (Allergan)		In 15 mL.[1,2]

[1] Refrigerate.
[2] With 0.01% benzalkonium Cl, glycerin, and sodium chloride.
[3] With glycerin and 0.01% benzalkonium Cl.
[4] Refrigerate after opening.

MISCELLANEOUS LOCAL ANESTHETIC COMBINATIONS

For complete prescribing information, refer to the Topical Local Anesthetics group monograph.

Indications:

For procedures in which a topical ophthalmic anesthetic agent in conjunction with a disclosing agent is indicated: Corneal anesthesia of short duration (eg, tonometry, gonioscopy, removal of corneal foreign bodies); short corneal and conjunctival procedures.

Administration and Dosage:

Removal of foreign bodies or sutures; tonometry: 1 to 2 drops (in single instillations) in each eye before operating.

Deep ophthalmic anesthesia:

Proparacaine/Fluorescein – Instill 1 drop in each eye every 5 to 10 minutes for 5 to 7 doses. Use of an eye patch is recommended.

Benoxinate/Fluorescein – Instill 2 drops into each eye at 90-second intervals for 3 instillations.

Storage: Protect from light.

Rx	**Fluoracaine** (Akorn)	**Solution:** 0.5% propara-caine HCl and 0.25% fluore-scein sodium	In 5 mL.[1,2]
Rx	**Fluress** (Akorn)	**Solution:** 0.4% benoxinate HCl and 0.25% fluorescein sodium	In 5 mL with dropper.[3]

[1] Refrigerate.
[2] With glycerin, povidone, polysorbate 80, 0.01% thimerosal.
[3] With povidone, boric acid, 1% chlorobutanol.

MYDRIATICS AND CYCLOPLEGICS

Mydriatics are drugs that dilate the pupil. Adrenergic agonists are used for routine dilation of the pupil. Phenylephrine (eg, *Neo-Synephrine*) and epinephrine (eg, *Epifrin*) are the only direct-acting adrenergic agents available that produce mydriasis without cycloplegia. However, epinephrine is not used clinically for its mydriatic effects.

Anticholinergic agents administered topically to the eye for purposes of inhibiting accommodation are termed *cycloplegics*. Their primary use is for cycloplegic refraction and in the treatment of uveitis. Because these agents also inhibit action of the iris sphincter muscle, they are effective mydriatics. Of the cholinergic blocking agents, only tropicamide (eg, *Mydriacyl*) is used routinely for mydriasis. For most dilation procedures, the adrenergic or anticholinergic agents can be used alone or in combination for maximum mydriasis.

MYDRIATICS

Phenylephrine HCl

Phenylephrine is a synthetic alpha-receptor agonist that is structurally similar to epinephrine. Following topical application on the eye, it contracts the iris dilator muscle and smooth muscle of the conjunctival arterioles, causing pupillary dilation and "blanching" of the conjunctiva. Mueller's muscle of the upper eyelid may be stimulated, widening the palpebral fissure.

For pupillary dilation, concentrations of 2.5% and 10% are commercially available. Maximum dilation occurs within 45 to 60 minutes, depending on the concentration used or number of drops instilled. The pupil size usually returns to predrug levels within 4 to 6 hours. Because phenylephrine has little or no effect on the ciliary muscle, mydriasis occurs without cycloplegia.

Phenylephrine 1% solution can be used in diagnosis of Horner's syndrome. Significant mydriasis can occur in the eye with a postganglionic lesion as compared with one with a normal innervation.

The mydriatic response to phenylephrine may be affected in situations that alter corneal epithelial integrity. Corneal abrasions or trauma from such procedures as tonometry or gonioscopy, as well as prior instillation of a topical anesthetic, can enhance its pharmacologic effect. Concentrations as small as 0.125%, as present in *otc* decongestants, can cause mydriasis if the corneal epithelium is damaged.

Because the topical instillation of phenylephrine can be accompanied by clinically significant ocular and systemic side effects, cardiovascular effects in particular, avoid use of the 10% concentration if possible. The 2.5% concentration is generally recommended for routine dilation, especially in infants and the elderly. Use the drug with caution in patients with cardiac disease, hypertension, arteriosclerosis, and diabetes. It is contraindicated in patients taking tricyclic antidepressants (eg, amitriptyline [eg, *Elavil*]), MAO inhibitors (eg, phenelzine [*Nardil*]), reserpine, guanethidine (*Ismelin*), and methyldopa (eg, *Aldomet*).

CYCLOPLEGIC MYDRIATICS

Commonly used cycloplegic mydriatics include the following: Atropine (eg, *Isopto Atropine*), homatropine (eg, *Isopto Homatropine*), scopolamine (eg, *Isopto Hyoscine*), cyclopentolate (eg, *Cyclogyl*), and tropicamide (eg, *Tropicacyl*).

Objective and subjective refractive procedures are employed to determine the nature of the refractive error. Under normal circumstances, this is best accomplished without interference from topically applied drugs that might adversely affect examination results. However, under some circumstances, the instillation of cycloplegics may enable a more accurate refractive examination.

Use in Esotropia

Children with strabismus, especially esotropia, should receive a cycloplegic examination. It is important to uncover the full amount of hyperopia in young patients with suspected accommodative esotropia so that plus lenses can relieve the effort placed on the accommodative-convergence system. Some clinicians use cycloplegics in children who exhibit myopia for the first time to rule out accommodative spasm (pseudomyopia) as the underlying etiology. Patients who are unresponsive or inconsistent in their responses to subjective refraction will often benefit from cycloplegia. Cycloplegic refraction also is indicated to confirm the refractive amount in patients who exhibit symptoms of malingering or conversion reaction. Refraction of young children and infants is usually more accurate and easier with cycloplegics because these patients may fixate any distance during the examination. Patients with suspected latent hyperopia will also benefit from cycloplegic refraction.

Contraindications: Cycloplegics cause pupillary dilation; therefore, they are contraindicated in patients with extremely narrow anterior chamber angles or a history of angle-closure glaucoma. Use atropine with caution in patients with Down's syndrome and in patients receiving systemic anticholinergic drugs. Patients allergic to atropine can usually be given scopolamine, which will enable similar examination results.

Drug selection: Atropine provides the most effective cycloplegia of any currently available anticholinergic drug and is indicated for the cycloplegic retinoscopy of infants and children up to 4 years of age with suspected accommodative esotropia. The use of atropine allows determination of the maximum amount of hyperopia.

Cyclopentolate has become the drug of choice for the cycloplegic refraction of strabismic patients over 4 years of age and nonstrabismic patients of any age. Although atropine is still preferred for patients < 4 years of age with suspected accommodative esotropia, there is a trend toward the use of cyclopentolate in these patients.

Clinical procedures: The use of atropine for the refractive examination of patients with suspected accommodative esotropia requires that the medication be instilled at home for 1 to 3 days prior to the office visit. This allows time for maximum cycloplegia to occur.

MYDRIATICS AND CYCLOPLEGICS

Cyclopentolate is used in the practitioner's office and is instilled 30 to 60 minutes prior to refractive examination. Once maximum cycloplegia has occurred, retinoscopy or subjective refraction is performed. Considerable skill and judgment are required to interpret the findings and prescribe a useful refractive correction.

Use in Uveitis

Uveitis is an inflammation of the iris, ciliary body, or choroid of the eye. The inflammation can be limited to the anterior structures or the posterior structures of the eye, or both; the clinical features depend on the site of involvement. Uveitis can be classified based on the anatomic site of inflammation. For example, uveitis involving the iris only is termed iritis. Another method to classify the uveal inflammation is based on whether it affects the anterior or posterior structures of the eye. Uveitis can also be classified as either granulomatous or nongranulomatous. Any clinical classification system has considerable overlap, but these classifications provide the opportunity to differentiate various clinical presentations and predict the natural course of the uveal inflammation.

Etiology: Uveitis is thought to be an immune-complex disease with T-cell antigen dysfunction playing a major role. Idiopathic anterior uveitis is the most common clinical presentation. Human leukocyte antigen (HLA) studies are being undertaken to identify individuals who might be predisposed to recurrent episodes of uveitis or whose uveitis might be associated with other conditions. Systemic disorders are often associated with uveitis and include collagen diseases such as rheumatoid arthritis, ankylosing spondylitis, and systemic lupus erythematosus. Other systemic causes include metabolic diseases, granulomatous diseases, and infectious diseases such as herpes zoster and herpes simplex.

Diagnosis: The signs and symptoms of uveitis depend largely on the anatomic site of inflammation. Anterior uveitis is characterized by conjunctival hyperemia, the distribution of which often follows a circumcorneal pattern. The pupil is frequently miotic, and there is almost always an anterior chamber reaction manifested by cells and flare. The intraocular pressure may be reduced, and there are often keratic precipitates on the corneal endothelium as seen with the slit lamp. Symptoms include ocular pain, photophobia, and blurred vision. Consider cases of anterior uveitis that are bilateral, recurrent, or resistant to treatment for more extensive diagnostic evaluation for the presence of underlying systemic disease.

Posterior uveitis is characterized by little or no pain, and although there can be some anterior chamber reaction, inflammation of the vitreous (vitritis) is most prominent. If the macula is involved or if the vitreous is sufficiently hazy to diminish vision, visual acuity will be affected.

Drug selection: Cycloplegics are useful in the treatment of anterior uveitis because they often prevent posterior synechiae. Cycloplegia places the ciliary body and iris at rest, reducing many of the associated symptoms, and cycloplegics also reduce the anterior chamber reaction. Cyclopentolate, homatropine, and atropine are the most commonly used cycloplegic agents for the treatment of uveitis.

Topical corticosteroids are usually administered in conjunction with cycloplegic therapy. In severe cases, periocular or oral steroids may also be considered; immunosuppressive agents can be used in cases where corticosteroids may not be effective. If uveitic glaucoma ensues, antiglaucoma therapy is usually initiated.

Jimmy D. Bartlett, OD, DOS
University of Alabama at Birmingham

Siret D. Jaanus, PhD
Southern California College of Optometry

Thom Zimmerman, MD, PhD
University of Louisville

For More Information

Bartlett JD. Administration of and adverse reactions to cycloplegic agents. *Am J Optom Physiol Optics* 1978;55:227.

Bartlett JD, Jaanus SD, eds. Clinical Ocular Pharmacology, ed. 4. Boston: Butterworth-Heinemann, 2001.

Cremer SA, et al. Hydroxyamphetamine mydriasis in Horner's Syndrome. *Am J Ophthalmol* 1990;110:71.

Fraunfelder FT, Scafidi AF. Possible adverse effects from topical ocular 10% phenylephrine. *Am J Ophthalmol* 1978;85:862.

Gambill HD, et al. Mydriatic effect of four drugs determined by pupillograph. *Arch Ophthalmol* 1967;77:740.

Hendly DE, et al. Changing patterns of uveitis. *Am J Ophthalmol* 1987;103:131.

Larkin KM, Charap A, Cheetham JK, et al. Ideal concentration of tropicamide with hydroxyamphetamine 1% for routine pupillary dilation. *Ann Ophthalmol* 1989;21:340.

Manny RE, Fern KD, Zervas HJ, et al. 1% cyclopentolate hydrochloride: Another look at the time course of cycloplegia using an objective measure of the accommodative response. *Optom Vis Sci* 1993;70:651-65.

Montgomery DMI, Macewan CS. Pupil dilation with tropicamide. The effects on acuity, accommodation and refraction. *Eye* 1989;3:845.

Moore BD. Cycloplegic refraction of young children. *N Engl J Optom* 1988;41:10.

Paggiarino DA, Brancato LJ, Newton RE. The effect on pupil size and accommodation of sympathetic and parasympatholytic agents. *Ann Ophthalmol* 1993;25:244-53.

MYDRIATICS AND CYCLOPLEGICS

PHENYLEPHRINE HCl

Actions:

Pharmacology: Phenylephrine ophthalmic solution possesses predominantly α-adrenergic effects. In the eye, phenylephrine acts locally as a potent vasoconstrictor and mydriatic by constricting ophthalmic blood vessels and the radial muscle of the iris. The ophthalmic usefulness of phenylephrine is because of its rapid effect and moderately prolonged action.

Actions of different concentrations of phenylephrine are shown in the following table:

Phenylephrine HCl			
	Mydriasis/Vasoconstriction		
Strength of solution (%)	Maximal (min)	Recovery time (hrs)	Paralysis of accommodation
0.12	30 to 90	-	-
2.5	15 to 60	3	trace
10	10 to 60	6	slight

Although rare, systemic absorption of sufficient quantities of phenylephrine may lead to systemic α-adrenergic effects, such as rise in blood pressure, which may be accompanied by a reflex atropine-sensitive bradycardia.

Indications:

2.5% and 10%: Decongestant and vasoconstrictor and for pupil dilation in uveitis (posterior synechiae), open-angle glaucoma, refraction without cycloplegia, prior to surgery, ophthalmoscopic examination (funduscopy).

Contraindications:

Hypersensitivity to any component of the formulation; narrow-angle glaucoma or individuals with a narrow (occludable) angle who do not have glaucoma; in low birth weight infants and in some elderly adults with severe arteriosclerotic cardiovascular or cerebrovascular disease; during intraocular operative procedures when the corneal epithelial barrier has been disturbed.

Phenylephrine 10%: In infants, small children with low body weights, debilitated or elderly patients, and patients with aneurysms. The administration of phenylephrine is contraindicated in patients with long-standing, insulin-dependent diabetes, hypertensive patients receiving reserpine or guanethidine, advanced arteriosclerotic changes, idiopathic orthostatic hypotension, and in patients with a known history of organic cardiac disease.

In individuals with an intraocular lens implant, the administration of 10% phenylephrine is contraindicated because of the possibility of dislodging the lens.

Warnings:

Phenylephrine 10%: There have been rare reports of the development of serious cardiovascular reactions, including ventricular arrhythmias and myocardial infarctions. These episodes, some fatal, have usually occurred in elderly patients with preexisting cardiovascular diseases.

OPHTHALMIC DRUG FACTS

Elderly: Use with caution. Because of the strong action of phenylephrine 2.5% to 10% on the dilator muscle, older individuals also may develop transient pigment floaters in the aqueous humor 30 to 45 minutes following administration. The appearance may be similar to anterior uveitis or microscopic hyphema.

Rebound miosis occurs in some elderly patients. Subsequent instillation of phenylephrine may produce less mydriasis than the initial instillation. This may be of clinical importance when dilating pupils prior to retinal detachment or cataract surgery. Exercise caution not to overdose these patients.

Pregnancy: Category C. Safety for use has not been established. Use only if clearly needed and potential benefits to the mother outweigh potential hazards to the fetus.

Lactation: It is not known whether this drug is excreted in breast milk. Use caution when phenylephrine HCl is administered to a nursing woman.

Children: Safety and efficacy for use in children have not been established. Phenylephrine 2.5% has been used for a "one application method" in combination with a preferred rapid-acting cycloplegic (see Administration and Dosage). Phenylephrine 10% is contraindicated in infants.

Precautions:

Systemic absorption: Exceeding recommended dosages or applying phenylephrine 2.5% to 10% to an instrumented, traumatized, diseased, or postsurgical eye or adnexa, or to patients with suppressed lacrimation, as during anesthesia, may result in the absorption of sufficient quantities to produce a systemic vasopressor response.

A significant elevation in blood pressure is rare but has been reported following conjunctival instillation of recommended doses of phenylephrine 10%. Use with caution in children of low body weight, the elderly, and patients with insulin-dependent diabetes, hypertension, hyperthyroidism, generalized arteriosclerosis, or cardiovascular disease. Carefully monitor the posttreatment blood pressure of these patients and any patients who develop symptoms (see Contraindications).

The hypertensive effects of phenylephrine may be treated with an α-adrenergic blocking agent, such as phentolamine mesylate, 5 to 10 mg IV, repeated as necessary.

Narrow-angle glaucoma: Ordinarily, mydriatics are contraindicated in glaucoma patients. However, when temporary pupil dilation may free adhesions, or when intrinsic vessel vasoconstriction may lower IOP, this may temporarily outweigh danger from coincident dilation.

Corneal effects: If the corneal epithelium has been denuded or damaged, corneal clouding may occur if phenylephrine 10% is instilled. This may be especially serious following corneal epithelium removal during retinal detachment surgery or vitrectomy. The corneas of diabetic patients may manifest epithelial ulcerations as well as a slow rate of reepithelialization. Use of phenylephrine in such corneas may be especially hazardous.

Rebound congestion: Rebound congestion may occur with extended use of ophthalmic vasoconstrictors.

Sulfite sensitivity: Some of these products contain sulfites. Sulfites may cause allergic-type reactions (eg, hives, itching, wheezing, anaphylaxis) in certain susceptible persons. Although the overall prevalence of sulfite sensitivity in the general population is

MYDRIATICS AND CYCLOPLEGICS

low, it is seen more frequently in asthmatics or in atopic nonasthmatic persons. Specific products containing sulfites are identified in the product listings.

Drug Interactions:

Anesthetics: Use anesthetics that sensitize the myocardium to sympathomimetics (eg, cyclopropane or halothane) cautiously. Local anesthetics can increase ocular absorption of topical drugs. Exercise caution when applying prior to use of phenylephrine.

β-*adrenergic blocking agents:* Systemic side effects may occur more readily in patients taking these drugs. A severe hypertensive episode and fatal intracranial hemorrhage possibly associated with ophthalmic use of phenylephrine was reported in 1 patient taking propranolol for hypertension.

MAOIs: When given with, or up to 21 days after MAOIs, exaggerated adrenergic effects may result. Supervise and adjust dosage carefully. The pressor response of adrenergic agents may also be potentiated by tricyclic antidepressants, propranolol, reserpine, guanethidine, methyldopa, and anticholinergics (see Adverse Reactions).

Adverse Reactions:

Ophthalmic: Transitory stinging on initial instillation; blurring of vision; mydriasis; increased redness; irritation; discomfort; punctate keratitis; lacrimation; increased IOP. May cause rebound miosis and decreased mydriatic response to therapy in the elderly.

Cardiovascular: Palpitations; tachycardia; cardiac arrhythmia; hypertension; collapse; extrasystoles; ventricular arrhythmias (ie, premature ventricular contractions); reflex bradycardia; coronary occlusion; subarachnoid hemorrhage; myocardial infarction; stroke; death associated with cardiac reactions. Headache or browache may occur.

> *Phenylephrine 10%* – Significant elevation of blood pressure is rare but can occur after conjunctival instillation. Exercise caution with elderly patients and children of low body weight. Carefully monitor the blood pressure of these patients. (See Warnings and Contraindications.) There have been rare reports of the development of serious cardiovascular reactions, including ventricular arrhythmias and myocardial infarctions. These episodes, some fatal, have usually occurred in elderly patients with preexisting cardiovascular diseases.

Miscellaneous: Headache; blanching; sweating; dizziness; nausea; nervousness; drowsiness; weakness; hyperglycemia.

Patient Information:

Potentially hazardous tasks: May cause temporary blurred vision. Observe caution while driving or performing other hazardous tasks.

If severe eye pain, headache, vision changes, acute eye redness, or pain with light exposure occur, discontinue use and consult a physician.

To avoid contamination, do not touch dropper tip to any surface. Replace cap after using.

Do not use if solution changes color or becomes cloudy.

Administration and Dosage:

Vasoconstrictors and pupil dilation: Instill a drop of topical anesthetic. Follow in a few minutes with 1 drop of the 2.5% or 10% phenylephrine. The anesthetic prevents stinging and consequent dilution of solution by lacrimation. It may be necessary to repeat the instillation after 1 hour, again preceded by a topical anesthetic.

Uveitis: The formation of synechiae may be prevented by using the 2.5% or 10% solution and atropine to produce wide dilation of the pupil. However, the vasoconstrictor effect of phenylephrine may be antagonistic to the increase of local blood flow in uveal infection.

To free recently formed posterior synechiae, instill 1 drop of the 2.5% or 10% solution to the upper surface of the cornea. Continue treatment the following day, if necessary. In the interim, apply hot compresses for 5 or 10 minutes, 3 times daily using 1 drop of 1% or 2% solution of atropine sulfate before and after each series of compresses.

Glaucoma: Instill 1 drop of 10% solution on the upper surface of the cornea as often as necessary. The 2.5% and 10% solutions have been used in conjunction with miotics in patients with open-angle glaucoma. Phenylephrine reduces the difficulties experienced by the patient because of the small field produced by miosis. Hence, there may be marked improvement in visual acuity after using phenylephrine with miotic drugs.

Surgery: When a short-acting mydriatic is needed for wide dilation of the pupil before intraocular surgery, the 2.5% or 10% solution may be instilled from 30 to 60 minutes before the operation.

Refraction: Prior to determination of refractive errors, the 2.5% solution may be used effectively with homatropine HBr, atropine sulfate, cyclopentolate, tropicamide HCl, or a combination of homatropine and cocaine HCl.

Adults – Instill 1 drop of the preferred cycloplegic in each eye; follow in 5 minutes with 1 drop phenylephrine 2.5% solution and in 10 minutes with another drop of the cycloplegic. In 50 to 60 minutes, the eyes are ready for refraction.

Because adequate cycloplegia is achieved at different time intervals after the necessary number of drops, different cycloplegics will require different waiting periods.

Children – Instill 1 drop of atropine sulfate 1% in each eye; follow in 10 to 15 minutes with 1 drop of phenylephrine 2.5% solution and in 5 to 10 minutes with a second drop of atropine sulfate 1%. In 1 to 2 hours, the eyes are ready for refraction.

For a "one application method," combine 2.5% phenylephrine solution with a cycloplegic, such as cyclopentolate, to elicit synergistic action. The additive effect varies depending on the patient. Therefore, when using a "one application method," it may be desirable to increase the concentration of the cycloplegic.

Ophthalmoscopic examination: Phenylephrine is rarely used alone for mydriasis. Maximum dilation is achieved in 45 to 60 minutes.

Diagnostic procedures: Heavily pigmented irides may require larger doses in all the following procedures:

Retinoscopy – When dilation of the pupil without cycloplegic action is desired, the 2.5% solution may be used alone.

MYDRIATICS AND CYCLOPLEGICS

Blanching test – Instill 1 to 2 drops of the 2.5% solution in the injected eye. After 5 minutes, examine for perilimbal blanching. If blanching occurs, the congestion is superficial and probably does not indicate iritis.

Stability: Prolonged exposure to air or strong light may cause oxidation and discoloration. Do not use if solution changes color, becomes cloudy, or contains a precipitate.

Rx	**Phenylephrine HCl** (Various, eg, Baush & Lomb, Falcon)	**Solution**: 2.5%	In 2, 5, and 15 mL.
Rx	**AK-Dilate** (Akorn)		In 2 and 15 mL.[1]
Rx	**Mydfrin 2.5%** (Alcon)		In 3 and 5 mL Drop-Tainers.[2]
Rx	**Neo-Synephrine** (Sanofi-Synthelabo)		In 15 mL.[3]
Rx	**Phenylephrine HCl** (Various, eg, Ciba Vision)	**Solution**: 10%	In 1, 2, and 5 mL.
Rx	**AK-Dilate** (Akorn)		In 2 and 5 mL.[1]
Rx	**Neo-Synephrine** (Sanofi-Synthelabo)		In 5 mL.[4]
Rx	**Neo-Synephrine Viscous** (Sanofi-Synthelabo)		In 5 mL.[5]

[1] With benzalkonium chloride.
[2] With 0.01% benzalkonium chloride, EDTA, sodium bisulfite.
[3] With 1:7500 benzalkonium chloride.
[4] With 1:10,000 benzalkonium chloride.
[5] With 1:10,000 benzalkonium chloride, methylcellulose.

CYCLOPLEGIC MYDRIATICS

Actions:

Pharmacology: Anticholinergic agents (cholinergic antagonists) block the responses of the sphincter muscle of the iris and the muscle of the ciliary body to cholinergic stimulation, producing pupillary dilation (mydriasis), and paralysis of accommodation (cycloplegia).

	Cycloplegic Mydriatics				
	Mydriasis		Cycloplegia		
Drug	Peak (minutes)	Recovery (days)	Peak (minutes)	Recovery (days)	Solution available
Atropine	30-40	7-10	60-180	6-12	0.5%-2%
Homatropine	40-60	1-3	30-60	1-3	2%-5%
Scopolamine	20-30	3-7	30-60	3-7	0.25%
Cyclopentolate	30-60	1	25-75	0.25-1	0.5%-2%
Tropicamide	20-40	0.25	20-35	h 0.25	0.25%-1%

Indications:

Mydriasis/Cycloplegia: For cycloplegic refraction and for dilating the pupil in inflammatory conditions of the iris and uveal tract. See individual monographs for specific indications.

Contraindications:

Primary glaucoma or a tendency toward glaucoma (eg, narrow anterior chamber angle); hypersensitivity to belladonna alkaloids or any component of the products; adhesions (synechiae) between the iris and the lens; children who have previously had a severe systemic reaction to atropine.

Warnings:

For topical ophthalmic use only: Not for injection.

Glaucoma: Determine the intraocular tension and the depth of the angle of the anterior chamber before and during use to avoid glaucoma attacks.

Elderly: Use these products with caution in the elderly and others where increased IOP may be encountered.

Pregnancy: Category C (atropine, cyclopentolate, homatropine). Safety for use during pregnancy has not been established. Give to a pregnant woman only if clearly needed.

Lactation: Atropine and homatropine may be detectable, in very small amounts, in breast milk. Although this is controversial, according to the American Academy of Pediatrics, these agents are compatible with breastfeeding. It is not known if cyclopentolate is excreted in breast milk. Exercise caution when administering to a nursing woman.

Children: Excessive use in children and in certain susceptible individuals may produce systemic toxic symptoms. Use with extreme caution in infants and small children.

> *Tropicamide and cyclopentolate* – May cause CNS disturbances, which may be dangerous in infants and children. Keep in mind the possibility of psychotic reaction and behavioral disturbance caused by hypersensitivity to anticholinergic drugs. Use with extreme caution. Increased susceptibility to cyclopentolate has been reported in infants, young children, and in children with spastic paralysis or brain damage. Feeding intolerance may follow ophthalmic use of this product in neonates. It is recommended that feeding be withheld for 4 hours after examination. Do not use in concentrations > 0.5% in small infants.

Precautions:

Systemic effects: Avoid excessive systemic absorption by compressing the lacrimal sac by digital pressure during and for 2 to 3 minutes after instillation.

Down's syndrome/children with brain damage: Use cycloplegics with caution. These patients may demonstrate a hyperreactive response to topical atropine.

Hazardous tasks: May produce drowsiness, blurred vision, or sensitivity to light (caused by dilated pupils); observe caution while driving or performing other tasks requiring alertness, coordination, or physical dexterity.

MYDRIATICS AND CYCLOPLEGICS

Sulfite sensitivity: Some of these products contain sulfites, which may cause allergic-type reactions (eg, hives, itching, wheezing, anaphylaxis) in certain susceptible people. Although the overall prevalence of sulfite sensitivity in the general population is probably low, it is seen more frequently in asthmatics or in atopic nonasthmatic people. Specific products containing sulfites are identified in the product listings.

Adverse Reactions:

Local: Increased intraocular pressure; transient stinging/burning; irritation with prolonged use (eg, allergic lid reactions, hyperemia, follicular conjunctivitis, blepharoconjunctivitis, vascular congestion, edema, exudate, eczematoid dermatitis).

Systemic: Dryness of the mouth and skin; blurred vision; photophobia with or without corneal staining; tachycardia; headache; parasympathetic stimulation; somnolence; visual hallucinations.

Other toxic manifestations of anticholinergic drugs include the following: Skin rash; abdominal distention in infants; unusual drowsiness; hyperpyrexia; vasodilation; urinary retention; diminished GI motility; decreased secretion in salivary and sweat glands, pharynx, bronchi, and nasal passages. Severe manifestations of toxicity include the following: Coma; medullary paralysis; death. Severe reactions are manifested by hypotension with progressive respiratory depression.

Cyclopentolate and tropicamide have been associated with psychotic reactions and behavioral disturbances in children. Ataxia, incoherent speech, restlessness, hallucinations, hyperactivity, seizures, disorientation as to time and place, and failure to recognize people have occurred with cyclopentolate. CNS disturbances also have occurred in children with tropicamide.

Overdosage:

Ocular: If ocular overdosage occurs, flush eye(s) with water or normal saline. Use of a topical miotic may be required. If accidentally ingested, induce emesis or gastric lavage.

Systemic: If symptoms develop (see Adverse Reactions), patients usually recover spontaneously when the drug is discontinued. In cases of severe toxicity, give physostigmine salicylate (see individual monograph in the Agents for Glaucoma chapter). Have atropine 1 mg available for immediate injection if physostigmine causes bradycardia, convulsions, or bronchoconstriction.

Cyclopentolate toxicity: Cyclopentolate toxicity may produce exaggerated symptoms (see Adverse Reactions). When administration of the drug product is discontinued, the patient usually recovers spontaneously. In case of severe manifestations of toxicity, the antidote of choice is physostigmine salicylate.

Children – Slowly inject physostigmine salicylate 0.5 mg IV. If toxic symptoms persist and no cholinergic symptoms are produced, repeat at 5-minute intervals to a maximum cumulative dose of 2 mg.

Adults and adolescents – Slowly inject physostigmine salicylate 2 mg IV. A second dose of 1 to 2 mg may be given after 20 minutes if no reversal of toxic manifestations has occurred.

Patient Information:

To avoid contamination, do not touch dropper tip to any surface. Replace cap after using.

May cause blurred vision. Do not drive or engage in any hazardous activities while the pupils are dilated.

May cause sensitivity to light. Protect eyes in bright illumination during dilation.

Keep out of the reach of children. These drugs should not be taken orally. Wash your hands and the child's hands following administration.

If eye pain occurs, discontinue use and consult physician immediately.

Individual drug monographs are on the following pages.

MYDRIATICS AND CYCLOPLEGICS

ATROPINE SULFATE

For complete prescribing information, refer to the Cycloplegic Mydriatrics group monograph.

Indications:

Mydriasis/Cycloplegia: For cycloplegic refraction or pupil dilation in acute inflammatory conditions of iris and uveal tract.

Administration and Dosage:

Solution:

> *Adults - Uveitis* – Instill 1 or 2 drops into the eye(s) up to 4 times daily.

> *Children - Uveitis* – Instill 1 or 2 drops of 0.5% solution into the eye(s) up to 3 times daily.

> *Refraction* – Instill 1 or 2 drops of 0.5% solution into the eye(s) twice daily for 1 to 3 days before examination.

Ointment: Apply a small amount in the conjunctival sac up to 3 times daily.

Compress the lacrimal sac by digital pressure during and for 2 to 3 minutes after instillation.

Individuals with heavily pigmented irides may require larger doses.

Storage: Keep away from heat.

Rx	**Atropine Sulfate Ophthalmic** (Various, eg, Bausch & Lomb, Fougera)	**Ointment:** 1%	In 3.5 and UD 1 g.
Rx	**Isopto Atropine** (Alcon)	**Solution:** 0.5%	In 5 mL Drop-Tainers.[1]
Rx	**Atropine Sulfate** (Various, eg, Alcon, Bausch & Lomb, Fougera, Ivax)	**Solution:** 1%	In 2, 5, and 15 mL and UD 1 mL.
Rx	**Atropine Care** (Akorn)		In 2, 5, and 15 mL.[2]
Rx	**Atropisol** (Novartis)		In 1 mL Dropperettes.[3]
Rx	**Isopto Atropine** (Alcon)		In 5 and 15 mL Drop-Tainers.[1]

[1] With 0.01% benzalkonium chloride, 0.5% hydroxypropyl methylcellulose, boric acid.
[2] With 0.01% benzalkonium chloride, hydroxypropyl methylcellulose, boric acid.
[3] With benzalkonium chloride, EDTA, boric acid.

OPHTHALMIC DRUG FACTS

HOMATROPINE HYDROBROMIDE

For complete prescribing information, refer to the Cycloplegic Mydriatics group monograph.

Indications:

Mydriasis/Cycloplegia: A moderately long-acting mydriatic and cycloplegic for refraction, and in the treatment of inflammatory conditions of the uveal tract. For preoperative and postoperative states when mydriasis is required.

Lens opacity: As an optical aid in some cases of axial lens opacities.

Administration and Dosage:

Uveitis: Instill 1 or 2 drops into the eye(s) up to every 3 to 4 hours.

Refraction: Instill 1 or 2 drops into the eye(s); repeat in 5 to 10 minutes if necessary.

Individuals with heavily pigmented irides may require larger doses.

Children: Use only the 2% strength.

Compress the lacrimal sac by digital pressure during and for 2 to 3 minutes after instillation.

Storage: Store at 8° to 24°C (46° to 75°F).

Rx	Isopto Homatropine (Alcon)	Solution: 2%	In 5 and 15 mL Drop-Tainers.[1]
Rx	Homatropine HBr (Various, eg, Alcon, Ciba Vision)	Solution: 5%	In 1, 2, and 5 mL.
Rx	AK-Homatropine (Akorn)		In 5 mL.
Rx	Isopto Homatropine (Alcon)		In 5 and 15 mL Drop-Tainers.[2]

[1] With 0.01% benzalkonium chloride, 0.5% hydroxypropyl methylcellulose, polysorbate 80.
[2] With 0.005% benzethonium chloride, 0.5% hydroxypropyl methylcellulose.

SCOPOLAMINE HYDROBROMIDE (Hyoscine Hydrobromide)

For complete prescribing information, refer to the Cycloplegic Mydriatics group monograph.

Indications:

Mydriasis/Cycloplegia: For cycloplegia and mydriasis in diagnostic procedures.

Iridocyclitis: For preoperative and postoperative states in the treatment of iridocyclitis.

MYDRIATICS AND CYCLOPLEGICS 53

Administration and Dosage:

Uveitis: Instill 1 or 2 drops into the eye(s) up to 4 times daily.

Refraction: Instill 1 or 2 drops into the eye(s) 1 hour before refracting.

Compress the lacrimal sac by digital pressure during and for 2 to 3 minutes after instillation.

Storage: Protect from light. Store at 8° to 27°C (46° to 80°F).

Rx	Isopto Hyoscine (Alcon)	Solution: 0.25%	In 5 and 15 mL Drop-Tainers.[1]

[1] With 0.01% benzalkonium chloride, 0.5% hydroxypropyl methylcellulose.

CYCLOPENTOLATE HYDROCHLORIDE

For complete prescribing information, refer to the Cycloplegic Mydriatics group monograph.

Indications:

Mydriasis/Cycloplegia: For mydriasis and cycloplegia in diagnostic procedures.

Administration and Dosage:

Adults: Instill 1 or 2 drops of 0.5%, 1%, or 2% solution into eye(s). Repeat in 5 to 10 minutes, if necessary. Complete recovery usually occurs in 24 hours.

Children: Instill 1 or 2 drops of 0.5%, 1%, or 2% solution into each eye. Follow in 5 to 10 minutes with a second application of 0.5% or 1% solution, if necessary.

Small infants: Instill 1 drop of 0.5% solution into each eye. Observe patient closely for ≥ 30 minutes following instillation.

Compress the lacrimal sac by digital pressure during and for 2 to 3 minutes after instillation.

Individuals with heavily pigmented irides may require higher strengths.

Storage: Store at 8° to 27°C (46° to 80°F).

Rx	Cyclogyl (Alcon)	Solution: 0.5%	In 2, 5, and 15 mL Drop-Tainers.[1]
Rx	Cyclopentolate HCl (Various, eg, Bausch & Lomb)	Solution: 1%	In 2, 5, and 15 mL.
Rx	AK-Pentolate (Akorn)		In 2, 5, and 15 mL.[1]
Rx	Cyclogyl (Alcon)		In 2, 5, and 15 mL.[1]
Rx	AK-Pentolate (Akorn)	Solution: 2%	In 2, 5, and 15 mL white opaque dropper bottles.
Rx	Cyclogyl (Alcon)		In 2, 5, and 15 mL Drop-Tainers.[1]

[1] With 0.01% benzalkonium chloride, EDTA, boric acid.

TROPICAMIDE

For complete prescribing information, refer to the Cycloplegic Mydriatics group monograph.

Indications:

Mydriasis/Cycloplegia: For mydriasis and cycloplegia for diagnostic purposes.

Administration and Dosage:

Refraction: Instill 1 or 2 drops of 1% solution into the eye(s); repeat in 5 minutes. If patient is not seen within 20 to 30 minutes, instill an additional drop to prolong mydriatic effect.

Examination of fundus: Instill 1 or 2 drops of 0.5% solution 15 to 20 minutes prior to examination. Compress the lacrimal sac by digital pressure during and for 2 to 3 minutes after instillation to avoid excessive absorption.

Individuals with heavily pigmented irides may require larger doses.

Storage: Store away from heat. Do not refrigerate.

Rx	**Tropicamide** (Various, eg, Bausch & Lomb, Falcon)	**Solution:** 0.5%	In 2 and 15 mL.
Rx	**Mydriacyl** (Alcon)		In 15 mL Drop-Tainers.[1]
Rx	**Tropicacyl** (Akorn)		In 2 and 15 mL.
Rx	**Tropicamide** (Various, eg, Falcon)	**Solution:** 1%	In 3 and 15 mL.
Rx	**Mydriacyl** (Alcon)		In 3 and 15 mL Drop-Tainers.[1]
Rx	**Tropicacyl** (Akorn)		In 2 and 15 mL.[2]

[1] With 0.01% benzalkonium chloride, EDTA.
[2] With 0.1% benzalkonium chloride, EDTA.

MYDRIATIC COMBINATIONS

These combinations induce mydriasis that is greater than that of either drug used alone at the concentrations present in these combination formulations. See individual monographs for complete prescribing information.

Indications:

Cyclomydril: Production of mydriasis.

Murocoll-2: For mydriasis, cycloplegia, and to break posterior synechiae in iritis.

Administration and Dosage:

Cyclomydril: Instill 1 drop into each eye every 5 to 10 minutes, not to exceed 3 times.

MYDRIATICS AND CYCLOPLEGICS

Murocoll-2:

Mydriasis – Instill 1 or 2 drops into eye(s); repeat in 5 minutes, if necessary.

Postoperatively – Instill 1 or 2 drops into the eye(s) 3 or 4 times daily.

Rx	**Cyclomydril** (Alcon)	**Solution:** 0.2% cyclopentolate HCl and 1% phenylephrine HCl.	In 2 and 5 mL Drop-Tainers.[1]
Rx	**Murocoll-2** (Bausch & Lomb)	**Drops:** 0.3% scopolamine HBr and 10% phenylephrine HCl.	In 5 mL.[2]

[1] With 0.01% benzalkonium chloride, EDTA, boric acid.
[2] With 0.01% benzalkonium chloride, sodium metabisulfite, EDTA.

Antiallergy and Decongestant Agents

Release of histamine, prostaglandins, leukotrienes, and other less well-defined mediators from the mast cell during an allergic reaction can cause a variety of uncomfortable symptoms and sometimes life-threatening complications. Drug therapy is often successful in satisfactorily relieving associated signs and symptoms, especially when ocular tissues are affected.

Type I hypersensitivity reactions, also known as anaphylactic, immediate, or IgE-mediated reactions, occur when an antigen such as a drug or pollen is reintroduced into an individual who has been previously exposed to the antigen. Upon initial exposure to the antigen, IgE antibodies are produced that attach to mast cells and make the cells susceptible to rupture when the patient is again exposed to the same antigen. Disruption (degranulation) of mast cells causes a release of large quantities of inflammatory mediators, including histamine, prostaglandins, leukotrienes, and eosinophil chemotactic factor. Histamine activates H_1 receptors on blood vessels, causing vasodilation. These dilated blood vessels leak fluid, causing tissues to swell. Common symptoms and signs of local Type I reactions include redness, swelling, and itching. Such reactions occur in hay fever, allergic conjunctivitis, asthma, bee stings, and other chemical and toxin sensitivities (eg, penicillin). The following ocular diseases are characterized by Type I hypersensitivity reactions and may be treated with antihistamines or mast cell stabilizers.

ALLERGIC CONDITIONS

Seasonal Allergic Conjunctivitis

Allergic conjunctivitis can result from a variety of exogenous antigens and is often a component of more widespread allergic states. Airborne pollens, dust, and other environmental contaminants constitute the largest single group of agents responsible for the disorder. Ophthalmic drugs and their preservatives/excipients, which may cause allergic conjunctivitis, include neomycin, sulfonamides, atropine, and thimerosal. A careful patient history along with the typical appearance of conjunctival chemosis and hyperemia, together with itching and tearing, are necessary for the proper etiologic diagnosis.

Vernal Conjunctivitis

Affecting primarily adolescent males, vernal conjunctivitis is a bilateral inflammation involving the upper tarsal conjunctiva and sometimes the limbal conjunctiva. The disease is seasonal and has peak activity during the warm months of the year. It is characterized by the formation of large papillae having the appearance of cobble-stones on the upper tarsal conjunctiva. Papillary hypertrophy can occur at the limbus and is characterized by a gelatinous thickening of the superior limbus. Tear histamine levels are significantly higher than in normal patients. Symptoms include intense itching during warm months and often a thick, ropy discharge. If the cornea becomes involved, photophobia may be marked. Significant papillary involvement of the upper lids may result in ptosis.

Atopic Keratoconjunctivitis

Atopic keratoconjunctivitis represents a hypersensitivity state caused by predisposi-tional, constitutional, or hereditary factors rather than by acquired hypersensitivity to specific antigens. Patients usually have a personal or family history of allergy, espe-cially asthma or hay fever. Atopic dermatitis is characterized by patches of thickened, excoriated, lichenified skin that is usually dry and itchy. Ocular findings are charac-terized by conjunctival hyperemia and chemosis. Corneal involvement is not uncom-mon and may be evident as a classic shield ulcer or pannus.

Giant Papillary Conjunctivitis

Giant papillary conjunctivitis (GPC) is a specific conjunctival inflammatory reaction to materials on contact lenses (eg, protein), but has also been reported in patients wearing methylmethacrylate ocular prostheses. The condition is characterized by papillary hypertrophy and primarily affects the upper tarsal conjunctiva. Although the condition is similar in appearance to that of vernal conjunctivitis, it probably repre-sents a chronic conjunctival inflammatory reaction to denatured proteins that are adherent to the anterior lens surface. Lens bulk (thickness and diameter) may also play a part. Once the conjunctival changes reach a certain point, itching, lens instability, mucoid discharge, and contact lens intolerance occur.

DECONGESTANTS

The vasoconstrictor effect of the adrenergic agonists (ie, phenylephrine and the imida-zole derivatives) makes them useful as topical ocular decongestants. Following instil-lation, conjunctival vessels constrict within minutes, causing the eye to whiten. Minor ocular irritation can be temporarily relieved.

Because of the relatively low concentrations required for ocular decongestion, phenyl-ephrine and the imidazole derivatives generally do not cause systemic side effects. These products are designed for short-term use because they may mask symptoms of more serious ocular problems such as bacterial or other infections. If the condition does not respond to use of these products within 48 hours, a more serious condition should be suspected.

Phenylephrine

Phenylephrine (eg, *Neo-Synephrine*), a synthetic amine structurally similar to epineph-rine, has been used in *otc* products at concentrations of 0.12% or 0.125%, which cause vasoconstriction with little or no pupillary dilation in eyes with intact corneal epi-thelium. Because a potential for mydriasis does exist at low concentrations, phenyl-ephrine is contraindicated in eyes predisposed to angle-closure glaucoma. Prolonged or excessive use can result in rebound conjunctival hyperemia. The eye may become more congested and red as the effect of the drug begins to subside.

ANTIALLERGY AND DECONGESTANT AGENTS

Phenylephrine can exhibit variable effectiveness because it is subject to oxidation on exposure to air, light, or heat. The solution may show no evidence of discoloration. To prolong shelf-life, antioxidants such as sodium bisulfite may be added to the formulation.

Imidazole Derivatives

The imidazole derivatives, naphazoline (eg, *Naphcon*), tetrahydrozoline (eg, *Visine*), and oxymetazoline (eg, *Visine L.R.*), differ structurally from phenylephrine by replacement of the benzene ring with an unsaturated ring. Concentrations used for ocular vasoconstriction do not alter pupil size or raise intraocular pressure in the normal eye.

The imidazole derivatives do not differ significantly in their ability to relieve conjunctival congestion. After instillation, the blanching effect occurs within minutes and may last up to several hours. These agents are generally more stable in solution than phenylephrine, and have a longer shelf-life and duration of action. Imidazole derivatives are buffered to a pH of 6.2 and may sting upon initial instillation.

ANTIHISTAMINES, MAST CELL STABILIZERS, AND NSAIDS

Because many of the signs and symptoms associated with Type I hypersensitivity reactions are due to the release of histamine from mast cells, antihistamines can be effective in relieving at least some signs and symptoms and provide patient comfort. Several H_1-receptor antagonists, including levocabastine (*Livostin*) and emedastine (*Emadine*) have been formulated for topical ocular use.

Ketorolac tromethamine (*Acular*) is the first NSAID approved for topical ocular use in seasonal allergic conjunctivitis (see the Anti-inflammatory Agents chapter). It can alleviate the ocular itching as well as other signs and symptoms that accompany the reaction.

Mast cell stabilizers can also be useful for certain ocular allergic signs and symptoms. Cromolyn sodium (*Crolom*) and lodoxamide tromethamine (*Alomide*) are currently FDA-approved for the management of vernal keratoconjunctivitis. Nedocromil (*Alocril*) is approved for seasonal allergic conjunctivitis. This agent has a relatively fast onset of action (ie, ≈ 15 minutes) following institution. The dose is 2 times/day. Some agents have mast cell stabilizing properties as well as H_1-receptor antagonist activity. Examples include olopatadine (*Patanol*) and ketotifen (*Zaditor*), both effective with twice-daily administration.

COMBINATION PRODUCTS

In addition to vasoconstrictor substances, ocular decongestants may also contain preservatives, antihistamines, viscosity-increasing agents, buffers, and astringents. Because preservatives may induce allergic reactions in some patients, unit-dose preservative-free products are being formulated.

PHARMACOLOGIC MANAGEMENT

Antihistamines can be given with or without decongestants, and are administered topically or orally, depending on the degree of involvement. Mast cell stabilizers such as nedocromil (*Alocril*) and azelastine (*Optivar*) can provide immediate relief of itching and provide protection throughout the allergy season. Cromolyn sodium (*Crolom*) and pemirolast (*Alcomast*) are also effective and can even be used prophylactically. For severe reactions or when rapid relief of symptoms is warranted, topical, such as lotoprednol (*Alerex*), or oral corticosteroids may be justified. In addi-

OPHTHALMIC DRUG FACTS

tion, ketorolac tromethamine (*Acular*), a nonsteroidal anti-inflammatory drug, is indicated for the relief of ocular itching due to seasonal allergic conjunctivitis (see the Anti-inflammatory Agents chapter).

Jimmy D. Bartlett, OD, DOS
University of Alabama at Birmingham

Siret D. Jaanus, PhD
Southern California College of Optometry

For More Information

Abelson MB, Schaefer K. Conjunctivitis of allergic origin. *Surv Ophthalmol* 1993;38:115.

Abelson MA, Spitalny L. Combined analysis of two studies using the conjuctival allergen model to evaluate oloptadine, a new ophthalmic antiallergic agent with dual activity. *Am J Ophthalmol* 1998;125:797-804.

Bartlett JD, Jaanus SD, eds. Clinical Ocular Pharmacology, ed. 4. Boston: Butterworth-Heinemann, 2001.

Bartlett JD, Ross RN. Primary care of ocular allergy. *J Am Optom Assoc* 1990;61(6)(Suppl):S3-S46.

Bartlett JD, Swanson MW. Ophthalmic products. In: Covington T, ed. *Handbook of Non-Prescription Drugs*, ed. 10. Washington, DC: American Pharmaceutical Association, 1993:351.

Caldwell DR, Verin P, Hartwich-Young R, et al. Efficacy and safety of lodoxamide 0.1% vs cromolyn sodium 4% in patients with vernal keratoconjunctivitis. *Am J Ophthalmol* 1992;113:632-37.

Ciprandi G, Buscaglia S, et al. Drug treatment of allergic conjunctivitis. *Drugs* 1992;43:154.

Nobles S, McTavich D. Levocabastine: A study of its pharmacology, clinical efficacy and tolerability in the topical treatment of allergic rhinitis and conjunctivitis. *Drugs* 1995;50:1032-49.

Yanni JM, Stephens DJ, Parnell DW, et al. Preclinical efficacy of emadastine, a potent, selective antihistamine H_1 antagonist for topical ocular use. *J Ocul Pharmacol* 1994;10:665-75.

ANTIALLERGY AND DECONGESTANT AGENTS

DECONGESTANTS

Actions:

Pharmacology: The effects of sympathomimetic agents on the eye are concentration-dependent and include: Pupil dilation, increase in outflow of aqueous humor, and vasoconstriction (alpha-adrenergic effects).

Higher concentrations of drug (ie, phenylephrine 2.5% and 10%) cause vasoconstriction and pupillary dilation for diagnostic eye exams, during surgery, and to prevent synechiae formation in uveitis. Weak concentrations of phenylephrine (0.12%) and other alpha-adrenergic agonists (naphazoline; tetrahydrozoline) are used as ophthalmic decongestants (vasoconstriction of conjunctival blood vessels) and for symptomatic relief of minor eye irritations. Epinephrine is used for open-angle glaucoma and is not included in this monograph (see monograph in Agents for Glaucoma chapter).

Ophthalmic Vasoconstrictors			
Vasoconstrictor	Duration of action (hr)	Available concentration	Prescription status
Naphazoline	3 to 4	0.012%	otc
		0.02%	otc
		0.03%	otc
		0.1%	Rx
Oxymetazoline	4 to 6	0.025%	otc
Phenylephrine	0.5 to 1.5	0.12%	otc
	—	2.5%	Rx
	—	10%	Rx
Tetrahydrozoline	1 to 4	0.05%	otc

Indications:

Refer to individual product listings for specific indications.

Contraindications:

Hypersensitivity to any of these agents; narrow-angle glaucoma or anatomically narrow (occludable) angle with no glaucoma; prior to peripheral iridectomy in eyes capable of angle closure because mydriatic action may precipitate angle closure.

Phenylephrine 10%: Infants and patients with aneurysms.

Warnings:

Anesthetics: Discontinue prior to use of anesthetics that sensitize the myocardium to sympathomimetics (eg, cyclopropane, halothane).

Local anesthetics can increase absorption of topically applied drugs; exercise caution when applying prior to use of phenylephrine. However, use of a local anesthetic prior to phenylephrine 2.5% or 10% may prevent stinging and enhance ocular drug penetration.

Overuse: Overuse may produce rebound vasodilation and increased redness of the eye.

62   OPHTHALMIC DRUG FACTS

Phenylephrine 10%: There have been rare reports of the development of serious cardiovascular reactions, including ventricular arrhythmias and myocardial infarctions. These episodes, some fatal, usually have occurred in elderly patients with preexisting cardiovascular diseases.

Pregnancy: Category C. Safety for use in pregnancy is not established. Use only if clearly needed and if the potential benefits outweigh the potential hazards to the fetus.

Lactation: Safety for use during breastfeeding has not been established. Use caution when administering to a nursing woman.

Children: Safety and efficacy have not been established. Phenylephrine 10% is contraindicated in infants.

Precautions:

Special-risk patients: Use with caution in children of low body weight, the elderly, and in the presence of hypertension, diabetes, hyperthyroidism, cardiovascular abnormalities, or arteriosclerosis.

Narrow-angle glaucoma: Ordinarily, any mydriatic is contraindicated in patients with angle-closure glaucoma. However, when temporary pupil dilation may free adhesions, these advantages may temporarily outweigh danger from coincident pupil dilation.

Rebound congestion: Rebound congestion may occur with frequent or extended use of ophthalmic vasoconstrictors. Rebound miosis has occurred in older people 1 day after receiving phenylephrine; reinstillation produced a reduction in mydriasis.

Systemic absorption: Exceeding recommended dosages of these agents or applying phenylephrine 2.5% to 10% solutions to the instrumented, traumatized, diseased, or postsurgical eye or adnexa, or to patients with suppressed lacrimation, as during anesthesia, may result in the absorption of sufficient quantities to produce a systemic vasopressor response.

Pigment floaters: Older individuals may develop transient pigment floaters in the aqueous humor 30 to 45 minutes after instillation of phenylephrine. The appearance may be similar to anterior uveitis or to a microscopic hyphema.

Hazardous tasks: Phenylephrine may cause temporary blurred or unstable vision; observe caution while driving or performing other hazardous tasks.

Sulfite sensitivity: Some of these products contain sulfites that may cause allergic-type reactions (eg, hives, itching, wheezing, anaphylaxis) in certain susceptible people. Although the overall prevalence of sulfite sensitivity in the general population is low, it is seen more frequently in asthmatics or in atopic nonasthmatic people.

Drug Interactions:

Ophthalmic Sympathomimetic Drug Interactions			
Precipitant drug	Object drug*		Description
Anesthetics	Ophthalmic sympatho-mimetics	↑	Use with caution anesthetics that sensitize the myocardium to sympathomimetics (eg, cyclopropane, halothane). Local anesthetics can increase absorption of topical drugs; exercise caution when applying prior to use of phenylephrine.

ANTIALLERGY AND DECONGESTANT AGENTS

Ophthalmic Sympathomimetic Drug Interactions			
Precipitant drug	Object drug*		Description
Beta blockers	Ophthalmic sympatho-mimetics	↑	Systemic side effects may occur more readily in patients taking these drugs.
MAOIs	Ophthalmic sympatho-mimetics	↑	When given with, or up to 21 days after MAOIs, exaggerated adrenergic effects may result. Supervise and adjust dosage carefully.

* ↑ = Object drug increased.

Also consider drug interactions that may occur with systemic use of the sympatho-mimetics.

Adverse Reactions:

Ophthalmic: Transitory stinging on initial instillation; blurring of vision; mydriasis; increased redness; irritation; discomfort; punctate keratitis; lacrimation; increased IOP.

Phenylephrine may cause rebound miosis and decreased mydriatic response to therapy in older people.

Cardiovascular: Palpitation; tachycardia; cardiac arrhythmia; hypertension; collapse; extrasystoles; ventricular arrhythmias (ie, premature ventricular contractions); reflex bradycardia; coronary occlusion; subarachnoid hemorrhage; myocardial infarction; stroke; death associated with cardiac reactions. Headache or browache may occur.

> *Phenylephrine 10%* – Significant elevation of blood pressure is rare but can occur after conjunctival instillation. Exercise caution with elderly patients and children of low body weight. Carefully monitor the blood pressure of these patients. (See Warnings and Precautions.) There have been rare reports of the development of serious cardiovascular reactions, including ventricular arrhythmias and myocardial infarctions. These episodes, some fatal, have usually occurred in elderly patients with preexisting cardiovascular diseases.

Miscellaneous: Blanching; sweating; dizziness; nausea; nervousness; drowsiness; weakness; hyperglycemia.

Patient Information:

Do not use for > 48 to 72 hours without consulting a physician.

If irritation, blurring, or redness persists, or if severe eye pain, headache, vision changes, floating spots, dizziness, decrease in body temperature, drowsiness, acute eye redness, or pain with light exposure occur, discontinue use and consult a physician.

Do not use if you have glaucoma except under the advice of a physician.

Refer to the Dosage Forms and Administration chapter for more complete information.

Hazardous tasks: Phenylephrine may cause temporary blurred or unstable vision; observe caution while driving or performing other hazardous tasks.

Individual drug monographs are on the following pages.

PHENYLEPHRINE HCl

For complete prescribing information, refer to the Decongestants group monograph.

Indications:

0.12%: A decongestant to provide relief of minor eye irritations.

Administration and Dosage:

Minor eye irritations: Instill 1 or 2 drops of the 0.12% solution in eye(s) up to 4 times daily as needed.

Storage/Stability: Prolonged exposure to air or strong light may cause oxidation and discoloration. Do not use if solution changes color, becomes cloudy, or contains a precipitate.

otc	**AK-Nefrin** (Akorn)	**Solution**: 0.12%	In 15 mL.[1]
otc	**Prefrin Liquifilm** (Allergan)		In 20 mL.[2]
otc	**Relief** (Allergan)		Preservative free. In UD 0.3 mL.[3]
otc	**Zincfrin Solution** (Alcon)		In 15 mL Drop-Tainers.[4]

[1] With 0.005% benzalkonium chloride, 1.4% polyvinyl alcohol, EDTA.
[2] With 1.4% polyvinyl alcohol, 0.004% benzalkonium chloride, EDTA.
[3] With 1.4% polyvinyl alcohol, EDTA.
[4] With 0.01% benzalkonium chloride, polysorbate 80, and 0.25% zinc sulfate.

NAPHAZOLINE HCl

For complete prescribing information, refer to the Decongestants group monograph.

Indications:

Redness: To soothe, refresh, and remove redness caused by minor eye irritation such as smoke, smog, sun glare, allergies, or swimming.

Administration and Dosage:

Instill 1 or 2 drops into the conjunctival sac of affected eye(s) every 3 to 4 hours, up to 4 times daily.

Storage/Stability: Do not use if solution changes color or becomes cloudy.

otc	**20/20 Eye Drops** (S.S.S.)	**Solution**: 0.012%	In 15 mL.[1]
otc	**Allergy Drops** (Bausch & Lomb)		In 15 mL.[2]
otc	**Clear Eyes** (Ross)		In 15 and 30 mL.[3]
otc	**Clear Eyes ACR** (Ross)		In 15 and 30 mL.[4]
otc	**Naphcon** (Alcon)		In 15 mL.[5]

ANTIALLERGY AND DECONGESTANT AGENTS

otc	**VasoClear** (Novartis)	**Solution:** 0.02%	In 15 mL.[6]
otc	**VasoClear A** (Novartis)		In 15 mL.[7]
otc	**Allergy Drops Maximum Strength** (Bausch & Lomb)	**Solution:** 0.03%	In 15 mL.[8]
Rx	**Naphazoline HCl** (Various, eg, Major, Ivax, Qualitest)	**Solution:** 0.1%	In 15 mL.
Rx	**AK-Con** (Akorn)		In 15 mL.[5]
Rx	**Albalon** (Allergan)		In 15 mL.[9]
Rx	**Nafazair** (Bausch & Lomb)		In 15 mL.[5]
Rx	**Naphcon Forte** (Alcon)		In 15 mL Drop-Tainers.[5]
Rx	**Vasocon Regular** (Ciba Vision)		In 15 mL.[10]

[1] With 0.01% benzalkonium chloride, 0.4% glycerin, 0.25% zinc sulfate, EDTA.
[2] With 0.2% PEG-300, 0.01% benzalkonium chloride.
[3] With benzalkonium chloride, EDTA, 0.2% glycerin, boric acid.
[4] With benzalkonium chloride, EDTA, 0.25% zinc sulfate, 0.2% glycerin.
[5] With 0.01% benzalkonium chloride, EDTA.
[6] With 0.01% benzalkonium chloride, 0.25% polyvinyl alcohol, 1% PEG-400, EDTA.
[7] With 0.005% benzalkonium chloride, EDTA, 0.25% zinc sulfate, 0.25% polyvinyl alcohol, 1% PEG-400.
[8] With 0.01% benzalkonium chloride, 0.5% hydroxypropyl methylcellulose, EDTA.
[9] With 0.004% benzalkonium chloride, EDTA, 1.4% polyvinyl alcohol.
[10] With benzalkonium chloride, polyvinyl alcohol, EDTA, PEG-8000.

TETRAHYDROZOLINE HCl

For complete prescribing information, refer to the Decongestants group monograph.

Indications:

Redness: For relief of redness of the eye due to minor irritations.

Burning/Irritation: For temporary relief of burning and irritation caused by dryness of the eye or discomfort caused by minor irritations or to exposure to wind or sun.

Administration and Dosage:

Instill 1 or 2 drops into eye(s) up to 4 times a day.

Storage/Stability: Do not use if solution changes color or becomes cloudy.

otc	**Tetrahydrozoline HCl** (Rugby)	**Solution**: 0.05%	In 15 and 30 mL.
otc	**Collyrium Fresh** (Wyeth-Ayerst)		In 15 mL.[1]
otc	**Eyesine** (Akorn)		In 15 mL.[2]
otc	**Geneye** (Ivax)		In 15 and 22.5 mL.[3]
otc	**Murine Tears Plus** (Ross)		In 15 and 30 mL.[4]
otc	**Optigene 3** (Pfeiffer)		In 15 mL.[3]
otc	**Tetrasine** (Optopics)		In 15 and 22.5 mL.[5]
otc	**Tetrasine Extra** (Optopics)		In 15 mL.[6]
otc	**Visine** (Pfizer)		In 15, 22.5, and 30 mL.[3]
otc	**Visine A.C.** (Pfizer)		In 15 mL.[7]
otc	**Visine Advanced Relief** (Pfizer)		In 15 and 30 mL.[8]

[1] With 0.01% benzalkonium chloride, 0.1% EDTA, 1% glycerin.
[2] With 0.01% benzalkonium chloride, EDTA.
[3] With 0.01% benzalkonium chloride, 0.1% EDTA.
[4] With benzalkonium chloride, EDTA, 1.4% polyvinyl alcohol, 0.6% povidone.
[5] With benzalkonium chloride, EDTA.
[6] With 1% polyethylene glycol 400, benzalkonium chloride, EDTA.
[7] With 0.01% benzalkonium chloride, 0.1% EDTA, 0.25% zinc sulfate.
[8] With benzalkonium chloride, 1% polyethylene glycol 400, 1% povidone, 0.1% dextran 70, EDTA.

OXYMETAZOLINE HCl

For complete prescribing information, refer to the Decongestants group monograph.

Indications:

Redness: For the relief of redness of the eye caused by minor eye irritations.

Administration and Dosage:

Adults and children ≥ 6 years: Instill 1 or 2 drops in the affected eye(s) every 6 hours.

Storage/Stability: Do not use if solution changes color or becomes cloudy.

otc	**OcuClear** (Schering-Plough)	**Solution**: 0.025%	In 30 mL.[1]
otc	**Visine L.R.** (Pfizer)		In 15 and 30 mL.[1]

[1] With 0.01% benzalkonium chloride, 0.1% EDTA.

ANTIHISTAMINES

Actions:

Pharmacology: Antihistamines can be used alone or in combination with deconges-tants to provide relief of ocular irritation or congestion for the treatment of allergic or inflammatory ocular conditions. Antihistamines counteract the effects of histamine,

ANTIALLERGY AND DECONGESTANT AGENTS 67

a chemical released in the body in response to an antigen-antibody reaction that causes redness, itching, and irritation of tissues, and can cause watery eyes, runny nose, and sneezing.

Indications:

To provide relief of symptoms of allergic conjunctivitis (watering, itching eyes).

Contraindications:

Hypersensitivity to any component of the formulation; with monoamine oxidase (MAO) inhibitor use.

Warnings:

Elderly: The elderly may require lower doses. Antihistamines are more likely to cause dizziness, sedation, confusion, and decreased blood pressure in the elderly.

Pregnancy: Category C. Safety for use has not been established. Use only if clearly needed and if the potential benefits to the mother outweigh the potential hazards to the fetus.

Lactation: Antihistamines appear in breast milk. Breastfeeding should be discouraged while using these medications.

Children: Antihistamine overdosage in children may cause hallucinations, convulsions, and death. Antihistamines may decrease mental alertness. They produce hyperactivity in children. Use caution in children < 12 years of age.

Precautions:

Use with caution in the presence of asthma, coronary artery disease, digestive tract obstruction, enlarged prostate, glaucoma (narrow-angle), heart disease, hypertension, hyperthyroidism, irregular heartbeat, liver disease, peptic ulcer, pregnancy, urinary bladder obstruction.

Glaucoma: Because they produce angle closure, use with caution in people with narrow angle or a history of glaucoma.

Topical antihistamines: Topical antihistamines are potential sensitizers and may produce a local sensitivity reaction.

Drug Interactions:

Alcohol, sedatives (sleeping pills), tranquilizers, antianxiety medications, and narcotic pain relievers all are known to react with antihistamines. The following drugs and drug classes also interact with antihistamines: Anticoagulants, epinephrine, fluconazole, isocarboxazid, itraconazole, ketoconazole, macrolides, metronidazole, miconazole, phenelzine, procarbazine, selegiline, tranylcypromine.

Adverse Reactions:

Ophthalmic: Blurred and double vision; eye pain; dryness; sensitivity to light.

OPHTHALMIC DRUG FACTS

Systemic: Stomach ache; constipation; appetite changes; nausea; vomiting; diarrhea; drowsiness; dizziness; mental confusion; decreased coordination; fatigue; headache; sleeplessness; sleepiness; sore throat; pharyngitis; cough; dry nose, throat, and mouth; thickening of mucus in respiratory tract; wheezing; stuffiness.

Cardiovascular: Irregular heartbeat; palpitations; hypotension.

Miscellaneous: Difficult urination; urine retention; ringing in the ears; rash; hives; excessive perspiration; chills.

Patient Information:

May cause drowsiness or dizziness. Use caution while driving or performing tasks requiring mental alertness. Avoid alcohol and other sedatives, hypnotics, tranquilizers, etc.

Elderly patients are more likely to experience dizziness, sedation, decreased coordination, mental confusion, and fainting when they take antihistamines.

May produce unexpected excitation, restlessness, irritability, and insomnia in rare instances. This is most likely in children and elderly patients.

Do not use for several days before allergy skin testing.

To avoid contamination, do not touch tip of the container to any surface. Replace cap after using.

Individual drug monographs are on the following pages.

ANTIALLERGY AND DECONGESTANT AGENTS

KETOTIFEN FUMARATE

Actions:

Pharmacology: Ketotifen is a relatively selective, noncompetitive histamine H_1-receptor antagonist and mast cell stabilizer. Ketotifen inhibits the release of mediators from cells involved in hypersensitivity reactions. Decreased chemotaxis and activation of eosinophils has also been demonstrated.

In human conjunctival allergen challenge studies, ketotifen was significantly more effective than placebo in preventing ocular itching associated with allergic conjunctivitis. The onset of action occurs rapidly with an effect seen within minutes of administration.

Indications:

Allergic conjunctivitis: Temporary prevention of itching of the eye caused by allergic conjunctivitis.

Contraindications:

Hypersensitivity to any component of this product.

Warnings:

Route of Administration: For topical ophthalmic use only. Not for injection or oral use.

Pregnancy: Category C. It is not known whether ketotifen fumarate can cause fetal harm when administered to a pregnant woman or can affect reproductive capacity. There are no adequate and well-controlled studies in pregnant women. Use during pregnancy only if the potential benefits outweigh the potential hazards to the fetus.

Lactation: Ketotifen has been identified in the breast milk of rats following oral administration. It is not known whether topical ocular administration could result in sufficient systemic absorption to produce detectable quantities in breast milk. Caution should be exercised when ketotifen is administered to a nursing woman.

Children: Safety and effectiveness in pediatric patients < 3 years of age have not been established.

Adverse Reactions:

In controlled clinical studies, conjunctival injection, headaches, and rhinitis were reported at an incidence of 10% to 25%. The occurrence of these side effects was generally mild. Some of these events were similar to the underlying ocular disease being studied.

Ophthalmic: Allergic reaction, burning or stinging, conjunctivitis, discharge, dry eyes, eye pain, eyelid disorder, itching, keratitis, lacrimation disorder, mydriasis, photophobia, and rash (< 5%).

Miscellaneous: Flu syndrome; pharyngitis (< 5%).

Patient Information:

To prevent contaminating the dropper tip and solution, do not touch the eyelids or surrounding areas with the dropper tip of the bottle. Keep the bottle tightly closed when not in use.

Do not wear contact lenses if eyes are red. The preservative in ketotifen, benzalkonium chloride, may be absorbed by soft contact lenses. Ketotifen should not be used to treat contact lens-related irritation. Patients who wear contact lenses and whose eyes are not red should wait ≥ 10 minutes after instilling ketotifen before they insert their contact lenses.

Administration and Dosage:

The recommended dose is 1 drop in the affected eye(s) every 8 to 12 hours.

Storage/Stability: Store between 4° to 25°C (39° to 77°F).

Rx	**Zaditor** (Novartis)	**Solution:** 0.25 mg/mL (0.345 mg/mL ketotifen fumarate)	In 5 and 7 mL.[1]

[1] With 0.01% benzalkonium chloride, glycerol, sodium hydroxide/hydrochloric acid.

LEVOCABASTINE HCl

Actions:

Pharmacology: Levocabastine is a potent, selective histamine H_1-receptor antagonist for topical ophthalmic use. Antigen challenge studies performed 2 and 4 hours after initial drug instillation indicated activity was maintained for ≥ 2 hours.

Pharmacokinetics: After instillation in the eye, levocabastine is systemically absorbed. However, the amount of systemically absorbed levocabastine after therapeutic ocular doses is low (mean plasma concentrations in the range of 1 to 2 ng/mL).

Clinical Trials: Levocabastine instilled 4 times daily was significantly more effective than its vehicle in reducing ocular itching associated with seasonal allergic conjunctivitis.

Indications:

Allergic conjunctivitis: For the temporary relief of the signs and symptoms of seasonal allergic conjunctivitis.

Contraindications:

Hypersensitivity to any component of the product; while wearing soft contact lenses.

Warnings:

For ophthalmic use only: Not for injection.

ANTIALLERGY AND DECONGESTANT AGENTS 71

Carcinogenesis: In female mice, levocabastine doses of 5000 and 21,500 times the maximum recommended ocular human use level resulted in an increased incidence of pituitary gland adenoma and mammary gland adenocarcinoma possibly produced by increased prolactin levels. The clinical relevance of this finding is unknown with regard to the interspecies differences in prolactin physiology and the very low plasma concentrations of levocabastine following ocular administration.

Pregnancy: Category C. Levocabastine is teratogenic (polydactyly) in rats when given in doses 16,500 times the maximum recommended human ocular dose. Teratogenicity (polydactyly, hydrocephaly, brachygnathia), embryotoxicity, and maternal toxicity were observed in rats at 66,000 times the maximum recommended ocular human dose. There are no adequate and well-controlled studies in pregnant women. Use during pregnancy only if the potential benefits outweigh the potential hazards to the fetus.

Lactation: Based on determinations of levocabastine in breast milk after ophthalmic administration of the drug to one nursing woman, it was calculated that the daily dose of levocabastine in the infant was ≈ 0.5 mcg.

Children: Safety and efficacy in children < 12 years of age have not been established.

Adverse Reactions:

Mild, transient stinging and burning (15%); headache (5%); visual disturbances, dry mouth, fatigue, pharyngitis, eye pain/dryness, somnolence, red eyes, lacrimation/discharge, cough, nausea, rash/erythema, eyelid edema, dyspnea (1% to 3%).

Patient Information:

Shake well before using.

To prevent contaminating the dropper tip and suspension, take care not to touch the eyelid or surrounding area with the dropper tip of the bottle.

Keep bottle tightly closed when not in use. Do not use if the suspension has discolored. Store at controlled room temperature. Protect from freezing.

Administration and Dosage:

Shake well before using.

The usual dose is 1 drop instilled in the affected eye(s) 4 times daily. Treatment may be continued for up to 2 weeks.

Storage/Stability: Keep tightly closed when not in use. Do not use if the suspension has discolored. Store at controlled room temperature of 15° to 30°C (59° to 86°F). Protect from freezing.

Rx	**Livostin** (Novartis)	**Ophthalmic suspension:** 0.05%	In 2.5, 5, and 10 mL dropper bottles.[1]

[1] With 0.15 mg benzalkonium chloride, propylene glycol, EDTA.

EMEDASTINE DIFUMARATE

Actions:

Pharmacology: Emedastine is a relatively selective histamine H_1-antagonist. In vivo studies have shown concentration-dependent inhibition of histamine-induced increase in conjunctival vascular permeability in the conjunctiva following topical occular administration.

Pharmacokinetics: Following topical administration, emedastine has low systemic exposure.

Clinical Trials: Patients with allergic conjunctivitis treated with emedastine for 6 weeks gained relief of redness, itching, and other symptoms.

Indications:

Allergic Conjunctivitis: Temporary relief of the signs and symptoms of allergic conjunctivitis.

Contraindications:

Hypersensitivity to emedastine difumarate or any of its component products.

Warnings:

Topical (ophthalmic) use only: Not for injection or oral use.

Pregnancy: Category B. At 70,000 times the maximum recommended ocular human use level, emedastine difumarate increased the incidence of external, visceral, and skeletal anomalies in rats. There are no adequate and well-controlled studies in pregnant women. Use this drug during pregnancy only if clearly needed.

Lactation: Oral emedastine has been identified in rat milk. It is not known whether topical ocular administration could result in sufficient systemic absorption to produce detectable quantities in breast milk. Exercise caution when administering to a breast-feeding woman.

Children: Safety and efficacy in children < 3 years old have not been established.

Adverse Reactions:

Headache (11%); abnormal dreams, asthenia, bad taste, blurred vision, burning or stinging, corneal infiltrates, corneal staining, dermatitis, discomfort, dry eyes, foreign body sensations, hyperemia, keratitis, pruritus, rhinitis, sinusitis, tearing (< 5%).

Patient Information:

To prevent contaminating the dropper tip, take care not to touch the eyelids or surrounding areas with the dropper tip of the bottle.

Keep the bottle tightly closed when not in use. Do not use if the solution has become discolored.

ANTIALLERGY AND DECONGESTANT AGENTS 73

Do not wear contact lenses if eyes become red. Do not use emedastine to treat contact-lens related irritation. The preservative in emedastine, benzalkonium chloride, may be absorbed by soft contact lenses. Patients who wear soft contact lenses and whose eyes are not red should wait $\geq$ 10 minutes after instilling emedastine before inserting contacts.

Administration and Dosage:

One drop in the affected eye(s) up to 4 times a day.

Storage/Stability: Store at 4° to 30°C (39° to 86°F). Keep lid tightly closed.

Rx	**Emadine** (Alcon)	**Ophthalmic suspension:** 0.05%	In 5 mL opaque, plastic dispenser.[1]

[1] With 0.01% benzalkonium, tromethamine, sodium chloride, hydroxypropyl methylcellulose, hydrochloric acid/sodium hydroxide.

CROMOLYN SODIUM

Actions:

Pharmacology: In vitro and in vivo animal studies have shown that cromolyn inhibits the degranulation of sensitized mast cells that occurs after exposure to specific antigens. Cromolyn acts by inhibiting the release of histamine and other mediators from the mast cell.

Another activity demonstrated in vitro is the capacity of cromolyn to inhibit the degranulation of nonsensitized rat mast cells by phospholipase A and the subsequent release of chemical mediators. In another study, cromolyn did not inhibit the enzymatic activity of released phospholipase A on its specific substrate.

Cromolyn has no intrinsic vasoconstrictor, antihistaminic, or anti-inflammatory activity.

Pharmacokinetics: Cromolyn is poorly absorbed. When multiple doses of cromolyn ophthalmic solution are instilled into normal rabbit eyes, < 0.07% of the dose is absorbed into the systemic circulation (presumably by way of the eye, nasal passages, buccal cavity, and GI tract). Trace amounts (< 0.01%) of the dose penetrate into the aqueous humor, and clearance from this chamber is virtually complete within 24 hours after treatment is stopped.

In healthy volunteers, analysis of drug excretion indicates that $\approx$ 0.03% of cromolyn is absorbed following administration to the eye.

Indications:

Conjunctivitis: Treatment of vernal keratoconjunctivitis, vernal conjunctivitis, and vernal keratitis.

Contraindications:

Hypersensitivity to cromolyn or to any of the other ingredients.

Warnings:

Stinging/Burning: Patients may experience a transient stinging or burning sensation following instillation of cromolyn.

Duration/Frequency of therapy: The recommended frequency of administration should not be exceeded. Symptomatic response to therapy (decreased itching, tearing, redness, and discharge) is usually evident within a few days, but longer treatment for up to 6 weeks is sometimes required. Once symptomatic improvement has been established, continue therapy for as long as needed to sustain improvement.

Contact lens use: As with all ophthalmic preparations containing benzalkonium chloride, users of soft (hydrophilic) contact lenses should refrain from wearing lenses while under treatment with cromolyn ophthalmic solution. Wear can be resumed within a few hours after discontinuation of the drug.

Concomitant therapy: If required, corticosteroids may be used concomitantly with cromolyn ophthalmic solution.

Pregnancy: Category B. In animals receiving parenteral cromolyn, adverse fetal effects (increased resorption and decreased fetal weight) were noted only at the very high parenteral doses that produced maternal toxicity. There are no adequate and well-controlled studies in pregnant women. Use during pregnancy only if clearly needed.

Lactation: It is not known whether this drug is excreted in breast milk. Exercise caution when cromolyn is administered to a nursing woman.

Children: Safety and efficacy in children < 4 years of age have not been established.

Adverse Reactions:

The most frequently reported adverse reaction is transient ocular stinging or burning upon instillation. Other adverse reactions (infrequent) include: Conjunctival infection; wateriness; itchiness; dryness around the eye; puffiness; irritation; styes.

Patient Information:

Advise patients that the effect of cromolyn therapy is dependent on its administration at regular intervals, as directed.

Do not wear soft contact lenses while using cromolyn.

Administration and Dosage:

Instill 1 or 2 drops in each eye 4 to 6 times a day at regular intervals. One drop contains ≈ 1.6 mg cromolyn sodium.

Rx	**Cromolyn Sodium** (Various, eg, Akorn, Falcon, Teva)	**Solution:** 4%	In 10 and 15 mL.
Rx	**Crolom** (Bausch & Lomb)		In 2.5 and 10 mL bottles with controlled drop tip.
Rx	**Opticrom** (Allergan)		In 10 mL opaque polyethylene eye drop bottles.[1]

[1] With 0.01% benzalkonium chloride, 0.1% EDTA.

ANTIALLERGY AND DECONGESTANT AGENTS

LODOXAMIDE TROMETHAMINE

Actions:

Pharmacology: Lodoxamide is a mast cell stabilizer that inhibits, in vivo, the Type I immediate hypersensitivity reaction. Lodoxamide therapy inhibits the increases in cutaneous vascular permeability that are associated with reagin or IgE and antigen-mediated reactions. In vitro, lodoxamide stabilizes rodent mast cells, prevents release of mast cell inflammatory mediators, and inhibits eosinophil chemotaxis. Although lodoxamide's precise mechanism of action is unknown, the drug may prevent calcium influx into mast cells upon antigen stimulation.

Lodoxamide has no intrinsic vasoconstrictor, antihistaminic, cyclooxygenase inhibition, or other anti-inflammatory activity.

Pharmacokinetics: The disposition of lodoxamide was studied in 6 healthy adult volunteers receiving a 3 mg oral dose. Urinary excretion was the major route of elimination. The elimination half-life was 8.5 hours in urine. In a study in 12 healthy adult volunteers, topical administration of 1 drop in each eye 4 times per day for 10 days did not result in any measurable lodoxamide plasma levels at a detection limit of 2.5 ng/mL.

Indications:

Treatment of the ocular disorders referred to by the terms vernal keratoconjunctivitis, vernal conjunctivitis, and vernal keratitis.

Off-labeled use(s): Treatment of seasonal allergic conjunctivitis.

Contraindications:

Hypersensitivity to any component of this product.

Warnings:

For ophthalmic use only: Not for injection.

Contact lenses: As with all ophthalmic preparations containing benzalkonium chloride, instruct patients not to wear soft contact lenses during treatment with lodoxamide.

Pregnancy: Category B. There are no adequate and well-controlled studies in pregnant women. Use during pregnancy only if clearly needed.

Lactation: It is not known whether lodoxamide is excreted in breast milk. Exercise caution when administering to a nursing woman.

Children: Safety and efficacy in children < 2 years of age have not been established.

OPHTHALMIC DRUG FACTS

Precautions:

Burning/Stinging: Patients may experience a transient burning or stinging upon instillation of lodoxamide. Should these symptoms persist, advise the patient to contact their physician.

Adverse Reactions:

Ophthalmic: Transient burning, stinging, or discomfort upon instillation ($\approx$ 15%); ocular itching/pruritus, blurred vision, dry eye, tearing/discharge, hyperemia, crystalline deposits, foreign body sensation (1% to 5%); corneal erosion/ulcer, scales on lid/lash, eye pain, ocular edema/swelling, ocular warming sensation, ocular fatigue, chemosis, corneal abrasion, anterior chamber cells, keratopathy/keratitis, blepharitis, allergy, sticky sensation, epitheliopathy (< 1%).

Systemic: Headache (1.5%); heat sensation, dizziness, somnolence, nausea, stomach discomfort, sneezing, dry nose, rash (< 1%).

Overdosage:

Overdose of an oral preparation of 120 to 180 mg resulted in a temporary sensation of warmth, profuse sweating, diarrhea, lightheadedness, and a feeling of stomach distension; no permanent adverse effects were observed. Side effects reported following oral administration of 0.1 to 10 mg included a feeling of warmth or flushing, headache, dizziness, fatigue, sweating, nausea, loose stools, and urinary frequency/ urgency. Consider emesis in the event of accidental ingestion.

Administration and Dosage:

Adults and children > 2 years of age: Instill 1 to 2 drops in each affected eye 4 times daily for up to 3 months.

Rx **Alomide** (Alcon)	**Solution:** 0.1%	In 10 mL Drop-Tainers.

NEDOCROMIL SODIUM

Actions:

Pharmacology: Nedocromil is a mast cell stabilizer that inhibits the release of mediators from cells involved in hypersensitivity reactions. Decreased chemotaxis and decreased activation of eosinophils have also been demonstrated. In vitro studies with adult human bronchoalveolar cells showed that nedocromil sodium inhibits histamine release from a population of mast cells having been defined as belonging to the mucosal subtype and beta-glucuronidase release from macrophages.

Pharmacokinetics: Nedocromil exhibits low systemic absorption. When administered as a 2% ophthalmic solution in adult human volunteers, < 4% of the total dose was systemically absorbed following multiple dosing. Absorption is mainly through the nasolacrimal duct rather than through the conjunctiva. It is not metabolized and is eliminated primarily unchanged in urine (70%) and feces (30%). It has a pH of 4 to 5.5.

ANTIALLERGY AND DECONGESTANT AGENTS

Indications:

Treatment of itching associated with allergic conjunctivitis.

Contraindications:

Hypersensitivity to nedocromil or any component of this product.

Warnings:

Contact lenses: Users of contact lenses should refrain from wearing lenses while exhibiting the signs and symptoms of allergic conjunctivitis.

Carcinogenesis: A 2-year inhalation carcinogenicity study of nedocromil sodium at a dose of 24 mg/kg/day ($\approx$ 400 times the maximum recommended human daily ocular dose on a mg/kg basis) in Wistar rats showed no carcinogenic potential.

Mutagenesis: Nedocromil showed no mutagenic potential in the Ames Salmonella/microsome plate assay, mitotic gene conversion in *Saccharomyces cerevisiae*, mouse lymphoma forward mutation, and mouse micronucleus assays.

Fertility impairment: Reproduction and fertility studies in mice and rats showed no effects on male and female fertility at a subcutaneous dose of 100 mg/kg/day (> 1600 times the maximum recommended human daily ocular dose).

Elderly: No overall differences in safety or efficacy have been observed between elderly and younger patients.

Pregnancy: Category B. There are no adequate and well-controlled studies in pregnant women. Use during pregnancy only if clearly needed.

Lactation: After IV administration to lactating rats, nedocromil was excreted in milk. It is not known whether this drug is excreted in human breast milk. Exercise caution when administering to a nursing woman.

Children: Safety and efficacy in children < 3 years of age have not been established.

Adverse Reactions:

The most frequently reported adverse reaction was headache ($\approx$ 40%). Other adverse reactions include: Ocular burning, irritation and stinging, unpleasant taste, nasal congestion (10% to 30%); asthma, conjunctivitis, eye redness, photophobia, rhinitis (1% to 10%).

Patient Information:

Avoid placing nedocromil solution directly on the cornea (the area just over the pupil), because it is especially sensitive. The administration of eye drops will be more comfortable if placed just inside the lower eyelid.

To avoid contamination of the solution, do not touch the dropper tip to the eye, fingers, or any other surface. Replace cap after use. It is recommended that any remaining contents be discarded after the treatment period prescribed by the physician.

OPHTHALMIC DRUG FACTS

Do not use with any other ocular medication unless directed by a physician. Do not wear contact lenses during treatment with nedocromil.

Administration and Dosage:

The recommended dosage is 1 or 2 drops in each eye twice a day. Nedocromil should be used at regular intervals.

Treatment should be continued throughout the period of exposure (ie, until the pollen season is over or until exposure to the offending allergen is terminated), even when symptoms are absent.

Storage/Stability: Store between 2° to 25°C (36° to 77°F). Store in original carton.

Rx	**Alocril** (Allergan)	**Solution:** 2%	In 5 mL bottle with a controlled dropper tip.[1]

[1] With 0.01% benzalkonium chloride, 0.5% sodium chloride, 0.05% edetate disodium.

PEMIROLAST POTASSIUM

Actions:

Pharmacology: Pemirolast is a mast cell stabilizer that inhibits the in vivo Type I immediate hypersensitivity reaction. In vitro and in vivo studies have demonstrated that pemirolast inhibits the antigen-induced release of inflammatory mediators (eg, histamine, leukotriene C_4, D_4, E_4) from human mast cells. In addition, pemirolast inhibits the chemotaxis of eosinophils into ocular tissue and blocks the release of mediators from human eosinophils. Although the precise mechanism of action is unknown, the drug has been reported to prevent calcium influx into mast cells upon antigen stimulation.

Pharmacokinetics: Topical ocular administration of 1 to 2 drops of pemirolast in each eye 4 times daily in 16 healthy volunteers for 2 weeks resulted in detectable concentrations in the plasma. The mean peak plasma level of 4.7 $\pm$ 0.8 ng/mL occurred at 0.42 $\pm$ 0.05 hours and the mean t½ was 4.5 $\pm$ 0.2 hours. When a single 10 mg pemirolast dose was taken orally, a peak plasma concentraion of 0.723 mcg/mL was reached. Following topical administration, $\approx$ 10% to 15% of the dose was excreted unchanged in the urine.

Clinical Trials: In clinical environmental studies, pemirolast was significantly more effective than placebo after 28 days in preventing ocular itching associated with allergic conjunctivitis.

Indications:

Prevention of itching of the eye due to allergic conjunctivitis. Symptomatic response to therapy (decreased itching) may be evident within a few days but frequently requires longer treatment (up to 4 weeks).

Contraindications:

Hypersensitivity to any component of this product.

ANTIALLERGY AND DECONGESTANT AGENTS

Warnings:

For topical ophthalmic use only. Not for injection or oral use.

Mutagenesis: Pemirolast was not mutagenic or clastogenic when tested in a series of bacterial and mammalian tests for gene mutation and chromosomal injury in vitro, nor was it clastogenic when tested in vivo in rats.

Fertility impairment: Pemirolast had no effect on mating and fertility in rats at oral doses up to 250 mg/kg ($\approx$ 20,000-fold the human dose at 2 drops/eye, 40 mcL/drop, 4 times daily for a 50 kg adult). A reduced fertility and pregnancy index occurred in the F_1 generation when F_0 dams were treated with 400 mg/kg pemirolast during late pregnancy and lactation period ($\approx$ 30,000-fold the human dose).

Pregnancy: Category C. Pemirolast caused an increased incidence of thymic remnant in the neck, interventricular septal defect, fetuses with wavy rib, splitting of thoracic vertebral body, and reduced numbers of ossified sternebrae, sacral and caudal vertebrae, and metatarsi when rats were given oral doses $\geq$ 250 mg/kg ($\approx$ 20,000-fold the human dose at 2 drops/eye, 40 μL/drop, 4 times daily for a 50 kg adult) during organogenesis. Increased incidence of dilation of renal pelvis/ureter in the fetuses and neonates was also noted when rats were given an oral dose of 400 mg/kg pemirolast ($\approx$ 30,000-fold the human dose). There are no adequate and well-controlled studies in pregnant women. Use during pregnancy only if the benefit outweighs the risk.

Lactation: Pemirolast is excreted in the milk of lactating rats at concentrations higher than those in plasma. It is not known whether pemirolast is excreted in breast milk. Exercise caution when administering to a nursing woman.

Children: Safety and efficacy in pediatric patients < 3 years of age have not been established.

Adverse Reactions:

The most common adverse reactions were: Headache, rhinitis, cold/flu symptoms (10% to 25%). These side effects were generally mild.

Ophthalmic: Burning, dry eye, foreign body sensation, ocular discomfort (< 5%).

Miscellaneous: Allergy, back pain, bronchitis, cough, dysmenorrhea, fever, sinusitis, sneezing/nasal congestion (< 5%).

Patient Information:

To prevent contaminating the dropper tip and solution, do not touch the eyelids or surrounding areas with the dropper tip. Keep the bottle tightly closed when not in use.

Do not wear contact lenses if eye is red. Pemirolast should not be used to treat contact lens-related irritation. The preservative in this solution, lauralkonium chloride, may be absorbed by soft contact lenses. Patients who wear soft contact lenses and whose eyes are not red should wait $\geq$ 10 minutes after instilling the solution before inserting their contact lenses.

OPHTHALMIC DRUG FACTS

80

Administration and Dosage:

The recommended dose is 1 to 2 drops in each affected eye 4 times daily.

Storage/Stability: Store at 15° to 25°C (59° to 77°F).

Rx	**Alamast** (Santen)	**Solution:** 0.1%	In 10 mL bottles with a controlled dropper tip.[1]

[1] With 0.005% lauralkonium chloride, glycerin, dibasic sodium phosphate, monobasic sodium phosphate, phosphoric acid, or sodium hydroxide.

OLOPATADINE HCl

Actions:

Pharmacology: Olopatadine is a relatively selective H_1-receptor antagonist that inhibits, in vivo and in vitro, the Type I immediate hypersensitivity reaction. It has no effect on alpha-adrenergic, dopamine, muscarinic type 1 and 2, and serotonin receptors.

Pharmacokinetics: Olopatadine was shown to have low systemic exposure in humans following topical ocular administration. Olopatadine was evaluated in 2 studies of normal volunteers given 0.15% solution once every 12 hours for 2 weeks. The plasma concentrations were generally below 0.5 ng/mL. Higher concentrations were typically found within 2 hours of dosing and ranged from 0.5 to 1.3 ng/mL. Urinary excretion was the primary route of elimination. The half-life was ≈ 3 hours. Approximately 60% to 70% of the parent drug was recovered in the urine, with mono-desmethyl and N-oxide detected at low concentrations.

Olopatadine 0.1% was significantly more effective than its vehicle in preventing ocular itching associated with allergic conjunctivitis when challenged with an antigen initially and up to 8 hours after dosing.

Indications:

Allergic conjunctivitis: For the temporary prevention of itching of the eye.

Contraindications:

Hypersensitivity to any component of this product.

Warnings:

For topical ophthalmic use only. Not for injection.

Pregnancy: Category C. Rats treated at doses 93,750 times and rabbits treated at doses 62,500 times the maximum recommended ocular human use level showed a decrease in the number of live fetuses. There are no adequate and well-controlled studies in pregnant women. Use during pregnancy only if the potential benefits outweigh the potential hazards to the fetus.

Lactation: Olopatadine has been identified in the milk of nursing rats following oral administration. It is not known whether topical ocular administration could result in

ANTIALLERGY AND DECONGESTANT AGENTS

sufficient systemic absorption to produce detectable quantitites in human breast milk. Exercise caution when administering to a nursing woman.

Children: Safety and efficacy in pediatric patients < 3 years of age have not been established.

Adverse Reactions:

Ophthalmic: Burning or stinging; dry eye; foreign body sensation; hyperemia; keratitis; lid edema; pruritis.

Systemic: Headache (7%); asthenia; cold syndrome; pharyngitis; rhinitis; sinusitis; taste perversion.

Patient Information:

To prevent contaminating the dropper tip and solution, take care not to touch the eyelids or surrounding areas with the dropper tip of the bottle.

Administration and Dosage:

The recommended dose is 1 to 2 drops in each affected eye 2 times per day every 6 to 8 hours.

Storage/Stability: Keep bottle tightly closed when not in use. Store between 4° to 30°C (39° to 86°F) .

Rx	**Patanol** (Alcon)	**Ophthalmic solution:** 0.1%[1]	In 5 mL Drop-Tainers.

[1] With 0.01% benzalkonium chloride.

AZELASTINE HCl

Actions:

Pharmacology: Azelastine HCl is a relatively selective histamine H_1 antagonist and an inhibitor of the release of histamine and other mediators from cells (eg, mast cells) involved in the allergic response. Based on in vitro studies using human cell lines, inhibition of other mediators involved in allergic reactions (eg, leukotrienes and PAF) has been demonstrated with azelastine HCl. Decreased chemotaxis and activation of eosinophils has also been demonstrated.

Pharmacokinetics: Systemic absorption of azelastine following ocular administration is relatively low. A study in symptomatic patients receiving one drop of azelastine 0.06 to 0.12 mg in each eye 2 to 4 times daily demonstrated plasma concentrations of azelastine generally to be between 0.02 and 0.25 ng/mL after 56 days of treatment. Three of 19 patients had quantifiable amounts of N-desmethylazelastine that ranged from 0.25 to 0.87 ng/mL at day 56.

Based on IV and oral administration, the elimination half-life, steady-state volume of distribution and plasma clearance were 22 hours, 14.5 L/kg and 0.5 L/hr/kg, respectively. Approximately 75% of an oral dose of radiolabeled azelastine was excreted in feces with < 10% as unchanged azelastine. Azelastine is oxidatively metabolized to the principal metabolite, N-desmethylazelastine, by the cytochrome P450 enzyme sys-

OPHTHALMIC DRUG FACTS

tem. In vitro studies in human plasma indicate that the plasma protein binding of azelastine and N-desmethylazelastine are ≈ 88% and 97%, respectively. It has a pH of ≈ 5 to 6.5 and an osmolality of ≈ 271 to 312 mOsmol/L.

Clinical Trials: In a conjunctival antigen challenge study, azelastine was more effective than its vehicle in preventing itching associated with allergic conjunctivitis. Azelastine had a rapid (within 3 minutes) onset of effect and a duration of action of ≈ 8 hours for the prevention of itching.

In environmental studies, adult and pediatric patients with seasonal allergic conjunctivitis were treated with azelastine for 2 to 8 weeks. In these studies, azelastine was more effective than its vehicle in relieving itching associated with allergic conjunctivitis.

Indications:

Allergic conjunctivitis: Treatment of itching of the eye associated with allergic conjunctivitis.

Contraindications:

Known or suspected hypersensitivity to any of its components.

Warnings:

For ocular use only. Not for injection or oral use.

Carcinogenesis: Azelastine administered orally for 24 months was not carcinogenic in rats and mice at doses up to 30 mg/kg/day and 25 mg/kg/day, respectively. Based on a 30 mcL drop size, these doses were ≈ 25,000 and 21,000 times higher than the maximum recommended ocular human use level of 0.001 mg/kg/day for a 50 kg adult.

Mutagenesis: Azelastine showed no genotoxic effects in the Ames test, DNA repair test, mouse lymphoma forward mutation assay, mouse micronucleus test, or chromosomal aberration test in rat bone marrow.

Fertility impairment: Reproduction and fertility studies in rats showed no effect on male or female fertility at oral doses up to 25,000 times the maximum recommended ocular human use level. At 68.6 mg/kg/day (57,000 times the maximum recommended ocular human use level), the duration of the estrous cycle was prolonged and copulatory activity and the number of pregnancies were decreased. The numbers of corpora lutea and implantations were decreased; however, the implantation ratio was not affected.

Elderly: No overall differences in safety or efficacy have been observed between elderly and younger adult patients.

Pregnancy: Category C. Azelastine has been shown to be embryotoxic, fetotoxic, and teratogenic (external and skeletal abnormalities) in mice at an oral dose of 68.6 mg/kg/day (57,000 times the recommended ocular human use level). At an oral dose of 30 mg/kg/day (25,000 times the recommended ocular human use level), delayed ossification (undeveloped metacarpus) and the incidence of the 14th rib were increased in rats. At 68.6 mg/kg/day (57,000 times the recommended ocular human use level), azelastine caused resorption and fetotoxic effects in rats. The relevance to humans of these skeletal findings noted at only high drug exposure levels is unknown.

ANTIALLERGY AND DECONGESTANT AGENTS

83

There are no adequate and well-controlled studies in pregnant women. Azelastine should be used during pregnancy only if the potential benefit to the mother justifies the potential risk to the fetus.

Lactation: It is not known whether azelastine is excreted in human breast milk. Because many drugs are excreted in human milk, exercise caution when administering to a nursing woman.

Children: Safety and efficacy have not been established in pediatric patients < 3 years of age.

Adverse Reactions:

In controlled multiple-dose studies where patients were treated for up to 56 days, the most frequently reported adverse reactions were transient eye burning/stinging ($\approx$ 30%), headaches ($\approx$ 15%), and bitter taste ($\approx$ 10%). The occurrence of these events was generally mild.

The following events were reported in 1% to 10% of patients: Asthma, conjunctivitis, dyspnea, eye pain, fatigue, influenza-like symptoms, pharyngitis, pruritus, rhinitis, and temporary blurring. Some of these events were similar to the underlying disease being studied.

Patient Information:

Do not touch the dropper tip to any surface, the eyelids, or surrounding areas to prevent contaminating the dropper tip and the solution. Keep bottle tightly closed when not in use. This product is sterile when packaged.

Do not wear contact lens if the eye is red. Azelastine should not be used to treat contact lens-related irritation. The preservative in azelastine, benzalkonium chloride, may be absorbed by soft contact lenses. Patients who wear soft contact lenses and whose eyes are not red, should wait at least 10 minutes after instilling azelastine before they insert their contact lenses.

Administration and Dosage:

The recommended dose is 1 drop instilled into each affected eye twice a day.

Storage/Stability: Store upright between 2° and 25°C (36° and 77°F).

Rx	**Optivar** (Muro Pharmaceutical)	**Solution:** 0.05%	In 10 mL containers with a LDPE dropper tip.[1]

[1] 0.125 mg benzalkonium chloride, disodium edetate dihydrate, hydroxypropylmethylcellulose, sorbital solution, sodium hydroxide.

OPHTHALMIC DECONGESTANT/ANTIHISTAMINE COMBINATIONS

In these combinations:

Phenylephrine HCl, naphazoline HCl, and *tetrahydrozoline* have decongestant actions. See individual monographs for further information.

Hydroxypropyl methylcellulose and *polyvinyl alcohol* increase the viscosity of the solution, thereby increasing contact time.

84 — OPHTHALMIC DRUG FACTS

Zinc sulfate is an astringent.

Pheniramine maleate and *antazoline* are antihistamines.

Indications:

Itching/Redness: Temporary relief of the minor eye symptoms of itching and redness caused by pollen, animal hair, etc.

Warnings:

Antihistamines: Topical antihistamines are potential sensitizers and may produce a local sensitivity reaction. Because they may produce angle closure, use with caution in people with a narrow angle or a history of glaucoma.

Administration and Dosage:

Recommendations vary. Refer to manufacturer package insert for instructions.

		Decongestant	Antihistamine	
otc	**Naphcon-A Solution** (Alcon)	naphazoline HCl 0.025%	pheniramine maleate 0.3%	In 15 mL Drop-Tainers.[1]
otc	**Opcon-A Solution** (Bausch & Lomb)	naphazoline HCl 0.027%	pheniramine maleate 0.315%	In 15 mL.[2]
otc	**Vasocon-A Solution** (Novartis)	naphazoline HCl 0.05%	antazoline phosphate 0.5%	In 15 mL.[3]

[1] With 0.01% benzalkonium chloride, 0.01% EDTA.
[2] With 0.5% hydroxypropyl methylcellulose, 0.01% benzalkonium chloride, 0.1% EDTA, boric acid.
[3] With 0.01% benzalkonium chloride, PEG-8000, polyvinyl alcohol, EDTA.

Anti-inflammatory Agents

CORTICOSTEROIDS

Since their introduction into ocular therapy, corticosteroids have been useful in the control of inflammatory and immunologic diseases of the eye. The anti-inflammatory effects of corticosteroids are nonspecific, and they inhibit inflammation without regard to cause. In general, corticosteroids appear to be more effective in acute rather than chronic conditions. Degenerative diseases are usually completely refractory to corticosteroid therapy. Corticosteroids are generally not considered appropriate therapy for mild ocular allergies because other modalities can be effective (see the Antiallergy and Decongestant Agents chapter).

The beneficial effects of these agents on inflammation are numerous and include the following:

- Reduction in capillary permeability and cellular exudation;
- Inhibition of degranulation of mast cells, basophils, and neutrophils. Stabilization of intracellular membranes of these cells inhibits release of hydrolytic enzyme and other mediators of inflammation such as histamines, bradykinins, and platelet-activating factor;
- Suppression of lymphocyte proliferation;
- Inhibition of phospholipase A synthesis, resulting in decreased synthesis of prostaglandins and leukotrienes; and
- Inhibition of cell-mediated immune responses.

Clinical use and experimental data indicate that corticosteroids differ in their ability to suppress inflammation. This has been attributed, in part, to differences in their ability to penetrate the corneal epithelium. Acetate and alcohol formulations are sparingly soluble in water and are formulated for topical ocular use as suspensions. Phosphate derivatives are highly soluble in aqueous media and are formulated as solutions. The suspension formulations of acetate and alcohol derivatives exhibit biphasic solubility and can therefore better penetrate the lipid-rich layers of the cornea. It has also been suggested that corticosteroid particles in suspension persist in the cul-de-sac for longer periods of time and thus contact of the drug with the ocular surface is prolonged. For topical ocular use, prednisolone (eg, *AK-Pred*), fluorometholone (eg, *FML Liquifilm, Flarex*), and dexamethasone (eg, *Decadron Phosphate*) can be effective in inflammations involving the lids, conjunctiva, cornea, iris, and ciliary body. In severe forms of anterior uveitis, topical therapy may require supplementation with periocular injection or systemic corticosteroids.

Chorioretinitis and optic neuritis are usually treated with systemic or periocular administration, or both. Medrysone (*HMS*), which appears to exhibit limited corneal pen-

86

etration, is recommended for minor reactions involving the lids and conjunctiva. Its efficacy has not been demonstrated in iritis or uveitis.

More recently, a group of compounds with similar anti-inflammatory activity but less propensity to raise intraocular pressure has been synthesized. The first to become available are loteprednol etabonate and rimexolone (*Vexol*). Rimexolone is presently indicated for treatment of anterior uveitis and for postoperative inflammation following cataract surgery. Loteprednol etabonate is a product of the so-called "soft drug" design developed by Bodor to enhance drug efficacy and minimize adverse effects. Although loteprednol is structurally similar to prednisolone, the ketone group at position 20 is absent. This modification in the molecule allows for the synthetic production of a therapeutically active, but metabolically unstable, compound that is rapidly inactivated following administration.

Loteprednol etabonate has shown clinical efficacy for various inflammatory conditions affecting the eye, including giant papillary conjunctivitis, postoperative inflammation, and seasonal allergic conjunctivitis. The relatively low incidence, transient nature, and reversibility of ocular pressure increase reported thus far with loteprednol and rimexolone indicate that they can provide an additional treatment choice for ocular inflammatory condition. Loteprednol 0.5% *(Lotemax)* has also shown clinical efficacy in giant papillary conjunctivitis, whereas loteprednol 0.2% (*Alrex*) has been approved for seasonal allergic conjunctivitis.

The use of corticosteroids in ocular disease remains largely empirical, but some general guidelines include the following:

- ♦ Type and location of inflammation determine which route of administration is appropriate;
- ♦ Dosage is largely determined by clinical experience and should be reevaluated at frequent intervals during therapy;
- ♦ Therapy should be reduced gradually, not discontinued abruptly;
- ♦ The minimal effective dose should be used for the shortest time necessary;
- ♦ Individualize dosage; and
- ♦ Maintain close supervision to assess the effects of therapy on the disease course and possible adverse effects to the patient.

Patient compliance with the drug regimen is important in resolution of the inflammation. Patients should not discontinue use of medication at their own discretion. If suspensions are employed, the patient must shake the bottle sufficiently to maintain the proper concentration of drug.

Adverse effects can occur with all routes of administration and all preparations currently in use. Incidence of adverse effects appears to rise significantly as dosages are increased. Short-term topical ocular therapy usually does not produce significant ocular or systemic side effects.

NONSTEROIDAL ANTI-INFLAMMATORY AGENTS

Nonsteroidal anti-inflammatory drugs (NSAIDs), also referred to as the "aspirin-like" drugs, include the salicylates, as well as indole, pyrazolone and propionic acid derivatives, and the fenamates. Following oral administration, these agents relieve discomfort associated with rheumatoid arthritis and lupus erythematosus, and reduce fever and alleviate pain that accompanies injury or inflammation.

The mechanism of action of the NSAIDs involves inhibition of cyclo-oxygenase, an enzyme important in synthesis of prostaglandins from their precursor, arachidonic

ANTI-INFLAMMATORY AGENTS

acid. NSAIDs do not inhibit phospholipase A or the lipoxygenase enzyme, which generate the leukotrienes and related compounds that are also involved in the inflammatory response.

Prostaglandins are 20-carbon, unsaturated fatty acid derivatives that are subdivided into groups, designated by letters such as D, E, and F. Evidence indicates that they also act as mediators of inflammation in ocular structures. Prostaglandins can cause vasodilation of ocular blood vessels, disrupt the blood-aqueous barrier, and induce neovascularization and miosis. Some of the prostaglandins such as $PGF_{2\alpha}$ and PGD_2 can lower intraocular pressure whereas others (eg, PGF_2) can raise it.

The topical ocular use of NSAIDs includes maintenance of pupillary dilation during surgery and control of inflammation, photophobia, and pain after cataract extraction and following argon laser trabeculoplasty and photorefractive procedures. Also, reactions associated with nonsurgically induced inflammatory disorders of the eye, such as allergic conjunctivitis and cystoid macular edema, respond to topical ocular application. At present, 4 topical ocular solution formulations are available: Flurbiprofen (eg, *Ocufen*), suprofen (*Profenal*), diclofenac (eg, *Voltaren*), and ketorolac (*Acular*).

Siret D. Jaanus, PhD
Southern California College of Optometry

For More Information

Bartlett JD, Jaanus SD, eds. Clinical Ocular Pharmacology, ed. 4. Boston: Butterworth-Heinemann, 2001.

Bito LZ. Prostaglandins. Old concepts and new perspectives. *Arch Ophthalmol* 1987;105:1036.

Bodor N. The application of soft drug approaches to the design of safer steroids. In: Christophers E, ed. *Topical Corticosteroid Therapy. A novel approach to safer drugs*. New York: Raven Press, 1988.

Dell SJ, Lowry GM, Northcutt JA, et al. A randomized, double-marked, placebo-controlled parallel study of 0.2% Loteprednol etabonate in patients with seasonal allergic conjunctivitis. *J. Allergy Clin Immunol* 1998;102:241-55.

Flach AJ. Nonsteroidal anti-inflammatory drugs in ophthalmology. *Int Ophthalmol Clin* 1993;33:1.

Foster CS, et al. Efficacy and safety of rimexolone 1% ophthalmic suspension vs 1% prednisolone acetate in the treatment of uveitis. *Am J Ophthalmol* 1996;122:171-82.

Franzie JP, Leibowitz HM. Steroids. *Int Ophthalmol Clin* 1993;33:9.

Friedlander MH, Howes J. A double-masked, placebo-controlled evaluation of the efficacy and safety of Loteprednol etabonate in the treatment of giant papillary conjunctivitis. *Am J Opthalmol* 1997;123:455.

Leibowitz HM, Kupferman A. Anti-inflammatory medications. *Int Ophthalmol Clin* 1980;20:117.

Masferrer JL, Kulkarni PS. Cyclooxygenase-2 inhibitors: a new approach to the therapy of ocular inflammation. *Surv Ophthalmol* 1997;41:35-40.

The Loteprednol Etabonate Post operative Study group 2. A double-masked, placebo-controlled evaluation of 0.5% Loteprednol etabonate in the treatment of post operative inflammation. *Opthalmology* 1998;105:1780-86.

Urban RC, Cotlier E. Corticosteroid-induced cataracts. *Surv Ophthalmol* 1986;31:102.

CORTICOSTEROIDS, TOPICAL

Actions:

Pharmacology: Topical corticosteroids exert an anti-inflammatory action. Aspects of the inflammatory process such as hyperemia, cellular infiltration, vascularization, and fibroblastic proliferation are suppressed. Steroids inhibit inflammatory response to inciting agents of mechanical, chemical, or immunological nature. Topical corticosteroids are effective in acute inflammatory conditions of conjunctiva, sclera, cornea, lids, iris, ciliary body, and anterior segment of the globe; and in ocular allergic conditions. They inhibit edema and capillary dilation. In ocular disease, route depends on site and extent of disorder.

The mechanism of the anti-inflammatory action is thought to be potentiation of epinephrine vasoconstriction, stabilization of lysosomal membranes, retardation of macrophage movement, prevention of kinin release, inhibition of lymphocyte and neutrophil function, inhibition of prostaglandin synthesis, and, in prolonged use, decrease of antibody production.

Inhibiting fibroblastic proliferation may prevent symblepharon formation in chemical and thermal burns. Decreased scarring with clearer corneas after topical corticosteroids is a result of inhibiting fibroblast proliferation and vascularization.

Indications:

Inflammatory conditions: Treatment of steroid-responsive inflammatory conditions of the palpebral and bulbar conjunctiva, lid, cornea, and anterior segment of the globe, such as the following: Allergic conjunctivitis; nonspecific superficial keratitis; superficial punctate keratitis; herpes zoster keratitis; iritis; cyclitis; and selected infective conjunctivitis when the inherent hazard of steroid use is accepted to obtain a diminution in edema and inflammation. Rimexolone is also indicated for postoperative inflammation following ocular surgery.

Corneal injury: Also used for corneal injury from chemical, radiation, or thermal burns or penetration of foreign bodies.

Graft rejection: May be used to suppress graft rejection after keratoplasty.

Anterior uveitis.

Contraindications:

Acute superficial herpes simplex keratitis; fungal diseases of ocular structures; vaccinia, varicella, and most other viral diseases of the cornea and conjunctiva; mycobacterial infection of the eye (eg, ocular tuberculosis); diseases caused by microorganisms; hypersensitivity, or following uncomplicated removal of a superficial corneal foreign body.

Medrysone: Not for use in iritis and uveitis; its efficacy has not been demonstrated.

Warnings:

Moderate-to-severe inflammation: Use higher strengths for moderate-to-severe inflammations. In difficult cases of anterior segment eye disease, systemic therapy may be required. When deeper ocular structures are involved, use systemic therapy.

ANTI-INFLAMMATORY AGENTS 89

Ocular damage: Prolonged use may result in glaucoma, elevated IOP, optic nerve damage, defects in visual acuity and fields of vision, posterior subcapsular cataract formation, or secondary ocular infections from pathogens liberated from ocular tissues. Check IOP and lens frequently. In diseases causing thinning of cornea or sclera, perforation has occurred with topical steroids.

Mustard gas keratitis or Sjögren's keratoconjunctivitis: Topical steroids not effective.

Infections: Acute, purulent, untreated eye infection may be masked or activity enhanced by steroids. Fungal infections of the cornea have occurred with long-term local steroid applications. Therefore, suspect fungal invasion in any persistent corneal ulceration where a steroid has been, or is being used.

Stromal herpes simplex keratitis treatment with steroid medication requires great caution; frequent slit-lamp microscopy is mandatory.

Pregnancy: Category C. Use only when clearly needed and when potential benefits to the mother outweigh potential hazards to the fetus.

Lactation: It is not known whether topical steroids are excreted in breast milk. Exercise caution when administering to a nursing mother.

Children: Safety and efficacy have not been established in children.

Precautions:

Sulfite sensitivity: Some of these products contain sulfites that may cause allergic-type reactions (eg, hives, itching, wheezing, anaphylaxis) in certain susceptible people. Although the overall prevalence of sulfite sensitivity in the general population is low, it is seen more frequently in asthmatics or in atopic nonasthmatic people. Specific products containing sulfites are identified in the product listings.

Adverse Reactions:

Glaucoma (elevated IOP) with optic nerve damage, loss of visual acuity, and field defects; posterior subcapsular cataract formation; secondary ocular infection from pathogens, including herpes simplex liberated from ocular tissues; perforation of globe; exacerbation of viral and fungal corneal infections; transient stinging or burning; blurred vision; discharge; discomfort; ocular pain; foreign body sensation; hyperemia; pruritus (rimexolone). Rarely, filtering blebs have occurred with steroid use after cataract surgery.

Other ocular adverse reactions occurring in < 1% of patients included sticky sensation; increased fibrin; dry eye; conjunctival edema; corneal staining; keratitis; tearing; photophobia; edema; irritation; corneal ulcer; browache; lid margin crusting; corneal edema; infiltrate; corneal erosion.

Miscellaneous: Headache; aggravation or worsening of hypertension; rhinitis; pharyngitis; taste perversion.

Systemic: Systemic side effects may occur with extensive use.

Patient Information:

Medical supervision during therapy is recommended.

90 OPHTHALMIC DRUG FACTS

To avoid contamination, do not touch applicator tip to any surface. Replace cap after use.

If improvement of the condition being treated does not occur within several days, or if pain, itching, or swelling of the eye occurs, notify the physician. Do not discontinue use without consulting physician. Take care not to discontinue prematurely.

Refer to the Dosage Forms and Routes of Administration chapter for more complete information on administration and use.

Administration and Dosage:

Treatment duration varies with type of lesion and may extend from a few days to several weeks, depending on therapeutic response. Relapse may occur if therapy is reduced too rapidly; taper over several days. Relapses, more common in chronic active lesions than in self-limited conditions, usually respond to retreatment.

Suspensions and solutions: Refer to specific product labeling, because dosage depends on product and indication. Suspension must be vigorously shaken (5X) before instillation or the active ingredient will remain on the bottom of the bottle.

Generally, instill 1 or 2 drops into the conjunctival sac every hour during the day and every 2 hours during the night. When a favorable response is observed, reduce dosage to 1 drop every 4 hours. Later, 1 drop 3 or 4 times daily may suffice to control symptoms. Shake suspension well before use. For postoperative inflammation, instill 1 to 2 drops 4 times daily beginning 24 hours after surgery; continue throughout the first 2 weeks of the postoperative period.

Ointments: Apply a thin coating ($\approx$ 0.5 to 1 inch) in the lower conjunctival sac 3 or 4 times a day. When a favorable response is observed, reduce the number of daily applications to 2, and, later, to 1 as a maintenance dose if sufficient to control symptoms.

Ointments are particularly convenient when an eye pad is used and may be the preparation of choice when prolonged contact of drug with ocular tissues is needed.

For product information on Steroid/Antibiotic Combinations, see the Anti-infective Agents chapter.

Individual drug monographs are on the following pages.

ANTI-INFLAMMATORY AGENTS

DEXAMETHASONE

Complete prescribing information is found in the Corticosteroids group monograph.

Administration and Dosage:

Storage: Store upright at 8° to 27°C (46° to 80°F).

Rx	**Dexamethasone Sodium Phosphate** (Various, eg, Bausch & Lomb, Schein)	**Solution:** 0.1% dexamethasone phosphate (as sodium phosphate)	In 5 mL.
Rx	**AK-Dex** (Akorn)		In 5 mL.[1]
Rx	**Decadron Phosphate** (Merck)		In 5 mL Ocumeters.[2]
Rx	**Maxidex** (Alcon)	**Suspension:** 0.1% dexamethasone	In 5 and 15 mL Drop-Tainers.[3]
Rx	**Dexamethasone Sodium Phosphate** (Bausch & Lomb)	**Ointment:** 0.05% dexamethasone phosphate (as sodium phosphate)	In 3.5 g.
Rx	**AK-Dex** (Akorn)		In 3.5 g.[4]

[1] With 0.01% benzalkonium chloride, EDTA, hydroxyethylcellulose.
[2] With polysorbate 80, EDTA, 0.1% sodium bisulfite, 0.25% phenylethanol, 0.02% benzalkonium chloride.
[3] With 0.01% benzalkonium chloride, EDTA, 0.5% hydroxypropyl methylcellulose, polysorbate 80.
[4] With lanolin anhydrous, parabens, PEG-400, white petrolatum, mineral oil.

LOTEPREDNOL ETABONATE

Complete prescribing information is found in the Corticosteriods group monograph.

Administration and Dosage:

Storage: Store upright at 15° to 25°C (59° to 77°F); do not freeze.

Rx	**Alrex** (Bausch & Lomb)	**Suspension:** 0.2% loteprednol etabonate	In 5 and 10 mL.
Rx	**Lotemax** (Bausch & Lomb)	**Suspension:** 0.5% loteprednol etabonate[1]	In 2.5, 5, 10, and 15 mL.

[1] With EDTA, glycerin, povidone, tyloxapol.

FLUOROMETHOLONE

Complete prescribing information is found in the Corticosteroids group monograph.

Administration and Dosage:

Storage: Store at or below 25°C (77°F); protect from freezing.

OPHTHALMIC DRUG FACTS

Rx	Fluorometholone (Various, eg, Bausch & Lomb, Falcon)	Suspension: 0.1% fluoro-metholone alcohol	In 5, 10, and 15 mL.
Rx	Fluor-Op (Novartis)		In 5, 10, and 15 mL.[1]
Rx	FML (Allergan)		In 1, 5, 10, and 15 mL.[1]
Rx	Flarex (Alcon)	Suspension: 0.1% fluoro-metholone acetate	In 2.5, 5, and 10 mL Drop-Tainers.[2]
Rx	eFLone (Novartis)		In 5 and 10 mL.[2]
Rx	FML Forte (Allergan)	Suspension: 0.25% fluoro-metholone alcohol	In 2, 5, 10, and 15 mL.[3]
Rx	FML S.O.P. (Allergan)	Ointment: 0.1%	In 3.5 g.[4]

[1] With 0.004% benzalkonium chloride, EDTA, polysorbate 80, 1.4% polyvinyl alcohol.
[2] With 0.01% benzalkonium chloride, EDTA, hydroxyethylcellulose, tyloxapol.
[3] With 0.005% benzalkonium chloride, EDTA, polysorbate 80, 1.4% polyvinyl alcohol.
[4] With 0.0008% phenylmercuric acetate, white petrolatum, mineral oil, petrolatum, lanolin alcohol.

MEDRYSONE

Complete prescribing information is found in the Corticosteroids group monograph.

Administration and Dosage:

Storage: Protect from freezing.

Rx	HMS (Allergan)	Suspension: 1%	In 5 and 10 mL.[1]

[1] With 0.004% benzalkonium chloride, EDTA, 1.4% polyvinyl alcohol, hydroxypropyl methylcellulose.

PREDNISOLONE

Complete prescribing information is found in the Corticosteroids group monograph.

Administration and Dosage:

Storage: Protect from freezing.

Rx	Pred Mild (Allergan)	Suspension: 0.12% pred-nisolone acetate	In 5 and 10 mL.[1]
Rx	Econopred (Alcon)	Suspension: 0.125% pred-nisolone acetate	In 5 and 10 mL Drop-Tainers.[2]
Rx	AK-Pred (Akorn)	Solution: 0.125% predniso-lone sodium phosphate	In 5 mL.[3]
Rx	Inflamase Mild (Novartis)		In 3, 5, and 10 mL.[4]
Rx	Econopred Plus (Alcon)	Suspension: 1% predniso-lone acetate	In 5 and 10 mL Drop-Tainers.[2]
Rx	Pred Forte (Allergan)		In 1, 5, 10, and 15 mL.[1]
Rx	Prednisolone Acetate Ophthal-mic (Falcon)		In 5 and 10 mL.[2]

ANTI-INFLAMMATORY AGENTS

Rx	**Prednisolone Sodium Phosphate** (Various, eg, Bausch & Lomb)	**Solution:** 1% prednisolone sodium phosphate	In 5, 10, and 15 mL.
Rx	**AK-Pred** (Akorn)		In 5 and 15 mL.[3]
Rx	**Inflamase Forte** (Novartis)		In 3, 5, 10, and 15 mL.[4]

[1] With benzalkonium chloride, EDTA, polysorbate 80, hydroxypropyl methylcellulose, sodium bisulfite.
[2] With 0.01% benzalkonium chloride, EDTA, polysorbate 80, hydroxypropyl methylcellulose, glycerin.
[3] With 0.01% benzalkonium chloride, EDTA, hydroxypropyl methylcellulose, sodium bisulfite.
[4] With 0.01% benzalkonium chloride and EDTA.

RIMEXOLONE

Complete prescribing information is found in the Corticosteroids group monograph.

Administration and Dosage:

Storage: Store upright between 4° and 30°C (40° and 86°F).

Rx	**Vexol** (Alcon)	**Suspension:** 1%	In 5 and 10 mL Drop-Tainers.[1]

[1] With 0.01% benzalkonium chloride, polysorbate 80, EDTA in carbapol gel.

NONSTEROIDAL ANTI-INFLAMMATORY AGENTS (NSAIDS)

Actions:

Pharmacology: Flurbiprofen, suprofen, diclofenac, and ketorolac are NSAIDs available as ophthalmic solutions. Flurbiprofen and suprofen are phenylalkanoic acids, diclofenac is a phenylacetic acid, and ketorolac tromethamine is a member of the pyrrolo-pyrolle group; they have analgesic, antipyretic, and anti-inflammatory activity. Their mechanism of action is believed to be through inhibition of the cyclo-oxygenase enzyme that is essential in the biosynthesis of prostaglandins.

In animals, certain prostaglandins are mediators of intraocular inflammation. Prostaglandins produce disruption of the blood-aqueous humor barrier, vasodilation, increased vascular permeability, leukocytosis, and increased intraocular pressure (IOP).

Prostaglandins also appear to play a role in the miotic response produced during ocular surgery by constricting the iris sphincter independently of cholinergic mechanisms. NSAIDs inhibit the miosis induced during the course of cataract surgery.

Nonsteroidal Anti-Inflammatory Ophthalmic Agents			
Ophthalmic NSAID	Trade name (manufacturer)	Solution concentration	Ophthalmic indication
Flurbiprofen	*Ocufen* (Allergan)	0.03%	Inhibition of intraoperative miosis
Suprofen	*Profenal* (Alcon)	1%	
Diclofenac	*Voltaren* (Ciba Vision)	0.1%	Treatment of postoperative inflammation in patients who have undergone cataract extraction and for the temporary relief of pain and photophobia in patients undergoing corneal retractive surgery.

OPHTHALMIC DRUG FACTS

Nonsteroidal Anti-Inflammatory Ophthalmic Agents			
Ophthalmic NSAID	Trade name (manufacturer)	Solution concentration	Ophthalmic indication
Ketorolac	Acular (Allergan)	0.5%	Temporary relief of ocular itching caused by seasonal allergic conjunctivitis; treatment of postoperative inflammation in patients who have undergone cataract extraction.

Indications:

Flurbiprofen, suprofen: Inhibition of intraoperative miosis.

Diclofenac: Treatment of postoperative inflammation in patients who have undergone cataract extraction and for the temporary relief of pain and photophobia in patients undergoing corneal retractive surgery.

Ketorolac: Temporary relief of ocular itching caused by seasonal allergic conjunctivitis; treatment of postoperative inflammation in patients who have undergone cataract extraction.

Off-labeled uses:

Diclofenac: Anti-inflammatory treatment following argon laser trabeculoplasty, treatment of seasonal allergic conjunctivitis, pain associated with radial keratotomy, and photorefractive keratectomy.

Flurbiprofen: Inflammation after cataract or glaucoma laser surgery and uveitis syndromes.

Ketorolac: Treatment of pain associated with corneal surgery or trauma; topical treatment of cystoid macular edema.

Suprofen: Topical treatment of contact lens-associated GPC.

Contraindications:

Hypersensitivity to the drugs or any component of the products.

Suprofen: Epithelial herpes simplex keratitis (dendritic keratitis).

Diclofenac, ketorolac: Patients wearing soft contact lenses (see Precautions).

Warnings:

Cross-sensitivity: The potential for cross-sensitivity to acetylsalicylic acid, phenylacetic acid derivatives, and other NSAIDs exists. Therefore, use caution when treating individuals who have previously exhibited sensitivities to these drugs.

Bleeding tendencies: Systemic absorption occurs with drugs applied ocularly. With some NSAIDs, there exists the potential for increased bleeding time due to interference with thrombocyte aggregation. There have been reports that ocularly applied NSAIDs may cause increased bleeding of ocular tissues (including hyphemas) in conjunction with ocular surgery. Use with caution in surgical patients with known bleeding tendencies or in patients taking drugs known to cause bleeding (eg, anticoagulants).

ANTI-INFLAMMATORY AGENTS

Pregnancy: Category C (flurbiprofen, ketorolac, suprofen); *Category B* (diclofenac). Flurbiprofen is embryocidal, delays parturition, prolongs gestation, reduces weight, and slightly retards fetal growth in rats at daily oral doses of $\geq$ 0.4 mg/kg ($\approx$ 185 times the human daily topical dose).

Oral doses of ketorolac at 1.5 mg/kg (8.8 mg/m^2), which is half of the human oral exposure, administered after gestation day 17 caused dystocia and higher pup mortality in rats. Because of the known effects of prostaglandin-inhibiting drugs on the fetal cardiovascular system, avoid the use of ketorolac during late pregnancy.

Oral doses of suprofen of up to 200 mg/kg/day in animals resulted in an increased incidence of fetal resorption associated with maternal toxicity. There was an increase in stillbirths and a decrease in postnatal survival in pregnant rats treated with $\geq$ 2.5 mg/kg/day.

Oral diclofenac in mice and rats crosses the placental barrier. In rats, maternally toxic doses were associated with dystocia, prolonged gestation, and reduced fetal weights, growth, and survival. Because of the known effects of prostaglandin-inhibiting drugs on the fetal cardiovascular system, avoid the use of ophthalmic diclofenac during late pregnancy.

There are no adequate and well-controlled studies in pregnant women. Use during pregnancy only if the potential benefits to the mother outweigh the potential hazards to the fetus.

Lactation: It is not known whether flurbiprofen is excreted in breast milk. Because of the potential for serious adverse reactions in nursing infants, decide whether to discontinue nursing or to discontinue the drug, taking into account the importance of the drug to the mother.

Suprofen is excreted in breast milk after a single oral dose. Based on measurements of plasma and milk levels in women taking oral suprofen, the milk concentration is $\approx$ 1% of the plasma level. Because systemic absorption may occur from topical ocular administration, consider discontinuing nursing while on suprofen; its safety in human neonates has not been established.

Exercise caution while ketorolac is administered to a nursing woman.

Children: Safety and efficacy for use in children have not been established.

Precautions:

Wound healing: Wound healing may be delayed with the use of flurbiprofen and diclofenac.

Contact lenses: Patients wearing hydrogel soft contact lenses who have used diclofenac concurrently have experienced ocular irritation manifested by redness and burning.

Ketorolac – Do not administer while patient is wearing contact lenses.

Drug Interactions:

Acetylcholine chloride and carbachol: Although clinical and animal studies revealed no interference, and there is no known pharmacological basis for an interaction, both of these drugs have reportedly been ineffective when used in patients treated with flurbiprofen or suprofen.

OPHTHALMIC DRUG FACTS

Adverse Reactions:

Sterile infiltrates are increasingly seen when NSAIDS are used. In incisional of photoarefractive surgery without concommitant low dose steroids. The epithelial defect appears to predispose to this adverse effect.

Most frequent: Transient burning and stinging upon instillation (diclofenac 15%, ketorolac ≈ 40%); other minor symptoms of ocular irritation.

Suprofen: Discomfort; itching; redness; allergy, iritis, pain, chemosis, photophobia, irritation, punctate epithelial staining (< 0.5%).

Diclofenac: Keratitis (28%, although most cases occurred in cataract studies prior to drug therapy); elevated IOP (15%, although most cases occurred postsurgery and prior to drug therapy); dry eye complaints (12% in patients undergoing incisional refractive surgery); discharge; corneal deposits; corneal lesions; itching; irritation; blurred vision; fever; pain; insomnia. The following reactions occurred in ≤ 1%: Corneal edema; corneal opacity; eyelid disorder; iritis; injection and lacrimation disorder; asthenia; chills; facial edema; vomiting; viral infection; anterior chamber reaction; ocular allergy; nausea.

Ketorolac: Ocular irritation, allergic reactions; superficial keratitis; superficial ocular infections. The following adverse reactions occurred rarely: Eye dryness; corneal infiltrates; corneal ulcer; visual disturbance (blurred vision).

Overdosage:

Overdosage will not ordinarily cause acute problems. If accidentally ingested, drink fluids to dilute.

Individual drug monographs are on the following pages.

ANTI-INFLAMMATORY AGENTS 97

DICLOFENAC SODIUM

Complete prescribing information is found in the NSAIDs group monograph.

Administration and Dosage:

Cataract surgery: Instill 1 drop in the affected eye 4 times daily, beginning 24 hours after cataract surgery and continuing throughout the first 2 weeks of the postoperative period.

Incisional refractive surgery: Within 1 hour prior to incisional refractive surgery, instill 1 drop to the operative eye(s). Instill a second drop within 15 minutes after surgery. Instill 1 drop to the operative eye(s) 4 times daily beginning 4 to 6 hours after surgery and continuing for up to 3 days as needed.

Storage: Store at 15° to 30°C (59° to 86°F). Protect from light.

Rx	Diclofenac Sodium Ophthalmic (Various, eg, Falcon, Geneva)	Solution: 0.1%	In 15 mL.
Rx	Voltaren (Novartis)		In 2.5 and 5 mL dropper bottles.[2]

[1] With Mannitol.
[2] With 1 mg/mL EDTA, boric acid, polyoxyl 35 castor oil, 2 mg/mL sorbic acid, tromethamine.

FLURBIPROFEN SODIUM

Complete prescribing information is found in the NSAIDs group monograph.

Administration and Dosage:

Instill 1 drop approximately every 30 minutes, beginning 2 hours before surgery (total of 4 drops).

Storage: Store at room temperature.

Rx	Ocufen (Allergan)	Solution: 0.03%	In 2.5, 5, and 10 mL dropper bottles.[1]
Rx	Flurbiprofen Sodium Ophthalmic (Various, eg, Bausch & Lomb)		In 2.5 mL.[1]

[1] With 1.4% polyvinyl alcohol, 0.005% thimerosal, EDTA.

KETOROLAC TROMETHAMINE

Complete prescribing information is found in the NSAIDs group monograph.

Administration and Dosage:

Relief of ocular itching: Instill 1 drop (0.25 mg) 4 times a day.

Postoperative inflammation: Instill 1 drop (0.25 mg) in the affected eye(s) 4 times daily beginning 24 hours after cataract surgery and continuing through the first 2 weeks of the postoperative period.

OPHTHALMIC DRUG FACTS

Storage: Store at controlled room temperature 15° to 30°C (59° to 86°F). Protect from light.

Rx	**Acular** (Allergan)	**Solution**: 0.5%	In 5 mL dropper bottles.[1]
Rx	**Acular PF** (Allergan)		In 12 single-use 0.4 mL vials.[2]

[1] With 0.01% benzalkonium chloride, 0.1% EDTA, octoxynol 40.
[2] With 0.5% ketorolac tromethamine.

SUPROFEN

Complete prescribing information is found in the NSAIDs group monograph.

Administration and Dosage:

On the day of surgery, instill 2 drops into the conjunctival sac at 3, 2, and 1 hour prior to surgery. Two drops may be instilled into the conjunctival sac every 4 hours, while awake, the day preceding surgery.

Storage: Store at room temperature.

Rx	**Profenal** (Alcon)	**Solution**: 1%	In 2.5 mL Drop-Tainers.[1]

[1] With 0.005% thimerosal, 2% caffeine, EDTA.

ARTIFICIAL TEAR SOLUTIONS AND OCULAR LUBRICANTS

Availability of synthetic polymers suitable for ocular use has resulted in development of artificial tear solutions, ointments, and other formulations to help alleviate ocular discomfort and maintain integrity of the surface epithelium. Ideally, formulations for dry eyes should be compatible with and substitute for components of the tear film, including lipid, aqueous, and mucin layers.

SOLUTIONS

Lubricant preparations formulated as artificial tear solutions usually contain inorganic electrolytes, preservatives, and water-soluble polymeric systems. Sodium chloride (NaCl), potassium chloride (KCl), various other ions, and boric acid help maintain tonicity and pH of the formulations. Preservatives, including benzalkonium chloride, chlorobutanol, thimerosal, EDTA, methylparaben, and propylparaben, are included in multidose preparations to prevent bacterial contamination. Methylcellulose and its derivatives, polyvinyl alcohol (PVA), povidone (PVP), dextran, and propylene glycol can enhance viscosity and promote tear film stability. A more recent advance in artificial tear formulations is the introduction of preservative-free preparations. These formulations can prevent adverse ocular surface effects in patients who use artificial tears frequently or for prolonged periods of time.

In addition to polymers, lipids and vitamins have also been incorporated into ocular lubricants. Retinyl, the alcohol form of vitamin A, is available as a solution for topical use on the eye. The formulation *Viva-Drops* contains vitamin A, polysorbate 80, and EDTA. Definitive data on the benefits of vitamin-containing formulations in dry eye disorders are not available and large-scale, well-controlled masked studies are lacking regarding efficacy of vitamin A or its derivatives in patients with ocular surface disease. Awaiting FDA approval is a topical cyclosporine formulation, which will be available as *Restadis*.

Artificial tear solutions should be administered at dosage frequencies of 4 to 6 hours. However, depending on the severity of the clinical signs and symptoms, they may be used as often as hourly or only occasionally. It is highly recommended that the prescriber of the artificial tear product recommend a specific dosage schedule for the patient, particularly at the start of therapy.

OINTMENTS

Petrolatum, lanolin, and mineral oil ointments are the second most frequent approach for ocular lubrication. When placed on the eye, they dissolve at the temperature of the ocular tissue and disperse with the tear fluid. A major advantage is that ointments appear to be retained in the cul-de-sac longer than artificial tear solutions.

Ointments are usually applied directly to the inferior conjunctival sac as a 0.25- to 0.5-inch ribbon. An alternative method is to place the ointment on a cotton-tipped applicator and apply it to the lid margins and lashes. Blurring of vision and possible irritation are minimized with this method of instillation. Recently, manufacturers have begun to formulate preservative-free ointment preparations. These preparations are less toxic and less allergenic than those containing preservatives.

Ophthalmic lubricant ointments are generally preferred for bedtime use. Depending on the clinical signs and patient symptoms, they may also be used as often as necessary during the day. Because ointments may block access of solution to the ocular surface, solutions should be instilled prior to application.

SOLID DEVICES

Another approach to relief of dry eye symptoms is use of a preservative-free, water-soluble, polymeric insert (*Lacrisert*). The cylindrical rod, which contains 5 mg hydroxypropylcellulose, is placed in the lower cul-de-sac. It then imbibes fluid and swells. As it dissolves, the polymer is released to the ocular surface for 12 to 24 hours.

The device can be beneficial in dry eye syndromes such as keratitis sicca. It is generally comfortable, but some disadvantages are associated with its use. Manual dexterity is required for placement in the cul-de-sac, and the cost to the patient is greater than use of solutions and ointments. A common patient complaint is blurred vision as the rod dissolves, causing the tear film to thicken. Adding fluid drops to the eye (eg, isotonic saline) following insertion of the pellet can reduce viscosity and minimize visual complaints.

PUNCTAL PLUGS

Mechanical occlusion of the lacrimal punctum has become an accepted method to block tear drainage and thereby prolong action of natural tears as well as artificial tear preparations. Several types of punctal plugs are currently used including a silicone-based plug and a temporary absorbable collagen implant.

The *Freeman* punctal plug is usually inserted directly into the inferior punctum. The procedure may require topical anesthesia and punctal dilation prior to placement.

The temporary punctal/canalicular collagen implant consists of collagen inserts packaged at the edge of a foam strip. The implants are placed halfway into the punctal opening and advanced into the horizontal canaliculus with the aid of a jeweler's forceps and magnification. The procedure can be done with or without an anesthetic. Following placement, the implant swells, impeding tear flow up to 14 days before the implants are totally absorbed.

Punctal occlusion can benefit patients whose symptoms are not relieved by topical therapy alone. Although rare, punctal occlusion can lead to epiphora.

Siret D. Jaanus, PhD
Southern California College of Optometry

ARTIFICIAL TEAR SOLUTIONS AND OCULAR LUBRICANTS

For More Information

Bartlett JD, Jaanus SD, eds. Clinical Ocular Pharmacology, ed. 4. Boston: Butterworth-Heinnemann, 2001.

Bernal DL, Ubels JL. Quantitative evaluation of the corneal epithelial barrier: Effect of artificial tears and preservatives. *Curr Eye Res* 1991;10:645.

Holly FJ. Tear film physiology. *Int Ophthalmol Clin* 1987;27:2.

Lemp MA. Recent developments in dry eye management. *Surv Ophthalmol* 1987;94:1299.

Marquardt R. Therapy of the dry eye. In: Lemp MA, Marquardt R, eds. The Dry Eye. Berlin: Springer-Verlag, 1992; chapter 6.

Norn MS, Opauszki A. Effects of ophthalmic vehicles on the stability of the precorneal tear film. *Acta Ophthalmol* 1977;55:23.

Tuberville AW, et al. Punctal occlusion in tear deficiency syndromes. *Ophthalmology* 1982;89:1170.

Werblin TP, et al. The use of slow-release artificial tears in the long-term management of keratitis sicca. *Ophthalmology*1981;88:78.

Tabbara KF, Wagoner MD. Diagnosis and management of dry-eye syndrome. *Int Ophthalmol Clin* 1996;36:61-75.

ARTIFICIAL TEAR SOLUTIONS

Actions:

Pharmacology: These products contain the following: Balanced amounts of salts to maintain ocular tonicity (0.9% NaCl equivalent); buffers to adjust pH; viscosity agents to prolong eye contact time; preservatives for sterility. See the Dosage Forms and Routes of Administration chapter for a description and listing of these ingredients.

Indications:

Ophthalmic lubricants: These products offer tear-like lubrication for the relief of dry eyes and eye irritation associated with deficient tear production and exposure to wind, sun, or other irritants. Also used as ocular lubricants for artificial eyes.

Contraindications:

Hypersensitivity to any component of the product.

Patient Information:

To avoid contamination, do not touch the tip of the container or dropper to any surface. Close container immediately after use.

If headache, eye pain, vision changes, or irritation occurs, if redness continues, or if the condition worsens or persists for > 3 days, discontinue use and consult a physician.

May cause mild stinging or temporary blurred vision.

Some of these products should not be used with soft contact lenses. Check package label.

Administration and Dosage:

Instill 1 to 2 drops into eye(s) 3 or 4 times daily, as needed.

otc	**20/20 Tears** (S.S.S. Company)	**Solution:** 1.4% PVA, 0.01% benzalkonium Cl, 0.05% EDTA, KCl, NaCl	Thimerosal free. In 15 mL.
otc	**Akwa Tears** (Akorn)	**Solution:** 1.4% PVA, 0.005% benzalkonium Cl, EDTA, NaCl, sodium phosphate,	In 15 mL.
otc	**AquaSite** (Novartis)	**Solution:** 0.2% PEG-400, 0.1% dextran 70, polycarbophil, EDTA, NaCl, sodium hydroxide	Preservative free. In 6 mL (single-use 24s).
otc	**Artificial Tears** (Various, eg, Rugby, United)	**Solution:** 1.4% PVA, NaCl, EDTA, 0.01% benzalkonium Cl, KCL.	In 15 mL.
otc	**Bion Tears** (Alcon)	**Solution:** 0.1% dextran 70, 0.3% hydroxypropyl methylcellulose 2910, carbon dioxide, hydrochloric acid, sodium hydroxide	Preservative free. In 0.45 mL (UD 28s).
otc	**Celluvisc** (Allergan)	**Solution:** 1% carboxymethylcellulose, calcium chloride, KCl, NaCl, sodium lactate	Preservative free. In 0.1 mL (UD 30s and 50s).

ARTIFICIAL TEAR SOLUTIONS AND OCULAR LUBRICANTS 103

otc	**Dry Eye Therapy** (Bausch & Lomb)	**Solution:** 0.3% glycerin, KCl, NaCl, sodium citrate, sodium phosphate	Preservative free. In 3 mL.
otc	**GenTeal** (Novartis)	**Solution:** 0.3% hydroxypropyl methylcellulose, boric acid, NaCl, phosphoric acid, sodium perborate	In 15 and 25 mL.
otc	**HypoTears** (Novartis)	**Solution:** 1% PVA, 1% PEG-400, 0.01% benzalkonium Cl, dextrose, EDTA	In 15 and 30 mL.
otc	**HypoTears PF** (Novartis)	**Solution:** 1% PVA, 1% PEG-400, dextrose, EDTA	Preservative free. In 0.5 mL (UD 30s).
otc	**Isopto Plain** (Alcon)	**Solution:** 0.5% hydroxypropyl methylcellulose 2910, 0.01% benzalkonium Cl, NaCl, sodium citrate, sodium phosphate	In 15 mL Drop-Tainers.
otc	**Isopto Tears** (Alcon)		In 15 and 30 mL.
otc	**Just Tears** (Blairex)	**Solution:** 1.4% PVA, benzalkonium Cl, EDTA, KCl, NaCl	In 15 mL.
otc	**Liquifilm Tears** (Allergan)	**Solution:** 1.4% PVA, 0.5% chlorobutanol, NaCl	In 15 and 30 mL.
otc	**Moisture Eyes** (Bausch & Lomb)	**Solution:** 1% propylene glycol, 0.3% glycerin, 0.01% benzalkonium Cl	In 15 and 30 mL.
otc	**Moisture Eyes Preservative Free** (Bausch & Lomb)	**Solution:** 0.95% propylene glycol, boric acid, EDTA, KCl, NaCl, sodium borate	In 0.6 mL (UD 32s).
otc	**Murine Tears** (Ross)	**Solution:** 0.6% PVP, 0.5% PVA, benzalkonium Cl, dextrose, EDTA, KCl, NaCl, sodium bicarbonate, sodium citrate, sodium phosphate	In 15 and 30 mL.
otc	**Murocel** (Bausch & Lomb)	**Solution:** 1% methylcellulose, propylene glycol, 0.028% methylparaben, 0.012% propylparaben, boric acid, NaCl, sodium borate	In 15 mL.
otc	**Nu-Tears II** (Optopics)	**Solution:** 1% PVA, 1% PEG-400, benzalkonium Cl, EDTA, dextrose	In 15 mL.
otc	**OcuCoat** (Lederle)	**Solution:** 0.1% dextran 70, 0.8% hydroxypropyl methylcellulose, 0.01% benzalkonium Cl, dextrose, KCl, NaCl, sodium phosphate	In 15 mL.
otc	**OcuCoat PF** (Lederle)	**Solution:** 0.1% dextran 70, 0.8% hydroxypropyl methylcellulose, dextrose, KCl, NaCl, sodium phosphate	Preservative free. In 0.5 mL (UD 28s).
otc	**Puralube Tears** (Fougera)	**Solution:** 1% PVA, 1% PEG 400, benzalkonium Cl, dextrose, EDTA	In 15 mL.
otc	**Refresh** (Allergan)	**Solution:** 1.4% PVA, 0.6% PVP, NaCl	Preservative free. In 0.3 mL (UD 30s and 50s).
otc	**Refresh Plus** (Allergan)	**Solution:** 0.5% carboxymethylcellulose sodium, calcium chloride, KCl, magnesium chloride, NaCl, sodium lactate	Preservative free. In 0.3 mL (UD 30s and 50s).
otc	**Refresh Tears** (Allergan)	**Solution:** 0.5% carboxymethylcellulose sodium, boric acid, calcium chloride, KCl, magnesium chloride, NaCl, stabilized oxychloro complex	In 15 mL.
otc	**Teargen** (Zenith-Goldline)	**Solution:** 1.4% PVA, 0.01% benzalkonium Cl, EDTA, NaCl, sodium phosphate	In 15 mL.

OPHTHALMIC DRUG FACTS

otc	**Teargen II** (Zenith-Goldline)	**Solution:** 0.4% hydroxypropyl methylcellulose 2910, 0.01% benzalkonium Cl, EDTA, KCl, NaCl, sodium phosphate	In 15 mL.
otc	**Tearisol** (Novartis)	**Solution:** 0.5% hydroxypropyl methylcellulose, 0.01% benzalkonium Cl, boric acid, EDTA, KCl, sodium carbonate	In 15 mL.
otc	**Tears Naturale** (Alcon)	**Solution:** 0.3% hydroxypropyl methylcellulose, 0.1% dextran 70, 0.01% benzalkonium Cl, EDTA, hydrochloric acid, KCl, NaCl, sodium hydroxide	In 15 and 30 mL.
otc	**Tears Naturale II** (Alcon)	**Solution:** 0.3% hydroxypropyl methylcellulose 2910, 0.1% dextran 70, 0.001% polyquaternium-1, KCl, NaCl, sodium borate	In 15 and 30 mL DropTainers.
otc	**Tears Naturale Free** (Alcon)	**Solution:** 0.3% hydroxypropyl methylcellulose 2910, 0.1% dextran 70	Preservative free. In 0.6 mL (UD 32s).
otc	**Tears Plus** (Allergan)	**Solution:** 1.4% PVA, 0.6% PVP, 0.5% chlorobutanol, NaCl	In 15 and 30 mL.
otc	**Tears Renewed** (Akorn)	**Solution:** 0.3% hydroxypropyl methylcellulose 2906, 0.1% dextran 70, 0.01% benzalkonium Cl, EDTA, hydrochloric acid, KCl, NaCl, sodium hydroxide	In 15 mL.
otc	**Thera Tears** (Advanced Vision)	**Solution:** 0.25% sodium carboxymethylcellulose, borate buffers, calcium chloride, KCl, magnesium chloride, NaCl, sodium bicarbonate, sodium phosphate	Preservative free. In 0.6 mL (UD 32s).
otc	**Ultra Tears** (Alcon)	**Solution:** 1% hydroxypropyl methylcellulose 2910, 0.01% benzalkonium Cl, NaCl, sodium citrate, sodium phosphate	In 15 mL.
otc	**Visine Tears** (Pfizer)	**Solution:** 1% PEG-400, 0.2% hydroxypropyl methycellulose, 0.2% glycerin, ascorbic acid, benzakonium Cl, boric acid, dextrose, disodium phosphate, glycine, KCl, magnesium chloride, NaCl, sodium borate, sodium citrate, sodium lactate	In 15 mL.
otc	**Viva-Drops** (Vision Pharm)	**Solution:** Polysorbate 80, citric acid, EDTA, mannitol, NaCl, pyruvate, retinyl palmitate, sodium citrate	Preservative free. In 10 and 15 mL.

OCULAR LUBRICANTS (Ointments and Gels)

Actions:

Pharmacology: These products serve as lubricants and emollients.

Indications:

Ophthalmic lubrication: Protection and lubrication of the eye.

Contraindications:

Hypersensitivity to any component of the products.

ARTIFICIAL TEAR SOLUTIONS AND OCULAR LUBRICANTS

Patient Information:

To avoid contamination, do not touch tube tip to any surface.

Do not use with contact lenses.

If eye pain, vision changes, or or irritation occurs, if redness continues, or if the condition worsens or persists for > 72 hours, discontinue use and contact a physician.

Refer to the Dosage Forms and Routes of Administration for more complete information.

Administration and Dosage:

Pull down the lower lid of affected eye(s) and apply a small amount (0.25 inch) of ointment to the inside of the eyelid.

Storage/Stability: Store at room temperature 15° to 30°C (59° to 86°F). Store away from heat.

otc	**Akwa Tears** (Akorn)	**Ointment:** White petrolatum, mineral oil, lanolin	Preservative free. In 3.5 g.
otc	**Artificial Tears** (Rugby)	**Ointment:** 83% white petrolatum, 15% mineral oil, lanolin oil	In 3.5 g.
otc	**Dry Eyes** (Bausch & Lomb)	**Ointment:** White petrolatum, mineral oil, lanolin	Preservative free. In 3.5 g.
otc	**Duratears Naturale** (Alcon)	**Ointment:** White petrolatum, anhydrous liquid lanolin, mineral oil	Preservative free. In 3.5 g.
otc	**HypoTears** (Novartis)	**Ointment:** White petrolatum, light mineral oil	Preservative and lanolin free. In 3.5 g.
otc	**Lacri-Lube NP** (Allergan)	**Ointment:** 57.3% white petrolatum, 42.5% mineral oil	Preservative free. In 0.7 g.
otc	**Lacri-Lube S.O.P.** (Allergan)	**Ointment:** 56.8% white petrolatum, 42.5% mineral oil, chlorobutanol, lanolin alcohols	In 0.7, 3.5, and 7 g.
otc	**Moisture Eyes PM** (Bausch & Lomb)	**Ointment:** 80% white petrolatum, 20% mineral oil	Preservative free. In 3.5 mg.
otc	**Puralube** (Fougera)	**Ointment:** White petrolatum, light mineral oil	In 3.5 g.
otc	**Refresh PM** (Allergan)	**Ointment:** 56.8% white petrolatum, 41.5% mineral oil, lanolin alcohols, NaCl	Preservative free. In 3.5 g.
otc	**Stye** (Del Pharm)	**Ointment:** 57.7% white petrolatum, 31.9% mineral oil, stearic acid, wheat germ oil, microcrystalline wax	In 3.5 g.
otc	**Tears Naturale P.M.** (Alcon)	**Ointment:** White petrolatum, anhydrous liquid lanolin, mineral oil	Preservative free. In 3.5 g.
otc	**Tears Renewed** (Akorn)	**Ointment:** White petrolatum, light mineral oil, lanolin oil	Preservative free. In 3.5 g.
otc	**GenTeal Gel** (Novartis)	**Gel:** 0.3% hydroxypropyl methylcellulose, 0.028% sodium perborate, carbopol 980, phosphoric acid, sorbitol	In 10 mL.

ARTIFICIAL TEAR INSERT

Actions:

Pharmacology: The hydroxypropyl cellulose insert acts to stabilize and thicken the precorneal tear film and prolong tear film breakup time, which is usually accelerated in patients with dry eye states. The insert also acts to lubricate and protect the eye.

Signs and symptoms resulting from moderate to severe dry eye syndromes, such as conjunctival hyperemia, corneal and conjunctival staining with rose bengal, exudation, itching, burning, foreign body sensation, smarting, photophobia, dryness, and blurred or cloudy vision are reduced. Progressive visual deterioration may be retarded, halted, or sometimes reversed.

Pharmacokinetics: Hydroxypropyl cellulose is a physiologically inert substance. Dissolution studies in rabbits showed that the inserts became softer within 1 hour after they were placed in the conjunctival sac. Most dissolved completely in 14 to 18 hours; with a single exception, all had disappeared by 24 hours after insertion. Similar dissolution of inserts was observed during prolonged use ($\leq$ 54 weeks).

Clinical Trials: In a multicenter crossover study, the 5 mg insert administered into the inferior cul-de-sac once a day during the waking hours was compared with artificial tears used $\geq$ 4 times daily. There was a prolongation of tear film breakup time and a decrease in foreign body sensation associated with dry eye syndrome in patients during treatment with inserts as compared with artificial tears. Improvement was greater in most patients who used the inserts.

Indications:

Dry eye syndromes, moderate to severe: Keratoconjunctivitis sicca (especially in patients who remain symptomatic after an adequate trial of artificial tear solutions); exposure keratitis; decreased corneal sensitivity; recurrent corneal erosions.

Contraindications:

Hypersensitivity to hydroxypropyl cellulose.

Adverse Reactions:

The following have occurred, but in most instances were mild and transient: Transient blurring of vision; ocular discomfort or irritation; matting or stickiness of eyelashes; photophobia; hypersensitivity; edema of the eyelids; hyperemia.

Patient Information:

May produce transient blurring of vision; exercise caution while operating hazardous machinery or driving a motor vehicle.

If improperly placed in the inferior cul-de-sac, corneal abrasion may result. Patient should practice insertion and removal in physician's office until proficiency is achieved.

Illustrated instructions are included in each package.

If symptoms worsen, remove insert and notify physician.

ARTIFICIAL TEAR SOLUTIONS AND OCULAR LUBRICANTS

Administration and Dosage:

Once daily, inserted into inferior cul-de-sac beneath the base of the tarsus, not in apposition to the cornea nor beneath the eyelid at the level of the tarsal plate. Individual patients may require twice-daily use for optimal results.

If not properly positioned, the insert will be expelled into the interpalpebral fissure, and may cause symptoms of a foreign body.

Occasionally, the insert is inadvertently expelled from the eye, especially in patients with shallow conjunctival fornices. Caution the patient against rubbing the eye(s), especially upon awakening, so as not to dislodge or expel the insert. If required, another insert may be used. If transient blurred vision develops, the patient may want to remove the insert a few hours after insertion.

Rx	**Lacrisert** (Merck & Co.)	**Insert:** 5 mg hydroxpropyl cellulose	Preservative free. In 60s with applicator.

PUNCTAL PLUGS

Actions:

Pharmacology: These flexible silicone plugs partially block the punctum and horizontal canaliculus to eliminate tear loss.

Indications:

Keratitis sicca (dry eye): Treatment of symptoms of dry eye (eg, redness, burning, reflex tearing, itching, foreign body sensation); after eye surgery to prevent complications due to dry eye; to enhance the efficacy of ocular medications; for patients experiencing dry eye-related contact lens problems.

Contraindications:

Hypersensitivity to silicone; eye infection.

Precautions:

Injection path: If injecting an anesthetic agent in the region of the canaliculus, maintain an $\approx$ 5 mm distance between the injection path and the angular vessels.

Dilation: Do not dilate punctal opening > 1.2 mm.

Irritation: If irritation caused by plug insertion persists longer than several days, reexamine the patient and consider plug removal.

Patient Information:

Do not press fingers on or near the eyelid. Use a cotton-tipped swab to remove "sleep" from the corner of eyes.

Do not attempt to replace a plug that has fallen out.

Relief may not occur immediately after insertion; some discomfort and tearing may occur for a few days.

Administration and Dosage:

Plugs must be inserted by a physician or doctor of optometry.

Rx	**EaglePlug** (Eagle Vision)	**Plug**: Silicone plug	In 0.4, 0.5, 0.6, 0.7, and 0.8 mm sizes (packs of 2 plugs).
Rx	**Eagle FlexPlug** (Eagle Vision)		In 0.4, 0.5, 0.6, 0.7, 0.8, and 0.9 mm sizes (single packs).
Rx	**Herrick Lacrimal Plug** (Lacri-medics)		In 0.3, 0.5, and 0.7 mm sizes (packs of 2 plugs).
Rx	**Ready-Set Punctum Plugs** (FCI Ophthalmics)		In 0.4, 0.5, 0.7, 0.8, and 1 mm sizes (packs of 2 plugs).
Rx	**Tears Naturale** (Alcon)		In 0.4, 0.5, 0.6, 0.7, and 0.8 mm sizes.
Rx	**Tearsaver** (Ciba Vision)		In 0.4, 0.5, 0.6, 0.7, and 0.8 mm sizes.

COLLAGEN IMPLANTS

Actions:

Pharmacology: These absorbable implants partially block the punctum and horizontal canaliculus, eliminating tear loss.

Indications:

Dry eyes: For the relief of dry eyes and secondary abnormalities such as conjunctivitis, corneal ulcer, pterygium, blepharitis, keratitis, red lid margins, recurrent chalazion, recurrent corneal erosion, filamentary keratitis, and other noninfectious external eye diseases; to enhance the effect of ocular medications; treatment of symptoms of dry eye (eg, redness, burning, reflex tearing, itching, foreign body sensation); after eye surgery to prevent complications; for patients experiencing dry eye-related contact lens problems.

Contraindications:

Tearing secondary to chronic dacryocystitis with mucopurulent discharge; allergy to bovine collagen; inflammation of eyelid; epiphoria.

Patient Information:

Relief may not occur immediately after insertion.

No removal is necessary; implants dissolve within 7 to 10 days.

Reexamination is usually required within 14 days.

ARTIFICIAL TEAR SOLUTIONS AND OCULAR LUBRICANTS

Successful treatment may indicate a need for permanent treatment (eg, nondissolvable silicone plugs).

Administration and Dosage:

Implants must be inserted by a physician or doctor of optometry. Placement of implants in all 4 canaliculi is recommended to prevent a false-negative response.

Rx	**Collagen Implant** (Lacrimedics)	**Implant:** Collagen implant	In 0.2, 0.3, 0.4, 0.5, and 0.6 mm sizes (72s).
Rx	**SoftPlug** (Oasis)		In 0.3 and 0.4 mm sizes (60s).
Rx	**Tears Naturale** (Alcon)		In 0.2, 0.3, and 0.4 mm sizes (60s).
Rx	**TearSaver** (Ciba Vision)		In 0.2, 0.3, 0.4, 0.5, and 0.6 mm sizes.
Rx	**Temporary Punctal/Canalicular Collagen Implant** (Eagle Vision)		In 0.2, 0.3, 0.4, 0.5, and 0.6 mm sizes (72s).

TYLOXAPOL (CLEANING/LUBRICANT FOR ARTIFICIAL EYES)

Actions:

Pharmacology: The cleaning/lubricant solution is a sterile, buffered isotonic solution formulated especially for artificial eye wearers. It contains the antibacterial agent benzalkonium chloride to kill most germs that are commonly found in the eye socket of artificial eye wearers. Tyloxapol, a detergent, liquifies the solid matter so that it is less irritating. Benzalkonium chloride, in addition to its germ-killing action, aids tyloxapol in wetting the artificial eye so that it is completely covered.

Indications:

Cleaner/Lubricant: To lubricate, clean, and wet artificial eyes to increase wearing comfort.

Contraindications:

Hypersensitivity to any component of the formulation.

Patient Information:

If irritation persists or increases, discontinue use and consult a physician. Keep container tightly closed. Keep out of the reach of children.

To avoid contamination, do not touch dropper tip to any surface. Replace cap after using.

Administration and Dosage:

Use drops as ordinary eyedrops are used. With the artificial eye in place, apply 1 or 2 drops 3 or 4 times daily. The artificial eye may be removed periodically if advised by a physician, and 2 or 3 drops applied to remove oily or mucous materials. The arti-

OPHTHALMIC DRUG FACTS

ficial eye is then rubbed between the fingers and rinsed with tap water. Then 1 or 2 drops may be applied to the artificial eye, either prior to or after reinsertion.

Storage/Stability: Store at 8° to 27°C (46° to 80°F).

| otc | **Enuclene** (Alcon) | **Solution:** 0.25%[1] | In 15 mL Drop-Tainers. |

[1] 0.02% benzalkonium Cl.

Anti-infective Agents

ANTIBIOTIC AGENTS

Topical systemic antibiotics may be utilized in the treatment of ocular infections. The most common ocular infections include blepharitis, conjunctivitis, dacryoadenitis, dacryocystitis, keratitis, orbital cellulitis, endophthalmitis, attendant sinusitis, and superficial erysipelas of the skin. Intravitreal antibiotics may be the treatment of choice for endophthalmitis.

The indigenous flora of the eyelids and conjunctiva are primarily *Staphylococcus aureus* and *Staphylococcus epidermidis*, which can overwhelm the ocular defenses and produce infection. Staphylococcal species are most commonly associated with acute papillary conjunctivitis, chronic blepharitis, dacryocystitis, impetigo, blepharoconjunctivitis, superficial keratitis, and endophthalmitis. Corneal ulcers are associated with gram-positive bacteria ≈ 75% of the time and gram-negative organisms 25% of the time. Broad spectrum coverage is now available from the fluoroquinolones for single antibiogen coverage of corneal ulcers obviating cultures if the infection responds promptly. Beware of the emerging prevalence of methicillin-resistant *S. aureus* strains (MRSA), which may now require vancomycin. Fungal organisms may be seen in up to 10% of corneal ulcers in Florida.

A purulent discharge and papillary conjunctivitis are associated with a bacterial infection. A serous discharge with conjunctival chemosis and itching is more frequently associated with conjunctival allergy. Conjunctival hemorrhages are associated with more virulent organisms such as streptococcus, haemophilus, or adenovirus. Infiltrative keratitis in the visual axis, decreased vision, hazing of the anterior chamber, or hypopyon are harbingers of imminent visual loss and require prompt microbiologic studies for organism identification and proper antibiotic selection. Similar fastidious cultures of the lids or conjunctiva are important for any chronic conjunctivitis.

The table on the following page reflects the sensitivity studies of the Department of Ophthalmology, University of South Florida, and antibiograms from regional institutions. Individual laboratory sensitivities may vary. See individual product inserts for more information on susceptible microorganisms.

Topical Ophthalmic Antibiotic Preparations

	Organism/Infection	Bacitracin[4]	Gramicidin	Polymyxin B[4]	Erythromycin[4]	Chloramphenicol[4]	Trimethoprim[4]	Oxytetracycline	Vancomycin[3,4]	Norfloxacin	Ciprofloxacin[4]	Ofloxacin[4]	Neomycin[4]	Gentamicin[4]	Tobramycin[4]	Amikacin[3,4]	Sodium Sulfacetamide[4]	Sulfisoxazole	Sulfamethoxazole[3]	Ampicillin[3]	Oxacillin[3,4]	Ticarcillin[3]	Cefotaxime[3]	Ceftazidime[3,4]	Cefuroxime[3]	Cephalothin[3,4]
Gram-Positive	Staphylococcus sp	✓	✓						✓	✓						✓									✓	✓
	S. aureus	✓	✓		✓				✓	✓			✓			✓		✓	✓		✓				✓	✓
	Streptococcus sp	✓	✓		✓			✓			✓	✓					✓	✓	✓							
	S. pneumoniae	✓	✓		✓	✓		✓	✓	✓	✓	✓					✓	✓	✓				✓			✓
	α-hemolytic streptococci (viridans group)	✓			✓	✓		✓			✓						✓	✓	✓	✓			✓		✓	✓
	β-hemolytic streptococci	✓												✓[1]	✓											
	S. pyogenes	✓			✓		✓				✓	✓		✓			✓									✓
	Corynebacterium sp	✓	✓			✓					✓		✓	✓	✓	✓										
Gram-Negative	Escherichia coli			✓		✓	✓	✓		✓	✓	✓	✓	✓	✓		✓	✓								
	Haemophilus aegyptius					✓	✓			✓				✓	✓		✓	✓								
	H. ducreyi					✓		✓		✓				✓	✓											
	H. influenzae or parainfluenzae		✓		✓	✓				✓	✓	✓								✓						
	Klebsiella sp					✓		✓		✓	✓	✓		✓	✓											
	K. pneumoniae			✓			✓	✓		✓	✓	✓		✓	✓											✓
	Neisseria sp	✓				✓					✓			✓	✓	✓										
	N. gonorrhoeae	✓			✓[2]					✓	✓	✓					✓									
	Proteus sp					✓	✓			✓	✓	✓	✓	✓	✓		✓	✓					✓	✓	✓	✓
	Acinetobacter calcoaceticus									✓	✓	✓		✓	✓								✓		✓	
	Enterobacter aerogenes			✓		✓	✓	✓		✓	✓	✓	✓	✓	✓	✓							✓		✓	
	Enterobacter sp					✓				✓	✓	✓	✓	✓	✓	✓	✓						✓			
	Serratia marcescens									✓	✓	✓		✓		✓										
	Moraxella sp	✓				✓		✓		✓	✓	✓	✓	✓	✓	✓	✓						✓	✓	✓	✓
	Chlamydia trachomatis			✓[2]						✓	✓						✓	✓								
	Pasteurella tularensis						✓	✓			✓			✓	✓	✓				✓			✓	✓	✓	✓
	Pseudomonas aeruginosa			✓						✓	✓	✓		✓	✓	✓							✓		✓	
	Bartonella bacilliformis							✓																		
	Bacteroides sp							✓																		
	Vibrio sp					✓		✓		✓	✓			✓	✓											
	Providencia sp									✓	✓															

[1] Increasing resistance has been seen.
[2] For prophylaxis.
[3] Not available as a commercial ophthalmic preparation.
[4] > 95% of ocular bacterial isolates sensitive.

ANTIFUNGAL AGENT

Natamycin (*Natacyn*) is the only topical ophthalmic antifungal agent available commercially. It is a tetraene polyene antibiotic derived from *Streptomyces natalensis*. It possesses in vitro activity against a variety of yeasts and filamentous fungi, including *Candida*, *Aspergillus*, *Cephalosporium*, *Fusarium*, and *Penicillium*.

Miconazole IV may be used topically if natamycin is not available. Amphotericin B 1% topical is a valuable alternative.

ANTIVIRAL AGENTS

The topical ophthalmic antiviral preparations appear to interfere with viral reproduction by altering DNA synthesis. Idoxuridine, vidarabine, and trifluridine are effective treatment for herpes simplex infections of the conjunctiva and cornea. Ganciclovir is indicated for use in immunocompromised patients with cytomegalovirus (CMV) retinitis and for prevention of CMV retinitis in transplant patients. Foscarnet and cidofovir are indicated for use only in AIDS patients with CMV retinitis.

Antiviral Agents for Ophthalmic Conditions			
Generic name	Trade name (manufacturer)	Preparations	Indications
Cidofovir	*Vistide* (Gilead)	Solution for Injection	Cytomegalovirus (CMV) retinitis
Fomivirsen sodium	*Vitravene* (Isis)	Solution for Injection	Cytomegalovirus (CMV) retinitis
Foscarnet sodium	*Foscavir* (Astra)	Solution for Injection	Cytomegalovirus (CMV) retinitis
Ganciclovir sodium	*Cytovene* (Syntex)	Reconstituted powder Capsules 250 mg	Cytomegalovirus (CMV) retinitis
	Vitrasert (Chiron Vision)	Implant	Cytomegalovirus (CMV) retinitis
Trifluridine	*Viroptic* (Monarch)	Solution 1%	Herpes simplex types 1 and 2; idoxuridine hypersensitivity; vidarabine-resistant keratitis
Vidarabine	*Vira-A* (Parke-Davis)	Ointment 3%	Herpes simplex types 1 and 2; idoxuridine-resistant herpes

Viral infection, especially epidemic keratoconjunctivitis (EKC), is more often associated with a follicular conjunctivitis, a serous conjunctival discharge, and preauricular lymphadenopathy. The exceptionally contagious organism causing EKC is not susceptible to antiviral therapy at this time. Pustular lesions of the nose and face, and spade-shaped fascicular keratitis in association with chronic blepharitis, suggesting acne rosacea, warrants a trial of systemic tetracycline (eg, *Achromycin V*) or doxycycline (eg, *Vibramycin*) as both an antibiotic and potentially anti-inflammatory regimen. (MMP = Matrix Metalloproteinase Inhibitor)

J. James Rowsey, MD
St. Luke's Cataract and Laser Institute Tarpon Springs, FL

For More Information

Bartlett JD, Jaanus SD, eds. *Clinical Ocular Pharmacology*, ed. 4. Boston: Butterworth-Heinemann, 2001.

Duane TD, ed. *Clinical Ophthalmology*. Philadelphia: Lippincott-Raven, 1997.

Kucers A, Bennett NM. *The Use of Antibiotics*, ed. 4. Philadelphia: J.B. Lippincott Company, 1987.

OPHTHALMIC DRUG FACTS

ANTIBIOTICS

Indications:

Ocular infections: Treatment of superficial ocular infections involving the conjunctiva or cornea (eg, conjunctivitis, keratitis, keratoconjunctivitis, corneal ulcers, blepharitis, blepharoconjunctivitis, acute meibomitis, dacryocystitis) caused by susceptible strains of microorganisms.

Erythromycin: Prophylaxis of ophthalmia neonatorum due to *Neisseria gonorrhoeae* or *Chlamydia trachomatis*.

Chloramphenicol: Use only in those serious infections for which less potentially dangerous drugs are ineffective or contraindicated (see Warnings).

For a listing of the microorganisms usually susceptible to the agents, refer to the Topical Ophthalmic Preparations table.

The table below lists common ocular conditions along with the antibiotics used most often to treat them. These antibiotics are preferred choices before cultures are available.

Antibiotic Treatment for Common Ocular Conditions			
	Blepharitis	Conjunctivitis	Keratitis
Bacitracin	X		
Polymixin B	X		
Sodium sulfacetamide	X		
Trimethoprim		X	
Vancomycin			X
Ciprofloxacin		X	X
Gentamicin			X
Tobramycin		X	
Amikacin		X	
Ofloxacin		X	X
Ceftazidime			X

Contraindications:

Hypersensitivity to any component of these products; history of hypersensitivity to other quinolones; epithelial herpes simplex keratitis (dendritic keratitis); vaccinia; varicella; mycobacterial infections of the eye; fungal diseases of the ocular structure; use of steroid combinations after uncomplicated removal of a corneal foreign body.

Warnings:

Ciprofloxacin and ofloxacin hypersensitivity reactions: Serious and occasionally fatal hypersensitivity (anaphylactic) reactions, some following the first dose, have been reported in patients receiving systemic quinolones, including ofloxacin. Some reactions were accompanied by cardiovascular collapse, loss of consciousness, angioedema (including laryngeal, pharyngeal, or facial edema), airway obstruction, dyspnea, urticaria, and itching. An occurrence of Stevens-Johnson syndrome, which progressed to toxic epidermal necrolysis, has been reported in a patient who was receiving topical ophthalmic ofloxacin. Discontinue drug if an allergic reaction occurs.

ANTI-INFECTIVE AGENTS 115

Serious acute hypersensitivity reactions may require immediate emergency treatment. Administer oxygen and airway management, including intubation, as clinically indicated.

Sensitization: Topical use of an antibiotic may contraindicate the drug's later systemic use in serious infections. For this reason, topical preparations containing antibiotics not ordinarily administered systemically are preferable. Products with neomycin sulfate may cause cutaneous/conjunctival sensitization.

Cross-sensitivity: Allergic cross-reactions may occur that could prevent future use of any or all of the following antibiotics: kanamycin, neomycin, paromomycin, streptomycin, and, possibly, gentamicin.

Hematopoietic toxicity: Hematopoietic toxicity has occurred occasionally with the systemic use of chloramphenicol and rarely with topical administration. It is generally a dose-related toxic effect on bone marrow, and is usually reversible on cessation of therapy. Rare cases of aplastic anemia, bone marrow hypoplasia, and death have been reported with prolonged (months to years) or frequent intermittent (over months and years) use of ocular chloramphenicol.

Corneal healing: Ophthalmic ointments may retard corneal epithelial healing.

Pregnancy: Category B (erythromycin, tobramycin). *Category C* (gentamicin, ciprofloxacin, norfloxacin, ofloxacin, polymyxin B). Safety for use during pregnancy has not been established. Use only when clearly needed and when the potential benefits to the mother outweigh the potential hazards to the fetus.

Lactation: It is not known whether ciprofloxacin, norfloxacin, or ofloxacin appears in breast milk following ophthalmic use. Exercise caution when administering ciprofloxacin to a nursing mother. Because of the potential for adverse reactions in nursing infants from norfloxacin, ofloxacin, chloramphenicol, and tobramycin, decide whether to discontinue nursing or discontinue the drug, taking into account the importance of the drug to the mother.

Children: Tobramycin is safe and effective in children. Safety and efficacy of fluoroquinolones in infants < 1 year of age, and of polymyxin B/trimethoprim in infants < 2 months of age have not been established.

Precautions:

Monitoring: Perform culture and susceptibility testing during treatment.

Systemic antibiotics: In all, except very superficial infections, supplement the topical use of antibiotics with appropriate systemic medication. Systemic aminoglycoside antibiotics require monitoring the total serum concentration (peak and trough). Recent studies suggest that intracameral antibiotics may be efficacious alone, for the treatment of endophthalmitis with minimally virulent organisms, with visual acuity > 20/400.

Crystalline precipitate: A white crystalline precipitate located in the superficial portion of the corneal defect was observed in ≈ 17% of patients on ciprofloxacin. Onset was within 1 to 7 days after starting therapy. The precipitate resolved in most patients within 2 weeks, and did not preclude continued use nor adversely affect the clinical course or outcome. Streptococcal corneal ulcers are often resistant to ciprofloxacin.

Superinfection: Do not use topical antibiotics in deep-seated ocular infections or in those that are likely to become systemic. Use of antibiotics (especially prolonged or

OPHTHALMIC DRUG FACTS

116

repeated therapy) may result in bacterial or fungal overgrowth of nonsusceptible organisms. Such overgrowth may lead to a secondary infection. Take appropriate measures if superinfection occurs.

Sulfite sensitivity: Some of these products contain sulfites, which may cause allergic-type reactions (eg, hives, itching, wheezing, anaphylaxis) in certain susceptible people. Although the overall prevalence of sulfite sensitivity in the general population is probably low, it is seen more frequently in asthmatics or in atopic nonasthmatic people. Specific products containing sulfites are identified in the product listings.

Adverse Reactions:

Sensitivity reactions such as transient irritation, burning, discomfort, redness, stinging, itching, inflammation, angioneurotic edema, urticaria, and vesicular and maculo-papular dermatitis have occurred in some patients.

Chloramphenicol:

> *Hematologic* – Hematological events (including aplastic anemia) have occurred (see Warnings).

Fluoroquinolones:

> *Miscellaneous* – White crystalline precipitates; lid margin crusting; crystals/scales; foreign body sensation; conjunctival hyperemia; bad/bitter taste in mouth; corneal staining; chemical conjunctivitis; keratopathy/keratitis; allergic reactions; lid and facial edema; tearing; photophobia; corneal infiltrates; nausea; decreased or blurred vision; chemosis; dryness; eye pain; dizziness (rarely).

Aminoglycosides:

> *Local* – Localized ocular toxicity and hypersensitivity, lid itching, lid swelling, and conjunctival erythema (< 3% with tobramycin); bacterial/fungal corneal ulcers; nonspecific conjunctivitis; conjunctival epithelial defects; conjunctival hyperemia (gentamicin). Similar reactions may occur with the topical use of other aminoglycoside antibiotics.

Overdosage:

Symptoms: Symptoms of tobramycin overdose include punctate keratitis, erythema, increased lacrimation, edema, and lid itching. These may be similar to adverse reactions.

Treatment: A topical overdose of ciprofloxacin may be flushed from the eyes with warm tap water.

Patient Information:

Tilt head back, place medication in conjunctival sac holding the dropper 1 inch from the eye, and close eyes. Apply light finger pressure on lacrimal sac for 1 minute following instillation.

May cause temporary blurring of vision or stinging following administration. Notify physician if stinging, burning, or itching becomes pronounced or if redness, irritation, swelling, decreasing vision, or pain persists or worsens.

ANTI-INFECTIVE AGENTS

To avoid contamination, do not touch tip of container to any surface. Replace cap after using.

In general, patients being treated for bacterial conjunctivitis should not wear contact lenses; however, if the physician considers contact lens use appropriate, wait ≥ 15 minutes after using any solutions containing benzalkonium chloride before inserting the lens, because benzalkonium chloride may be absorbed by the lens.

Quinolones: Discontinue use and notify physician at the first sign of a skin rash or other allergic reaction.

Administration and Dosage:

Administration and dosage varies for the individual products. Refer to the individual manufacturer inserts for complete information.

Individual drug monographs are on the following pages.

BACITRACIN

Complete prescribing information is found in the Ophthalmic Antibiotics group monograph.

Administration and Dosage:

Apply directly to conjunctival sac(s) 1 to 3 times daily.

Blepharitis: Carefully remove all scales and crusts and then spread ointment uniformly over lid margins.

Storage/Stability: Store at room temperature 15° to 30°C (59° to 86°F).

Rx	**Bacitracin** (Various, eg, Major, Goldline, Schein, URL, Zenith)	**Ointment:** 500 units/g	In 3.5 and 3.75 g.
Rx	**AK-Tracin** (Akorn)		Preservative free. In 3.5 g.[1]

[1] With white petrolatum, mineral oil.

POLYMYXIN B SULFATE

Complete prescribing information is found in the Ophthalmic Antibiotics group monograph.

Indications:

For treatment of infections of the eye caused by susceptible strains of *Pseudomonas aeruginosa.*

Administration and Dosage:

Dissolve 500,000 units polymyxin B sulfate in 20 to 50 mL sterile distilled water (Sterile Water for Injection, USP) or sterile physiologic saline (Sodium Chloride Injection, USP) for a 10,000 to 25,000 units/mL concentration.

For the treatment of P. aeruginosa infections of the eye: Administer a concentration of 0.1% to 0.25% (10,000 to 25,000 units/mL) 1 to 3 drops every hour, increasing the intervals as response indicates.

Consider continuous subpalpebral lavage for pseudomonas scleritis, sclero-keratitis, or perforating pseudomonoas ulcers.

Subconjunctival injection of up to 100,000 units/day may be used for the treatment of P. aeruginosa infections of the cornea and conjunctiva.

Avoid total systemic and ophthalmic instillations of over 25,000 units/kg/day.

Rx	**Polymyxin B Sulfate Sterile** (Bedford)	**Powder for solution:** 500,000 units	In 20 mL vials.

ANTI-INFECTIVE AGENTS   119

CHLORAMPHENICOL

Complete prescribing information is found in the Ophthalmic Antibiotics group monograph.

Use only in those serious infections for which less potentially dangerous drugs are ineffective or contraindicated (see Warnings).

Administration and Dosage:

Ointment: Place a small amount in the conjunctival sac(s) every 3 hours, or more often if required, day and night for the first 48 hours. Intervals between applications may be increased after the first 2 days. Since chloramphenicol is primarily bacteriostatic, continue therapy for 48 hours after an apparent cure has been obtained.

Solution (reconstituted): Instill 2 drops into the affected eye(s) every 3 hours, or more frequently if deemed advisable. Continue administration day and night for the first 48 hours, after which the interval between applications may be increased. Continue treatment for at least 48 hours after the eye appears normal.

Solution Preparation	
Strength of solution desired	Add sterile distilled water
0.5%	5 mL
0.25%	10 mL
0.16%	15 mL

Solution: Instill 1 or 2 drops 4 to 6 times a day for the first 72 hours, depending upon the severity of the condition. Intervals between applications may be increased after the first 2 days. Since the action of the drug is primarily bacteriostatic, continue therapy for 48 hours after an apparent cure has been attained.

Storage/Stability:

Ointment – Store at room temperature 15° to 30°C (59° to 86°F). Store away from heat.

Solution (reconstituted) – Store below 30°C (86°F). Reconstituted solutions remain stable at room temperature for 10 days.

Solution – Refrigerate at 2° to 8°C (36° to 46°F) until dispensed. Protect from light. Remove from refrigerator for dispensing; discard 21 days thereafter.

Rx	**Chloramphenicol** (Ivax)	**Solution**[1]: 5 mg/mL	In 7.5 mL.[2]
Rx	**AK-Chlor** (Akorn)		In 7.5 and 15 mL.[2]
Rx	**Chloromycetin** (Monarch)		In 15 mL.[3]
Rx	**Chloroptic** (Allergan)		In 2.5 and 7.5 mL.[4]

OPHTHALMIC DRUG FACTS

Rx	AK-Chlor (Akorn)	Ointment: 10 mg/g	In 3.5 g.[5]
Rx	Chloroptic S.O.P. (Allergan)		In 3.5 g.
Rx	Chloromycetin (Monarch)	Powder for solution: 25 mg/vial	Preservative free. In 15 mL with diluent.

[1] Refrigerate until dispensed.
[2] With 0.5% chlorobutanol, boric acid, sodium borate, hydroxypropyl methylcellulose, sodium hydroxide, hydrochloric acid.
[3] With propylene glycol.
[4] With 0.5% chlorobutanol, PEG-300, polyoxyl 40 stearate, sodium hydroxide or hydrochloric acid.
[5] With white petrolatum, mineral oil, polysorbate 60.

ERYTHROMYCIN

Complete prescribing information is found in the Ophthalmic Antibiotics group monograph.

Indications:

For the treatment of superficial ocular infections involving the conjunctiva or cornea caused by organisms susceptible to erythromycin.

For prophylaxis of ophthalmia neonatorum due to *Neisseria gonorrhoeae*. The Centers for Disease Control and the Committee on Drugs, the Committee on Infectious Diseases of the American Academy of Pediatrics, and the Committee on Fetus and Newborn recommend silver nitrate solution 1% in single-use ampules or single-use tubes of an ophthalmic ointment containing erythromycin 0.5% or tetracycline 1% as "effective and acceptable regimens for prophylaxis of gonococcal ophthalmia neonatorum." (For infants born to mothers with clinically apparent gonorrhea, give IV or IM injections of aqueous crystalline penicillin G: A single dose of 50,000 units for term infants or 20,000 units for infants of low birth weight. Topical prophylaxis alone is inadequate for these infants.)

For the prevention of neonatal conjunctivitis due to *chlamydia trachomatis*, condition that may develop one to several weeks after delivery in infants of mothers whose birth canals harbor the organism.

Administration and Dosage:

External ocular infections: Apply directly to the infected area ≥ 1 times daily, depending on the severity of the infection.

Prophylaxis of neonatal gonococcal or chlamydial conjunctivitis: Instill a thin line of ointment ≈ 0.5 to 1 cm in length into each conjunctival sac. Do not flush the ointment from the eye following application. Use a new tube for each infant. Administer to infants born by cesarian section and those delivered vaginally.

Storage/Stability: Store at room temperature 15° to 30°C (59° to 86°F).

Rx	Erythromycin (Various, eg, Akorn, Bausch & Lomb, Fougera, Rugby, Zenith Goldline)	Ointment: 5 mg/g	In 3.5 g.
Rx	Ilotycin (Dista)		In 3.5 g.[1]

[1] With white petrolatum, mineral oil.

ANTI-INFECTIVE AGENTS

GENTAMICIN SULFATE

Complete prescribing information is found in the Ophthalmic Antibiotics group monograph.

Administration and Dosage:

Solution: Instill 1 or 2 drops into the affected eye(s) every 4 hours. In severe infections, dosage may be increased to 2 drops once every hour.

This solution is not for injection. Do not inject subconjunctivally. Do not directly introduce into the anterior chamber.

Ointment: Apply a small amount to affected eye(s) 2 to 3 times daily.

Storage/Stability: Store at 2° to 30°C (36° to 86°F). Store away from heat.

Rx	Gentamicin Ophthalmic (Various, eg, Bausch & Lomb, Rugby, Schein, Zenith Goldline)	Solution: 3 mg/mL	In 5 and 15 mL.
Rx	Garamycin (Schering)		In 5 mL dropper bottles.[1]
Rx	Genoptic (Allergan)		In 1 and 5 mL dropper bottles.[2]
Rx	Gentacidin (Novartis)		In 3 and 5 mL dropper bottles.[1]
Rx	Gentak (Akorn)		In 5 and 15 mL dropper bottles.[1]
Rx	Gentamicin Ophthalmic (Various, eg, Novartis)	Ointment: 3 mg/g	In 3.5 g.
Rx	Garamycin (Schering)		In 3.5 g.[3]
Rx	Genoptic S.O.P. (Allergan)		In 3.5 g.[3]
Rx	Gentacidin (Novartis)		In 3.5 g.[4]
Rx	Gentak (Akorn)		In 3.5 g.[3]

[1] With 0.1 mg/mL benzalkonium chloride, sodium phosphate, NaCl.
[2] With benzalkonium chloride, 1.4% polyvinyl alcohol, EDTA, sodium phosphate dibasic, NaCl, hydrochloric acid or sodium hydroxide.
[3] With white petrolatum, parabens.
[4] With white petrolatum, mineral oil.

TOBRAMYCIN

Complete prescribing information is found in the Ophthalmic Antibiotics group monograph.

Administration and Dosage:

Solution:

> *Mild to moderate disease* – Instill 1 or 2 drops into the affected eye(s) every 4 hours. Not for injection into the eye.

> *Severe infections* – Instill 2 drops into the eye(s) hourly until improvement. Reduce treatment prior to discontinuation.

Ointment:

> *Mild to moderate disease* – Apply 0.5-inch ribbon into the affected eye(s) 2 or 3 times daily.

> *Severe infections* – Instill 0.5-inch ribbon into the affected eye(s) every 3 to 4 hours until improvement. Reduce treatment prior to discontinuation.

Storage/Stability: Store at 8° to 27°C (46° to 80°F).

Rx	**Tobramycin** (Various, eg, Bausch & Lomb, Steris)	**Solution**: 0.3%	In 5 mL bottle.
Rx	**AKTob** (Akorn)		In 5 mL.[1]
Rx	**Tobrex** (Alcon)		In 5 mL Drop-Tainers.[2]
Rx	**Tobrex** (Alcon)	**Ointment**: 3 mg/g	In 3.5 g.[3]

[1] With 0.01% benzalkonium chloride, boric acid, sodium sulfate, NaCl, tyloxapol.
[2] With 0.01% benzalkonium chloride, tyloxapol, boric acid, NaCl.
[3] With white petrolatum, mineral oil, 0.5% chlorobutanol.

CIPROFLOXACIN

Complete prescribing information is found in the Ophthalmic Antibiotics group monograph.

Administration and Dosage:

Not for injection into the eye.

Remove contact lenses before using.

For the treatment of corneal ulcers: Instill 2 drops into the affected eye(s) every 15 minutes for the first 6 hours and then 2 drops every 30 minutes for the remainder of the first day. On the second day, instill 2 drops every hour. On the third through the fourteenth day, instill 2 drops every 4 hours. Treatment may be continued after 14 days if corneal re-epithelialization has not occurred.

For the treatment of bacterial conjunctivitis: Instill 1 or 2 drops into the conjunctival sac(s) every 2 hours while awake for 2 days, and 1 or 2 drops every 4 hours while awake for the next 5 days.

Storage/Stability: Store at 2° to 30°C (36° to 86°F). Protect from light.

Rx	**Ciloxan** (Alcon)	**Solution**: 0.3% (equivalent to 3 mg base)	In 2.5, 5, and 10 mL Drop-Tainers.[1]
Rx	**Ciloxan** (Alcon)	**Ointment**: 0.3% (equivalent to 3 mg base)	In 3.5 g tube.[2]

[1] With 0.006% benzalkonium chloride, 4.6% mannitol, 0.05% EDTA.
[2] With mineral oil, white petrolatum.

NORFLOXACIN

Complete prescribing information is found in the Ophthalmic Antibiotics group monograph.

ANTI-INFECTIVE AGENTS

Administration and Dosage:

Bacterial conjunctivitis: Instill 1 or 2 drops into the affected eye(s) 4 times daily for up to 7 days. Depending on the severity of the infection, the dosage for the first day of therapy may be 1 or 2 drops every 2 hours during the waking hours.

Storage/Stability: Store at room temperature 15° to 30°C (59° to 86°F). Protect from light.

Rx	Chibroxin (Merck)	Solution: 3 mg/mL	In 5 mL Ocumeters.[1]

[1] With 0.0025% benzalkonium chloride, EDTA, NaCl.

OFLOXACIN

Complete prescribing information is found in the Ophthalmic Antibiotics group monograph.

Administration and Dosage:

Not for injection into the eye(s).

Bacterial conjunctivitis: Instill 1 to 2 drops every 2 to 4 hours for the first 2 days and then 4 times daily into the affected eye for up to 5 additional days.

Bacterial corneal ulcer: Instill 1 to 2 drops every 30 minutes while awake; awaken ≈ 4 and 6 hours after retiring and instill 1 to 2 drops for 2 days. Instill 1 to 2 drops while awake for the next 5 to 7 days. Instill 1 to 2 drops 4 times daily through treatment completion.

Storage/Stability: Store at 15° to 25°C (59° to 77°F).

Rx	Ocuflox (Allergan)	Solution: 0.3%	In 1, 5, and 10 mL.[1]

[1] With 0.005% benzalkonium chloride, NaCl.

LEVOFLOXACIN

Complete prescribing information is found in the Ophthalmic Antibiotics group monograph.

Administration and Dosage:

Gram-positive or gram-negative bacterial conjunctivitis: Days 1 and 2 instill 1 to 2 drops in the affected eye(s) every 2 hours while awake, up to 8 times per day. Days 3 through 7 instill 1 to 2 drops in the affected eye(s) every 4 hours while awake, up to 4 times per day.

Storage/Stability: Store at 15° to 25°C (59° to 77°F).

Rx	Quixin (Santen)	Solution: 0.5%	In 2.5 and 5 mL[1]

[1] With 0.005% benzalkonium chloride.

OPHTHALMIC DRUG FACTS

124

COMBINATION ANTIBIOTIC PRODUCTS

Complete prescribing information is found in the Ophthalmic Antibiotics group monograph.

	Product and distributor	Polymyxin B Sulfate (units/g or mL)	Neomycin Sulfate (mg/g or mL)	Bacitracin Zinc (units/g)	Other antibiotics	How supplied
Rx	**Triple Antibiotic Ophthalmic Ointment** (Various, eg, Fougera)	10,000	3.5	400		In 3.5 g.
Rx	**Bacitracin Neomycin Polymyxin B Ointment** (Various, eg, Fougera)					In 3.5 g.
Rx	**AK-Spore Ointment** (Akorn)					Preservative free. White petrolatum, mineral oil. In 3.5 g.
Rx	**Neosporin Ophthalmic Ointment** (GlaxoSmithKline)					White petrolatum. In 3.5 g.
Rx	**Neomycin Sulfate-Polymyxin B Sulfate-Gramicidin Solution** (Various, eg, Rugby, Steris Zenith Goldline)	10,000	1.75		0.025 mg/mL gramicidin	In 2 and 10 mL.
Rx	**AK-Spore Solution** (Akorn)					In 2 and 10 mL.[1]
Rx	**Neosporin Ophthalmic Solution** (GlaxoSmithKline)					In 10 mL Drop Dose.[1]
Rx	**Bacitracin Zinc and Polymyxin B Ointment** (Bausch & Lomb)	10,000		500		White petrolatum and mineral oil. In 3.5 g.
Rx	**AK-Poly-Bac Ointment** (Akorn)					Preservative free. White petrolatum, mineral oil. In 3.5 g.
Rx	**Polysporin Ophthalmic Ointment** (Monarch)					White petrolatum, mineral oil. In 3.5 g.
Rx	**Terramycin w/Polymyxin B Ointment** (Roerig)	10,000			5 mg/g oxytetra-cycline HCl	White and liquid petrolatum. In 3.5 g.
Rx	**Terak Ointment** (Akorn)					White and liquid petrolatum. In 3.5 g.
Rx	**Trimethoprim Sulfate and Polymyxin B Sulfate Ophthalmic Solution** (Bausch & Lomb)	10,000			1 mg/mL trimethoprim	In 10 mL.[2]
Rx	**Polytrim Ophthalmic Solution** (Allergan)	10,000			1 mg/mL trimethoprim	In 5 and 10 mL.[2]

[1] With 0.001% thimerosal, 0.5% alcohol, propylene glycol, polyoxyethylene polyoxypropylene.
[2] With 0.004% benzalkonium chloride, NaCl.

STEROID AND ANTIBIOTIC SOLUTIONS AND SUSPENSIONS

Indications:

Inflammatory conditions: For steroid-responsive inflammatory ocular conditions where a corticosteroid is indicated and bacterial infection or risk of infection exists.

For inflammatory conditions of the palpebral and bulbar conjunctiva, cornea, and anterior segment of the globe in which the inherent risk of steroid use in certain infective conjunctivitides is accepted to obtain a diminution in edema and inflammation. For chronic anterior uveitis and corneal injury from chemical, radiation or thermal burns, or penetration of foreign bodies.

Administration and Dosage:

Store suspensions upright and shake well before using.

Instill 1 or 2 drops into the affected eye(s) every 3 or 4 hours, or more frequently as required. Taper to discontinuation as inflammation subsides.

Do not prescribe > 20 mL initially; do not refill without further evaluation. For complete dosage instructions, see individual manufacturer inserts.

	Product and distributor	Steroid (per mL)	Antibiotic (per mL)	Other content	How supplied
Rx	**Neomycin/Polymyxin B Sulfate/Hydrocortisone** (Various, eg, Falcon, Bausch & Lomb)	1% hydrocortisone	Neomycin sulfate equivalent to 0.35% neomycin base and 10,000 units polymyxin B sulfate		In 7.5 and 10 mL.
Rx	**AK-Spore H.C. Ophthalmic Suspension** (Akorn)			0.001% thimerosal, cetyl alcohol, glyceryl monostearate, polyoxyl 40 stearate, propylene glycol, mineral oil, NaCl	In 7.5 mL.
Rx	**Cortisporin Suspension** (Monarch)				In 7.5 mL Drop Dose.
Rx	**Poly-Pred Suspension** (Allergan)	0.5% prednisolone acetate	Neomycin sulfate equivalent to 0.35% neomycin base, 10,000 units polymyxin B sulfate	1.4% polyvinyl alcohol, 0.001% thimerosal, polysorbate 80, propylene glycol	In 5 and 10 mL.

	Product and distributor	Steroid (per mL)	Antibiotic (per mL)	Other content	How supplied
Rx	**Pred-G Suspension** (Allergan)	1% prednisolone acetate	Gentamicin sulfate equivalent to 0.3% gentamicin base	1.4% polyvinyl alcohol, 0.005% benzalkonium chloride, EDTA, hydroxypropyl methylcellulose, polysorbate 80, NaCl	In 2, 5, and 10 mL.
Rx	**Neomycin Sulfate/ Dexamethasone Sodium Phosphate Solution** (Various, eg, Ivax, Zenith Goldline)	0.1% dexamethasone phosphate (as sodium phosphate)	Neomycin sulfate equivalent to 0.35% neomycin base		In 5 mL.
Rx	**NeoDecadron Solution** (Merck)			Polysorbate 80, EDTA, 0.2% benzalkonium Cl, 0.1% sodium bisulfite	In 5 mL Ocumeters.
Rx	**Neo-Dexameth** (Major)			0.01% benzalkonium Cl, EDTA, polysorbate 80, sodium bisulfite	In 5 mL.
Rx	**TobraDex Suspension** (Alcon)	0.1% dexamethasone	0.3% tobramycin	0.01% benzalkonium Cl, tyloxapol, EDTA, hydroxyethylcellulose, sodium sulfate, NaCl	In 2.5, 5, and 10 mL Drop-Tainers.
Rx	**Neomycin/Polymyxin B Sulfate/Dexamethasone Suspension** (Various, eg, Falcon)	0.1% dexamethasone	Neomycin sulfate equivalent to 0.35% neomycin base and 10,000 units polymyxin B sulfate		In 5 mL.
Rx	**AK-Trol Suspension** (Akorn)			0.004% benzalkonium chloride, polysorbate 20, 0.5% hydroxypropyl methylcellulose, NaCl	In 5 mL.
Rx	**Maxitrol Suspension** (Alcon)			0.5% hydroxypropyl methylcellulose, polysorbate 20, 0.004% benzalkonium chloride	In 5 mL Drop-Tainers.

[1] As a prepared solution.

STEROID AND ANTIBIOTIC OINTMENTS

Administration and Dosage:

Apply ointment to the affected eye(s) every 3 or 4 hours, depending on the severity of the condition.

Do not prescribe > 8 g initially, and do not refill the prescription until further evaluation. For complete dosage instructions, see individual manufacturer inserts.

	Product & Distributor	Steroid (per g)	Antibiotic (per g)	Other Content	How Supplied
Rx	**Bacitracin Zinc/Neomycin Sulfate/Polymyxin B Sulfate/ Hydrocortisone** (Various, eg, Fougera)	1% hydrocortisone	Neomycin sulfate equivalent to 0.35% neomycin base, 400 units bacitracin zinc, 10,000 units polymyxin B sulfate		In 3.5 g.
Rx	**AK-Spore H.C.** (Akorn)			White petrolatum, mineral oil	Preservative free. In 3.5 g.
Rx	**Cortisporin** (Monarch)			White petrolatum	In 3.5 g.
Rx	**Pred-G S.O.P.** (Allergan)	0.6% prednisolone acetate	Gentamicin sulfate equivalent to 0.3% gentamicin base	0.5% chlorobutanol, white petrolatum, mineral oil, petrolatum, lanolin alcohol	In 3.5 g.
Rx	**Neomycin/Polymyxin B Sulfate/Dexamethasone** (Various eg, Falcon, Bausch & Lomb)	0.1% dexamethasone	Neomycin sulfate equivalent to 0.35% neomycin base, 10,000 units polymyxin B sulfate		In 3.5 g.
Rx	**AK-Trol** (Akorn)			White petrolatum, lanolin oil, mineral oil, parabens	In 3.5 g.
Rx	**Dexacidin** (Novartis)			White petrolatum, mineral oil	In 3.5 g.

OPHTHALMIC DRUG FACTS

SULFONAMIDES

Actions:

Pharmacology: Sulfonamides are bacteriostatic against a wide range of susceptible gram-positive and gram-negative microorganisms. Through competition with para-aminobenzoic acid (PABA), they restrict synthesis of folic acid that bacteria require for growth.

Pharmacokinetics: Sulfonamides do not appear to be appreciably absorbed from mucous membranes.

Microbiology: Topically applied sulfonamides are considered active against susceptible strains of the following common bacterial eye pathogens: *Escherichia coli, Staphylococcus aureus, Streptococcus pneumoniae, Streptococcus* (viridans group), *Haemophilus influenzae, Klebsiella* sp, and *Enterobacter* sp.

Topically applied sulfonamides do not provide adequate coverage against *Neisseria* sp, *Serratia marcescens*, and *Pseudomonas aeruginosa*. A significant percentage of staphylococcal isolates are completely resistant to sulfa drugs.

Indications:

Ocular infections: For conjunctivitis, corneal ulcer, and other superficial ocular infections due to susceptible microorganisms.

Trachoma: As an adjunct to systemic sulfonamide therapy in the treatment of trachoma.

Contraindications:

Hypersensitivity to sulfonamides or any component of the product; infants < 2 months of age; in epithelial herpes simplex keratitis (dendritic keratitis), vaccinia, varicella, and many other viral diseases of the cornea and conjunctiva; mycobacterial infection or fungal diseases of the ocular structures; after uncomplicated removal of a corneal foreign body (steroid combinations).

Warnings:

Staphylococcus species: A significant percentage of isolates are resistant to sulfa drugs.

Hypersensitivity: Severe sensitivity reactions have been identified in individuals with no prior history of sulfonamide hypersensitivity (see Adverse Reactions).

Pregnancy: Category C. Safety for use during pregnancy has not been established. Use only when clearly needed and when potential benefits to the mother outweigh potential hazards to the fetus.

Lactation: Systemic sulfonamides are excreted in breast milk.

Children: Safety and efficacy not established. Contraindicated in infants < 2 months of age.

ANTI-INFECTIVE AGENTS

Precautions:

For topical ophthalmic use only: Not for injection.

Epithelial healing: Ophthalmic ointments may retard corneal wound healing.

Sensitization: Sensitization may occur when a sulfonamide is readministered, regardless of route. Cross-sensitivity between different sulfonamides may occur. If signs of sensitivity or other untoward reactions occur, discontinue use of the preparation.

PABA: PABA present in purulent exudates inactivates sulfonamides.

Dry eye: Use with caution in patients with severe dry eye.

Superinfection: Use of antibiotics (especially prolonged or repeated therapy) may result in bacterial or fungal overgrowth of nonsusceptible organisms. Such overgrowth may lead to a secondary infection. Take appropriate measures if this occurs.

Sulfite sensitivity: May cause allergic-type reactions (eg, hives, itching, wheezing, anaphylaxis) in certain susceptible persons. Although overall prevalence in the general population is probably low, it is more common in asthmatics or in atopic nonasthmatics. Specific products containing sulfites are identified in product listings.

Drug Interactions:

Silver preparations are incompatible with these solutions.

Adverse Reactions:

Headache; local irritation; itching; periorbital edema, burning, and transient stinging; bacterial and fungal corneal ulcers. As with all sulfonamide preparations, severe sensitivity reactions include rare occurrences of Stevens-Johnson syndrome, exfoliative dermatitis, toxic epidermal necrolysis, photosensitivity, fever, skin rash, GI disturbance, and bone marrow depression; fatalities have occurred.

Patient Information:

For topical use only.

To avoid contamination, do not touch tip of container to any surface.

Keep bottle tightly closed when not in use. Do not use if solution has darkened.

Notify physician if improvement is not seen after several days, if condition worsens, or if pain, increased redness, itching, or swelling of the eye occurs or persists for > 48 hours. Do not discontinue use without consulting physician.

Administration and Dosage:

Usual duration of treatment is 7 to 10 days.

130 OPHTHALMIC DRUG FACTS

Solutions:

Conjunctivitis or other superficial ocular infections – Instill 1 to 2 drops into the lower conjunctival sac(s) every 1 to 4 hours initially according to severity of infection. Dosages may be tapered by increasing the time interval between doses as the condition responds.

Trachoma – Instill 2 drops every 2 hours. Concomitant systemic sulfonamide therapy is indicated.

Ointments: Apply a small amount ($\approx$ 0.25 inch) into the lower conjunctival sac(s) 3 to 4 times daily and at bedtime. Dosages may be tapered by increasing the time interval between doses as the condition responds. Or apply 0.5 to 1 inch into the conjunctival sac(s) at night in conjunction with the use of drops during the day, or before an eye is patched.

Storage/Stability:

Solutions – Protect from light. On long standing, solutions will darken in color and should be discarded.

Ointments – Store away from heat.

SULFISOXAZOLE DIOLAMINE

Complete prescribing information is found in the Sulfonamides group monograph.

Rx	**Gantrisin** (Roche)	**Solution**: 4%	With 1:100,000 phenylmercuric nitrate. In 15 mL with dropper.

SULFACETAMIDE SODIUM

Complete prescribing information is found in the Sulfonamides group monograph.

Rx	**Sulster** (Akorn)	**Solution**: 1%	In 5 and 10 mL.
Rx	**Sulfacetamide Sodium** (Various, eg, Bausch & Lomb, Fougera, Geneva, Moore, Optopics, Rugby, Schein, Steris, URL, Zenith Goldline)	**Solution**: 10%	In 15 mL.
Rx	**AK-Sulf** (Akorn)		In 2, 5, and 15 mL.[1]
Rx	**Bleph-10** (Allergan)		In 2.5, 5, and 15 mL.[2]
Rx	**Ocusulf-10** (Optopics)		In 2, 5, and 15 mL.[3]
Rx	**Sodium Sulamyd** (Schering)		In 5 and 15 mL.[1]
Rx	**Sulf-10** (Novartis)		In 1 mL Dropperettes.[4]
Rx	**Sulfacetamide Sodium** (Various, eg, Schein, Steris)	**Solution**: 30%	In 15 mL.
Rx	**Sodium Sulamyd** (Schering)		In 15 mL.[5]

ANTI-INFECTIVE AGENTS

Rx	**Sulfacetamide Sodium** (Various, eg, Fougera, Moore, URL)	**Ointment:** 10%	In 3.5 g
Rx	**AK-Sulf** (Akorn)		In 3.5 g.[6]
Rx	**Bleph-10** (Allergan)		In 3.5 g.[7]
Rx	**IsoptoCetamide** (Alcon)		In 3.5 g.[8]
Rx	**Sodium Sulamyd** (Schering)		In 3.5 g.[9]

[1] With 3.1 mg sodium thiosulfate pentahydrate, 5 mg methylcellulose, 0.5 mg methylparaben, 0.1 mg propylparaben per mL.
[2] With 1.4% polyvinyl alcohol, 0.005% benzalkonium Cl, polysorbate 80, sodium thiosulfate, EDTA.
[3] With parabens, 1.4% polyvinyl alcohol, sodium thiosulfate.
[4] With sodium thiosulfate, 0.05 mg thimerosal, boric acid per mL.
[5] With 1.5 mg sodium thiosulfate pentahydrate, 0.5 mg methylparaben, 0.1 mg propylparaben per mL.
[6] With 0.5 mg methylparaben, 0.1 mg propylparaben, 0.25 mg benzalkonium Cl, petrolatum base per g.
[7] With 0.0008% phenylmercuric acetate, white petrolatum, mineral oil, petrolatum, lanolin alcohol.
[8] With 0.05% methylparaben, 0.01% propylparaben, white petrolatum, anhydrous liquid lanolin, mineral oil.
[9] With 0.5 mg methylparaben, 0.1 mg propylparaben, 0.25 mg benzalkonium Cl, petrolatum base per g.

SULFONAMIDE/DECONGESTANT COMBINATION

Complete prescribing information is found in the Sulfonamides group monograph.

In this combination, phenylephrine HCl, an alpha sympathetic receptor agonist, produces vasoconstriction.

Administration and Dosage:

Instill 1 or 2 drops into the lower conjunctival sac(s) every 2 or 3 hours during the day, less often at night.

Storage/Stability: Keep tightly closed. Protect from light.

Rx	**Vasosulf** (Ciba Vision)	**Solution:** 15% sodium sulfacetamide and 0.125% phenylephrine HCl	With sodium thiosulfate, poloxamer 188, parabens. In 5 and 15 mL.

STEROID AND SULFONAMIDE COMBINATIONS, SUSPENSIONS, AND SOLUTIONS

The information for steroid preparations and sulfonamide preparations must be considered when using these products. See individual monographs.

Indications:

Inflammation/Infection: For corticosteroid-responsive inflammatory ocular conditions where a corticosteroid is indicated and superficial bacterial ocular infection or a risk of infection exists.

Administration and Dosage:

Solutions/Suspensions: Instill 1 to 3 drops into the conjunctival sac(s) every 1 to 4 hours during the day and at bedtime until a favorable response is obtained.

132 OPHTHALMIC DRUG FACTS

Do not prescribe > 20 mL initially. Do not refill the prescription without further evaluation for steroid-induced glaucoma.

For complete dosage instructions, see individual manufacturer inserts.

Ointments: Apply a small amount ($\approx$ 0.25-inch ribbon) into the conjunctival sac(s) 3 or 4 times daily and once at bedtime (or once or twice at night) until a favorable response is obtained.

Do not prescribe > 8 g initially. Do not refill the prescription without further evaluation for steroid-induced glaucoma.

For complete dosage instructions, see individual manufacturer inserts.

Storage/Stability:

Solutions/Suspensions – Protect from light. Do not freeze. Shake suspensions well before using. Do not use if solution or suspension has darkened. Clumping may occur on long standing at high temperatures.

Ointments – Keep tightly closed. Store away from heat.

ANTI-INFECTIVE AGENTS

	Product and distributor	Steroid	Sulfonamide	Other content	How supplied
Rx	**FML-S Suspension** (Allergan)	0.1% fluorometholone	10% sodium sulfacetamide	EDTA, 1.4% polyvinyl alcohol, 0.006% benzalkonium chloride, polysorbate 80, povidone, sodium thiosulfate, NaCl	In 5 and 10 mL.
Rx	**Blephamide Suspension** (Allergan)	0.2% prednisolone acetate	10% sodium sulfacetamide	EDTA, 1.4% polyvinyl alcohol, polysorbate 80, sodium thiosulfate	In 5 and 10 mL.
Rx	**Isopto Cetapred Suspension** (Alcon)	0.25% prednisolone acetate	10% sodium sulfacetamide	0.5% hydroxypropyl methylcellulose 2910, EDTA, polysorbate 80, sodium thiosulfate, 0.025% benzalkonium chloride, 0.05% methylparaben, 0.01% propylparaben	In 5 and 15 mL Drop-Tainers.
Rx	**AK-Cide Suspension** (Akorn)	0.5% prednisolone acetate	10% sodium sulfacetamide	0.5% phenethyl alcohol, tyloxapol, sodium thiosulfate, 0.025% benzalkonium chloride and EDTA	In 5 mL dropper bottle.
Rx	**Metimyd Suspension** (Schering)			0.5% phenylethyl alcohol, 0.025% benzalkonium chloride, sodium thiosulfate, EDTA, tyloxapol	In 5 mL.
Rx	**Sulfacetamide Sodium and Prednisolone Sodium Phosphate** (Schein)	0.25% prednisolone sodium phosphate	10% sodium sulfacetamide	0.01% mg thimerosal, EDTA, boric acid	In 5 and 10 mL.
Rx	**Sulster Solution** (Akorn)			0.01% mg thimerosal, EDTA	In 5 and 10 mL.

STEROID AND SULFONAMIDE COMBINATIONS, OINTMENTS

	Product and distributor	Steroid	Sulfonamide	Other content	How supplied
Rx	**Blephamide S.O.P.** (Allergan)	0.2% prednisolone acetate	10% sodium sulfacetamide	0.0008% phenylmercuric acetate, mineral oil, white petrolatum, lanolin alcohol	In 3.5 g.
Rx	**Cetapred** (Alcon)	0.25% prednisolone acetate	10% sodium sulfacetamide	Mineral oil, white petrolatum, lanolin oil, 0.05% methylparaben, 0.01% propylparaben	In 3.5 g.
Rx	**AK-Cide** (Akorn)	0.5% prednisolone acetate	10% sodium sulfacetamide	0.05% methylparaben, 0.01% propylparaben, mineral oil, white petrolatum	In 3.5 g applicator tube.
Rx	**Metimyd** (Schering)			Mineral oil, white petrolatum, 0.05% methylparaben, 0.01% propylparaben	In 3.5 g.
Rx	**Vasocine** (Novartis)			Mineral oil, white petrolatum, 0.05% methylparaben, 0.01% propylpraben	In 3.5 g applicator tube.

ANTI-INFECTIVE AGENTS

ZINC SULFATE SOLUTION

Indications:

Astringent: A mild astringent for temporary relief of minor eye irritation.

Warnings:

Irritation/Eye pain: If irritation persists or increases, or if eye pain or a change in vision occurs, discontinue use and consult physician.

Administration and Dosage:

Instill 1 to 2 drops into eye(s) up to 4 times daily. If solution discolors or becomes cloudy, do not use.

otc	**20/20 Eye Drops** (S. S. S.)	**Solution**: 0.25%	In 15 mL.[1]
otc	**Clear Eyes ACR Eye Drops** (Ross)		In 15 and 30 mL.[2]
otc	**Vasoclear A Eye Drops** (Novartis)		In 15 mL.[3]
otc	**Visine AC** (Pfizer)		In 15 mL.[4]
otc	**Zincfrin** (Alcon)		In 15 mL.[5]

[1] With 0.4% glycerin, 0.012% naphazoline HCl, EDTA, KCl, and camphor.
[2] With 0.2% glycerin, 0.012% naphazoline HCl, benzalkonium chloride, boric acid, EDTA, NaCl, and sodium citrate.
[3] With 0.02% naphazoline HCl, 1% polyethylene glycol 40, 0.0025% PVA, NaCl, and EDTA.
[4] With 0.05% tetrahydrozoline HCl, EDTA, boric acid, NaCl and EDTA.
[5] With 0.12% phenylephrine HCl, 0.01% benzalkonium chloride, polysorbate 80, sodium cirate, and sodium hydroxide.

NATAMYCIN

Actions:

Pharmacology: Natamycin, a tetraene polyene antibiotic, is derived from *Streptomyces natalensis*. It possesses in vitro activity against a variety of yeast and filamentous fungi, including *Candida, Aspergillus, Cephalosporium, Fusarium,* and *Penicillium*. The mechanism of action appears to be through binding of the molecule to the fungal cell membrane. The polyenesterol complex alters membrane permeability, depleting essential cellular constituents. Although activity against fungi is dose-related, natamycin is predominantly fungicidal. It is not effective in vitro against gram-negative or gram-positive bacteria.

Pharmacokinetics: Topical administration appears to produce effective concentrations within the corneal stroma, but not in intraocular fluid. Absorption from the GI tract is very poor. Systemic absorption should not occur after topical administration.

Indications:

Fungal blepharitis, conjunctivitis, and keratitis: Caused by susceptible organisms. Natamycin is the initial drug of choice in *Fusarium solani* keratitis.

Contraindications:

Hypersensitivity to any component of the formulation.

Warnings:

Pregnancy: Catagory C. Safety for use during pregnancy has not been established. Use only when clearly needed and when potential benefits to the mother outweigh potential hazards to the fetus.

Lactation: It is not known if natamycin is excreted in breast milk. Use with caution in nursing women.

Children: Safety and efficacy have not been established

Precautions:

For topical use only: Not for injection. Conjunctival necrosis occurs if injected.

Fungal endophthalmitis: The effectiveness of topical natamycin as a single agent in fungal endophthalmitis has not been established.

Resistance: Failure of keratitis to improve following 7 to 10 days of administration suggests that the infection may be caused by a microorganism not susceptible to natamycin. Base continuation of therapy on clinical reevaluation and additional laboratory studies.

Toxicity: Adherence of the suspension to areas of epithelial ulceration or retention in the fornices occurs regularly. Should suspicion of drug toxicity occur, discontinue the drug.

Diagnosis/Monitoring: Determine initial and sustained therapy of fungal keratitis by the clinical diagnosis (laboratory diagnosis by smear and culture of corneal scrapings) and by response to the drug. Whenever possible, determine the in vitro activity of natamycin against the responsible fungus. Monitor tolerance to natamycin at least twice weekly.

Adverse Reactions:

One case of conjunctival chemosis and hyperemia, thought to be allergic in nature, was reported.

Patient Information:

Refer to the Dosage Forms and Routes of Administration chapter for more complete information.

ANTI-INFECTIVE AGENTS

Administration and Dosage:

Fungal keratitis: Instill 1 drop into the conjunctival sac(s) at 1- or 2-hour intervals. The frequency of application can usually be reduced to 1 drop 6 to 8 times daily after the first 3 to 4 days. Generally, continue therapy for 14 to 21 days, or until there is resolution of active fungal keratitis. In many cases, it may help to reduce the dosage gradually at 4- to 7-day intervals to ensure that the organism has been eliminated.

Fungal blepharitis and conjunctivitis: 4 to 6 daily applications may be sufficient.

Shake well before each use.

Storage/Stability: Store at room temperature 8° to 24°C (46° to 75°F) or refrigerate at 2° to 8°C (36° to 46°F). Do not freeze. Avoid exposure to light and excessive heat.

Rx **Natacyn** (Alcon)	**Suspension:** 5%	With 0.02% benzalkonium chloride. In 15 mL.

VIDARABINE (Adenine Arabinoside; Ara-A)

Actions:

Pharmacology: The antiviral mechanism of action has not been established. Vidarabine appears to interfere with the early steps of viral DNA synthesis. It is rapidly deaminated to arabinosylhypoxanthine (Ara-Hx), the principal metabolite. Ara-Hx also possesses in vitro antiviral activity less than that of vidarabine. In contrast to topical idoxuridine, vidarabine demonstrated less cellular toxicity in regenerating corneal epithelium of rabbits.

Pharmacokinetics:

> *Absorption* – Systemic absorption is not expected to occur following ocular administration and swallowing lacrimal secretions. In laboratory animals, vidarabine is rapidly deaminated in the GI tract to Ara-Hx.

> *Distribution* – Because of its low solubility, trace amounts of both vidarabine and Ara-Hx can be detected in the aqueous humor only if there is an epithelial defect in the cornea. If the cornea is normal, only trace amounts of Ara-Hx can be recovered from the aqueous humor.

Microbiology: Vidarabine possesses in vitro and in vivo antiviral activity against herpes simplex types 1 and 2, varicella-zoster and vaccinia viruses. Except for rhabdovirus and oncornavirus, it does not display antiviral activity against other RNA or DNA viruses, including adenovirus.

Indications:

Acute keratoconjunctivitis and recurrent epithelial keratitis: Due to herpes simplex virus types 1 and 2.

Superficial keratitis: Caused by herpes simplex virus that has not responded to topical trifluorothyamidine, or when toxic or hypersensitivity reactions to idoxuridine have occurred.

Contraindications:

Hypersensitivity to vidarabine; sterile trophic ulcers. Corticosteroids alone are normally contraindicated in herpes simplex virus eye infections.

Warnings:

Efficacy in other conditions: Vidarabine is not effective against RNA virus, adenoviral ocular infections, bacterial, fungal, or chlamydial infections of the cornea, or trophic ulcers. Effectiveness against stromal keratitis and uveitis due to herpes simplex virus has not been established.

Corticosteroids: Normally contraindicated in herpes simplex virus eye infections. If vidarabine is coadministered with topical corticosteroid therapy, consider corticosteroid-induced ocular side effects such as glaucoma or cataract formation and progression of bacterial or viral infection.

Temporary visual haze: May be produced with vidarabine.

Carcinogenesis: In female mice treated with IM vidarabine, there was an increase in liver tumor incidence; some male mice developed kidney neoplasia.

In rats, intestinal, testicular, and thyroid neoplasia occurred with greater frequency among the vidarabine-treated animals.

Mutagenesis: In vitro, vidarabine can be incorporated into mammalian DNA and can induce mutation. In vivo studies have not been conclusive; however, vidarabine may be capable of producing mutagenic effects in male germ cells.

Vidarabine has caused chromosome breaks and gaps when added to human leukocytes in vitro. While the significance is not fully understood, there is a well-known correlation between the ability of various agents to produce such effects and their ability to produce heritable genetic damage.

Pregnancy: Category C. A 10% ointment applied to 10% of the body surface during organogenesis induced fetal abnormalities in rabbits. The possibility of embryonic or fetal damage in pregnant women is remote. The topical ophthalmic dose is small, and the drug is relatively insoluble. Its ocular penetration is very low. However, a safe dose for a human embryo or fetus has not been established, and there are no adequate and well-controlled studies in pregnant women. Therefore, use only if the potential benefit to the mother outweighs the potential risk to the fetus.

Lactation: It is not known whether vidarabine is excreted in breast milk. Excretion of vidarabine in breast milk is unlikely because the drug is rapidly deaminated in the GI tract. However, it is still recommended that either nursing or the drug be discontinued, taking into account the importance of the drug to the mother.

Precautions:

Viral resistance: Vidarabine has not been observed, although this possibility exists.

Adverse Reactions:

Lacrimation; foreign body sensation; conjunctival infection; burning; irritation; superficial punctate keratitis; pain; photophobia; punctal occlusion; sensitivity.

ANTI-INFECTIVE AGENTS

Uveitis, stromal edema, secondary glaucoma, trophic defects, corneal vascularization and hyphema have occurred but may be disease-related.

Overdosage:

The rapid deamination to Ara-Hx should preclude any difficulty. No untoward effects should result from ingestion of the entire contents of a tube. Overdosage by ocular instillation is unlikely because any excess is quickly expelled from the conjunctival sac. Avoid too frequent administration.

Patient Information:

May cause sensitivity to bright light; this may be minimized by wearing sunglasses.

Notify physician if improvement is not seen after 7 days, if condition or pain worsens, or if a decrease in vision, burning, or irritation of the eye occurs. Do not discontinue use without consulting a physician.

Refer to the Dosage Forms and Routes of Administration chapter for more complete information.

Administration and Dosage:

Administer ≈ 0.5 inch of ointment into the lower conjunctival sac(s) 5 times daily at 3-hour intervals.

If there are no signs of improvement after 7 days, or if complete re-epithelialization has not occurred in 21 days, consider other forms of therapy. Some severe cases may require longer treatment.

After re-epithelialization has occurred, treat for an additional 7 days at a reduced dosage (such as twice daily) to prevent recurrence.

Concomitant therapy: Topical corticosteroids (prednisolone or dexamethasone) have been administered concurrently with vidarabine without an increase in adverse reactions, although their advantages and disadvantages must be considered (see Warnings).

Rx	**Vira-A** (Monarch)	**Ointment**: 3% vidarabine monohydrate (equivalent to 2.8% vidarabine)	In a liquid petrolatum base. In 3.5 g.

TRIFLURIDINE (Trifluorothymidine)

Actions:

Pharmacology: A fluorinated pyrimidine nucleoside with in vitro and in vivo activity against herpes simplex virus types 1 and 2, and vaccinia virus. Some strains of adenovirus are also inhibited in vitro. Trifluridine interferes with DNA synthesis in cultured mammalian cells. However, its antiviral mechanism of action is not completely known.

140   OPHTHALMIC DRUG FACTS

Pharmacokinetics:

Absorption – Intraocular penetration occurs after topical instillation. Decreased corneal integrity or stromal or uveal inflammation may enhance the penetration into the aqueous humor. Systemic absorption following therapeutic dosing appears negligible.

Indications:

Primary keratoconjunctivitis and recurrent epithelial keratitis: Due to herpes simplex virus types 1 and 2 in patients ≥ 6 years of age.

Epithelial keratitis: Epithelial keratitis that has not responded clinically to topical idox-uridine, or when ocular toxicity or hypersensitivity to idoxuridine has occurred. In a smaller number of patients resistant to topical vidarabine, trifluridine was also effective.

Contraindications:

Hypersensitivity reactions or chemical intolerance to trifluridine.

Warnings:

Efficacy in other conditions: The clinical efficacy in the treatment of stromal keratitis and uveitis due to herpes simplex or ophthalmic infections caused by vaccinia virus and adenovirus, or in the prophylaxis of herpes simplex virus keratoconjunctivitis and epithelial keratitis has not been established by well-controlled clinical trials. Not effective against bacterial, fungal, or chlamydial infections of the cornea or trophic lesions.

Dosage/Frequency: Do not exceed the recommended dosage or frequency of administration.

Mutagenesis: Trifluridine has exerted mutagenic, DNA-damaging, and cell-transforming activities in various standard in vitro test systems. Although the significance of these test results is not clear or fully understood, it is possible that mutagenic agents may cause genetic damage in humans.

Pregnancy: Category C. Fetal toxicity consisting of delayed ossification of portions of the skeleton occurred at dose levels of 2.5 and 5 mg/kg/day in rats and rabbits. In addition, both 2.5 and 5 mg/kg/day produced fetal death and resorption in rabbits. There are no adequate and well-controlled studies in pregnant women. Use during pregnancy only if the potential benefit to the mother justifies the risk to the fetus.

Lactation: It is unlikely that trifluridine is excreted in breast milk after ophthalmic instillation because of the relatively small dosage (≤ 5 mg/day), its dilution in body fluids, and its extremely short half-life (≈ 12 minutes). However, do not prescribe for nursing mothers unless the potential benefits outweigh the potential risks.

Children: Safety and effectiveness in pediatric patients < 6 years of age have not been established.

ANTI-INFECTIVE AGENTS

141

Precautions:

Viral resistance: Although documented in vitro, viral resistance has not been reported following multiple exposure to trifluridine; this possibility may exist.

Adverse Reactions:

The most frequent adverse reactions reported are mild, transient burning or stinging upon instillation (4.6%), and palpebral edema (2.8%). Other adverse reactions in decreasing order of reported frequency were: superficial punctate keratopathy; epithelial keratopathy; hypersensitivity reaction; stromal edema; irritation; keratitis sicca; hyperemia and increased intraocular pressure.

Overdosage:

Local: Overdosage by ocular instillation is unlikely because any excess solution is quickly expelled from the conjunctival sac.

Systemic: No untoward effects are likely to result from ingestion of the entire contents of a bottle. Single IV doses of 1.5 to 30 mg/kg/day in children and adults with neoplastic disease produce reversible bone marrow depression as the only potentially serious toxic effect and only after 3 to 5 courses of therapy.

Patient Information:

Transient stinging may occur upon instillation.

Notify physician if improvement is not seen after 7 days, if condition worsens, or if irritation occurs. Do not discontinue use without consulting physician.

Refer to the Dosage Forms and Routes of Administration chapter for more complete information.

Administration and Dosage:

Instill 1 drop onto the cornea of the affected eye(s) every 2 hours while awake, for a maximum daily dosage of 9 drops until the corneal ulcer has completely re-epithelialized. Following re-epithelialization, treat for an additional 7 days with 1 drop every 4 hours while awake, for a minimum daily dosage of 5 drops.

If there are no signs of improvement after 7 days, or if complete re-epithelialization has not occurred after 14 days, consider other forms of therapy. Avoid continuous administration for periods > 21 days because of potential ocular toxicity.

Storage/Stability: Store under refrigeration, 2° to 8°C (36° to 46°F).

Rx	**Viroptic** (Monarch)	**Solution:** 1%	In aqueous solution with NaCl and 0.001% thimerosal. In 7.5 mL Drop-Dose.

GANCICLOVIR (DHPG) CAPSULES AND POWDER FOR INJECTION

Warning:

The clinical toxicity of ganciclovir includes granulocytopenia, anemia, and thrombocytopenia. In animal studies, ganciclovir was carcinogenic, teratogenic, and caused aspermatogenesis.

Ganciclovir IV is indicated for use only in the treatment of cytomegalovirus (CMV) retinitis in immunocompromised patients and for the prevention of CMV disease in transplant patients at risk for CMV disease.

Because oral ganciclovir is associated with a risk of more rapid rate of CMV retinitis progression, use only in those patients for whom this risk is balanced by the benefit associated with avoiding daily IV infusions.

Actions:

Pharmacology: Ganciclovir, a synthetic guanine derivative active against CMV, is an acyclic nucleoside analog of 2'-deoxyguanosine that inhibits replication of herpes viruses in vitro and in vivo. Sensitive human viruses include CMV, herpes simplex virus-1 and -2, herpes virus type 6, Epstein-Barr virus, varicella-zoster virus, and hepatitis B virus.

Ganciclovir must be converted to the corresponding triphosphate in order to exert its antiviral activity. In herpes simplex virus-infected cells, the initial conversion to the monophosphate is catalyzed by a viral thymidine kinase. In contrast, in CMV-infected cells, a protein kinase homologue may be responsible for the initial phosphorylation of ganciclovir. Cellular kinases, in CMV-infected cells, subsequently phosphorylate ganciclovir monophosphate to the diphosphate and active triphosphate moieties. Levels of ganciclovir triphosphate are as much as 100-fold greater in CMV-infected cells than in uninfected cells, indicating a preferential phosphorylation of ganciclovir in virus-infected cells. Ganciclovir triphosphate, once formed, appears quite stable and persists for days in the CMV-infected cell. The antiviral activity of ganciclovir triphosphate is believed to be the result of inhibition of viral DNA synthesis by two known modes: (1) Competitive inhibition of viral DNA polymerases; and (2) direct incorporation into viral DNA, resulting in eventual termination of viral DNA elongation. The cellular DNA polymerase alpha is also inhibited, but at a higher concentration than required for inhibition of viral DNA polymerase.

The median concentration of ganciclovir that effectively inhibits the replication of either laboratory strains or clinical isolates of CMV (ED_{50}) has ranged from 0.02 to 3.48 mcg/mL. The relationship of in vitro sensitivity of CMV to ganciclovir and clinical response has not been established. Ganciclovir inhibits mammalian cell proliferation in vitro at higher concentrations: IC_{50} values range from 30 to 725 mcg/mL, with the exception of bone marrow-derived colony-forming cells that are more sensitive with IC_{50} values ranging from 0.028 to 0.7 mcg/mL.

Pharmacokinetics:

Absorption – The absolute bioavailability of oral ganciclovir under fasting conditions was ≈ 5% and following food it was 6% to 9%. When given with a meal containing 602 calories and 46.5% fat, the steady-state area under serum concentration vs time curve (AUC) increased and there was a significant prolongation of time to peak serum concentrations (see Drug Interactions).

ANTI-INFECTIVE AGENTS

143

At the end of a 1-hour IV infusion of 5 mg/kg, total AUC ranged between 22.1 and 26.8 mcg•hr/mL and C_{max} ranged between 8.27 and 9 mcg/mL.

Distribution – The steady-state volume of distribution after IV administration was 0.74 L/kg. Cerebrospinal fluid concentrations obtained 0.25 and 5.67 hours postdose in 3 patients who received 2.5 mg/kg ganciclovir IV every 8 or 12 hours ranged from 0.31 to 0.68 mcg/mL, representing 24% to 70% of the respective plasma concentrations. Binding to plasma proteins was 1% to 2% over ganciclovir concentrations of 0.5 and 51 mcg/mL.

Metabolism – Following oral administration of a single 1000 mg dose, 86% of the administered dose was recovered in the feces and 5% was recovered in the urine. No metabolite accounted for 1% to 2% recovered in urine or feces.

Excretion – When administered IV, ganciclovir exhibits linear pharmacokinetics over the range of 1.6 to 5 mg/kg and when administered orally, it exhibits linear kinetics up to a total daily dose of 4 g/day. Renal excretion of unchanged drug by glomerular filtration and active tubular secretion is the major route of elimination. In patients with normal renal function, 91.3% of IV ganciclovir was recovered unmetabolized in the urine. Systemic clearance of IV ganciclovir was 3.52 mL/min/kg while renal clearance was 3.2 mL/min/kg, accounting for 91% of the systemic clearance. After oral administration, steady state is achieved within 24 hours. Renal clearance following oral administration was 3.1 mL/min/kg. Half-life was 3.5 hours following IV administration and 4.8 following oral use.

Renal function impairment – Because the major elimination pathway for ganciclovir is renal, dosage must be reduced according to creatinine clearance (Ccr; see Administration and Dosage). The pharmacokinetics following IV administration were evaluated in 10 immunocompromised patients with renal impairment who received doses ranging from 1.25 to 5 mg/kg.

IV Ganciclovir Pharmacokinetics in Patients with Renal Impairment			
Ccr (mL/min)	Dose (mg/kg)	Clearance (mL/min)	Half-life (hours)
50-79 (n = 4)	3.2-5	128	4.6
25-49 (n = 3)	3-5	57	4.4
< 25 (n = 3)	1.25-5	30	10.7

The pharmacokinetics following oral administration were evaluated in 8 solid organ transplant recipients; dose was modified according to estimated Ccr.

Oral Ganciclovir in Patients with Renal Impairment			
Ccr (mL/min)	Dose (mg/kg)	AUC_{0-24} (mcg•hr/mL)	Half-life (hours)
50-69 (n = 4)	1000 mg q 8 hr	49.1 ± 2.2	NC[1]
25-49 (n = 1)	1000 mg every day	27.4	18.2
10-24 (n = 1)	500 mg every day	10.7	15.7
< 10 (n = 2)	500 mg 3 times weekly[2]	25.6 ± 5.9	NC[1]

[1] NC = Not calculated; half-life exceeded sampling interval.
[2] After hemodialysis.

Hemodialysis reduces plasma concentrations of ganciclovir ≈ 50% after IV and oral administration.

Race – The effects of race were studied in subjects receiving a dose regimen of 1000 mg every 8 hours. Although the numbers of blacks (16%) and Hispanics

(20%) were small, there appeared to be a trend toward a lower steady-state C_{max} and AUC_{0-8} in these subpopulations as compared with whites.

Children – At an IV dose of 4 or 6 mg/kg in 27 newborns (2 to 49 days of age), the pharmacokinetic parameters were, respectively, C_{max} of 5.5 and 7 mcg/mL, systemic clearance of 3.14 and 3.56 mL/min/kg, and half-life of 2.4 hours for both.

Clinical Trials:

IV – Immunocompromised patients – Of 314 immunocompromised patients enrolled in an open label study of the treatment of life- or sight-threatening CMV disease, 121 patients had a positive culture for CMV within 7 days prior to treatment.

		Virologic Response to IV Ganciclovir Treatment	
Culture source	No. patients cultured	No. (%) patients responding	Median days to response
Urine	107	93 (87%)	8
Blood	41	34 (83%)	8
Throat	21	19 (90%)	7
Semen	6	6 (100%)	15

Transplant recipients – In 149 CMV seropositive heart allograft recipients and 72 CMV culture positive allogeneic bone marrow transplant recipients, ganciclovir prevented recrudescence of CMV shedding in the heart allograft patients and suppressed CMV shedding in the bone marrow allograft patients.

	Patients with Positive CMV Cultures Following IV Ganciclovir			
	Heart allograft		Bone marrow allograft	
Time	Ganciclovir	Placebo	Ganciclovir	Placebo
Pretreatment	2%	8%	100%	100%
Week 2	3%	16%	6%	68%
Week 4	5%	43%	0%	80%

Oral – The antiviral activity of ganciclovir capsules was confirmed in 2 randomized, controlled trials comparing IV vs oral ganciclovir for the maintenance treatment of CMV retinitis in patients with acquired immunodeficiency syndrome (AIDS). Only a small proportion of patients remained culture-positive during maintenance therapy with either IV or oral ganciclovir. There were no statistically significant differences in the rates of positive cultures between the treatment groups. The antiviral effect of oral ganciclovir in the patients in the 2 studies is summarized in the following table:

	Patients with Positive CMV Following Oral Ganciclovir			
	Patients with newly diagnosed CMV retinitis[1]		Patients with stable, previously treated CMV retinitis[2]	
	IV	Oral	IV	Oral[3]
At start of maintenance	13.5%	24.3%	3%	3.6%
Anytime during maintenance	6.3%	9.1%	2.2%	7.1%

[1] 3 weeks of treatment with IV ganciclovir before start of maintenance.
[2] 4 weeks to 4 months treatment with IV ganciclovir before start of maintenance.
[3] Data from 6 times daily and 3 times daily regimens pooled.

Viral resistance – CMV resistance to ganciclovir in individuals with AIDS and CMV retinitis who have not previously been treated with ganciclovir does occur but appears to be infrequent. Viral resistance has been observed in patients receiving prolonged treatment with ganciclovir IV. However, because of the limited

ANTI-INFECTIVE AGENTS

number of viral isolates tested, it is difficult to estimate the overall frequency of reduced sensitivity in patients receiving ganciclovir. Nonetheless, consider the possibility of viral resistance in patients who show poor clinical response or experience persistent viral excretion during therapy. The principal mechanism of resistance to ganciclovir in CMV is the decreased ability to form the active triphosphate moiety. Mutations in the viral DNA polymerase also have been reported to confer viral resistance to ganciclovir. In 2 randomized controlled trials, the incidence of reduced sensitivity appeared to be no more common during treatment with oral ganciclovir than during IV treatment.

Indications:

IV:

> *CMV retinitis* – Treatment of CMV retinitis in immunocompromised patients, including patients with AIDS.

> *CMV disease* – Prevention of CMV disease in transplant recipients at risk for CMV disease.

Oral: Alternative to the IV formulation for maintenance treatment of CMV retinitis in immunocompromised patients, including patients with AIDS, in whom retinitis is stable following appropriate induction therapy and for whom the risk of more rapid progression is balanced by the benefit associated with avoiding daily IV infusions.

Off-labeled use(s): Ganciclovir also may be beneficial in some immunocompromised patients in the treatment of other CMV infections (eg, pneumonitis, gastroenteritis, hepatitis [see Warnings]).

Contraindications:

Hypersensitivity to ganciclovir or acyclovir.

Warnings:

CMV disease: Safety and efficacy have not been established for congenital or neonatal CMV disease nor for the treatment of established CMV disease other than retinitis nor for use in nonimmunocompromised individuals. The safety and efficacy of oral ganciclovir have not been established for treating any manifestation of CMV disease other than maintenance treatment of CMV retinitis.

Diagnosis of CMV retinitis: Diagnosis is ophthalmologic and should be made by indirect ophthalmoscopy. Other conditions in the differential diagnosis of CMV retinitis include candidiasis, toxoplasmosis, histoplasmosis, retinal scars, and cotton wool spots, any of which may produce a retinal appearance similar to CMV. The diagnosis may be supported by culture of CMV from urine, blood, throat, etc., but a negative CMV culture does not rule out CMV retinitis.

Retinal detachment: Retinal detatchment has been observed in subjects with CMV retinitis both before and after initiation of therapy with ganciclovir. Its relationship to therapy is unknown. Retinal detachment occurred in 11% of patients treated with IV ganciclovir and in 8% of patients treated with oral ganciclovir. Patients with CMV retinitis should have frequent ophthalmologic evaluations to monitor the status of their retinitis and to detect any other retinal pathology.

146   OPHTHALMIC DRUG FACTS

Hematologic: Do not administer if the absolute neutrophil count is < 500/mm³ or the platelet count is < 25,000/mm³. Granulocytopenia (neutropenia), anemia, and thrombocytopenia have been observed in patients treated with ganciclovir. The frequency and severity of these events vary widely in different patient populations (see Adverse Reactions). Therefore, use with caution in patients with pre-existing cytopenias or with a history of cytopenic reactions to other drugs, chemicals, or irradiation. Granulocytopenia usually occurs during the first or second week of treatment, but may occur at any time during treatment. Cell counts usually begin to recover within 3 to 7 days of discontinuing drug. Colony-stimulating factors have increased neutrophil and WBC counts in patients receiving IV ganciclovir for CMV retinitis.

Renal function impairment: Use ganciclovir with caution because the half-life and plasma/serum concentrations of ganciclovir will be increased because of reduced renal clearance (see Administration and Dosage).

Hemodialysis reduces plasma levels of ganciclovir by ≈ 50%.

Carcinogenesis: In mice, daily oral doses of 1000 mg/kg may have caused an increased incidence of tumors in the preputial gland of males, nonglandular mucosa of the stomach of males and females, and reproductive tissues (eg, ovaries, uterus, mammary gland, clitoral gland, vagina) and liver in females. A slightly increased incidence of tumors occurred in the preputial gland (males) and nonglandular mucosa (males and females) of the stomach in mice given 20 mg/kg/day. Consider ganciclovir a potential carcinogen in humans.

Mutagenesis: Ganciclovir caused point mutations and chromosomal damage in mammalian cells in vitro and in vivo. Because of the mutagenic and teratogenic potential of ganciclovir, advise women of childbearing potential to use effective contraception during treatment. Similarly, advise men to practice barrier contraception during and for ≥ 90 days following treatment with ganciclovir.

Fertility impairment: Animal data indicate that ganciclovir causes inhibition of spermatogenesis and subsequent infertility. Ganciclovir caused decreased fertility in male mice and hypospermatogenesis in mice and dogs. These effects were reversible at lower doses and irreversible at higher doses. Although data in humans have not been obtained regarding this effect, ganciclovir, at the recommended doses, may cause temporary or permanent inhibition of spermatogenesis. Animal data also indicate that suppression of fertility in females may occur. Ganciclovir caused decreased mating behavior, decreased fertility, and an increased incidence of embryolethality in female mice following IV doses ≈ 1.7 times the mean drug exposure in humans.

Elderly: The pharmacokinetic profile in elderly patients has not been established. Since elderly individuals frequently have a reduced glomerular filtration rate, pay particular attention to assessing renal function before and during administration of ganciclovir (see Administration and Dosage).

Pregnancy: Category C. Ganciclovir is embryotoxic in rabbits and mice following IV administration and teratogenic in rabbits. Fetal resorptions were present in ≥ 85% of rabbits and mice administered 2 times the human exposure. Effects observed in rabbits included the following: Fetal growth retardation, embryolethality, teratogenicity and maternal toxicity. Teratogenic changes included cleft palate, anophthalmia/microphthalmia, aplastic organs (kidney and pancreas), hydrocephaly, and brachygnathia. In mice, effects observed were maternal/fetal toxicity and embryolethality.

Daily IV doses given to female mice prior to mating, during gestation, and during lactation caused hypoplasia of the testes and seminal vesicles in the month-old male offspring, as well as pathologic changes in the nonglandular region of the stomach.

ANTI-INFECTIVE AGENTS

Ganciclovir may be teratogenic or embryotoxic at dose levels recommended for human use. There are no adequate and well-controlled studies in pregnant women. Use during pregnancy only if the potential benefits to the mother justify the potential risk to the fetus.

Lactation: It is not known whether ganciclovir is excreted in breast milk. However, because carcinogenic and teratogenic effects occurred in animals treated with ganciclovir, the possibility of serious adverse reactions from ganciclovir in nursing infants is considered likely. Instruct mothers to discontinue nursing if they are receiving ganciclovir. The minimum interval before nursing can safely be resumed after the last dose of ganciclovir is unknown.

Children: Safety and efficacy in children have not been established. The use of ganciclovir in children warrants extreme caution to the probability of long-term carcinogenicity and reproductive toxicity. Administer to children only after careful evaluation and only if the potential benefits of treatment outweigh the risks. Oral ganciclovir has not been studied in children < 13 years of age.

There has been very limited clinical experience using IV ganciclovir for the treatment of CMV retinitis in patients < 12 years of age. Two children (9 and 5 years of age) showed improvement or stabilization of retinitis for 23 and 9 months, respectively. These children received induction treatment with 2.5 mg/kg 3 times daily followed by maintenance therapy with 6 to 6.5 mg/kg once a day, 5 to 7 days per week. When retinitis progressed during once-daily maintenance therapy, both children were treated with the 5 mg/kg twice-daily regimen. Two other children (2.5 and 4 years of age) who received similar induction regimens showed only partial or no response to treatment. Another child, a 6-year-old with T-cell dysfunction, showed stabilization of retinitis for 3 months while receiving continuous infusions of IV ganciclovir at doses of 2 to 5 mg/kg/24 hours. Continuous infusion treatment was discontinued because of granulocytopenia.

Eleven of the 72 patients in the placebo-controlled trial in bone marrow transplant recipients were children, ranging from 3 to 10 years of age (5 treated with IV ganciclovir and 6 with placebo). Five of the pediatric patients treated with ganciclovir received 5 mg/kg IV twice daily for up to 7 days; 4 patients went on to receive 5 mg/kg once daily up to day 100 post-transplant. Results were similar to those observed in adult transplant recipients treated with IV ganciclovir. Two of the 6 placebo-treated pediatric patients developed CMV pneumonia vs none of the 5 treated with ganciclovir. The spectrum of adverse events in the pediatric group was similar to that observed in the adult patients.

The spectrum of adverse reactions reported in 120 immunocompromised pediatric clinical trial participants with serious CMV infections receiving IV ganciclovir were similar to those reported in adults. Granulocytopenia (17%) and thrombocytopenia (10%) were the most common adverse events reported.

Precautions:

Monitoring: Due to the frequency of neutropenia, anemia, and thrombocytopenia in patients receiving ganciclovir, it is recommended that complete blood counts and platelet counts be performed frequently, especially in patients in whom ganciclovir or other nucleoside analogs have previously resulted in leukopenia, or in whom neutrophil counts are < 1000/mm^3 at the beginning of treatment. Because dosing with ganciclovir must be modified in patients with renal impairment, and because of the incidence of increased serum creatinine levels that have been observed in transplant recipients treated with IV ganciclovir, patients should have serum creatinine or creatinine clearance values followed carefully.

148 OPHTHALMIC DRUG FACTS

Large doses/Rapid infusion: The maximum single dose administered was 6 mg/kg by IV infusion > 1 hour. Larger doses have resulted in increased toxicity. It is likely that more rapid infusions would also result in increased toxicity (see Overdosage).

Phlebitis/Pain at injection site: Initially, reconstituted solutions of IV ganciclovir have a high pH (pH 11). Despite further dilution in IV fluids, phlebitis or pain may occur at the site of IV infusion. Take care to infuse solutions containing ganciclovir only into veins with adequate blood flow to permit rapid dilution and distribution.

Hydration: Since ganciclovir is excreted by the kidneys and normal clearance depends on adequate renal function, ganciclovir administration should be accompanied by adequate hydration.

Photosensitivity: Photosensitization (photoallergy or phototoxicity) may occur; therefore, caution patients to take protective measures against exposure to ultraviolet or sunlight (ie, sunscreens, protective clothing) until tolerance is determined.

Drug Interactions:

Ganciclovir Drug Interactions			
Precipitant drug	Object drug*		Description
Ganciclovir	Cytotoxic drugs	↑	Cytotoxic drugs that inhibit replication of rapidly dividing cell populations such as bone marrow, spermatogonia, and germinal layers of skin and GI mucosa may have additive toxicity when administered concomitantly with ganciclovir. Therefore, consider the concomitant use of drugs such as dapsone, pentamidine, flucytosine, vincristine, vinblastine, adriamycin, amphotericin B, trimethoprim/sulfamethoxazole combinations, or other nucleoside analogs only if potential benefits outweigh the risks.
Imipenem-cilastatin	Ganciclovir	↑	Generalized seizures occurred in patients who received ganciclovir and imipenem-cilastatin. Do not use these drugs concomitantly unless the potential benefits outweigh the risks.
Nephrotoxic drugs	Ganciclovir	↑	Increases in serum creatinine were observed following concurrent use of ganciclovir and either cyclosporine or amphotericin B (see Warnings).
Probenecid	Ganciclovir	↑	Ganciclovir AUC increased 53% (range, -14% to 299%) in the presence of probenecid. Renal clearance of ganciclovir decreased 22% (range, -54% to -4%), which is consistent with an interaction involving competition for renal tubular secretion.
Ganciclovir	Didanosine	↑	Steady-state didanosine AUC increased 111% (range, 10% to 493%) when didanosine was administered either 2 hours prior to or simultaneously with ganciclovir. A decrease in steady-state ganciclovir AUC of 21% (range, -44% to 5%) was observed when didanosine
Didanosine	Ganciclovir	↓	was administered 2 hours prior to administration of ganciclovir, but ganciclovir AUC was not affected by the presence of didanosine when the 2 drugs were administered simultaneously.
Ganciclovir	Zidovudine	↑	Mean steady-state ganciclovir AUC decreased 17% (range, -52% to 23%) in the presence of zidovudine. Steady-state zidovudine AUC increased 19% (range, -11% to 74%) in the presence of ganciclovir. Because
Zidovudine	Ganciclovir	↓	both drugs can cause granulocytopenia and anemia, many patients will not tolerate combination therapy at full dosage.

* ↑ = Object drug increased. ↓ = Object drug decreased.

Drug/Food interactions: When ganciclovir was administered orally with food at a total daily dose of 3 g/day (either 500 mg every 3 hours 6 times daily or 1000 mg 3 times daily), the steady-state absorption as measured by AUC and C_{max} were similar fol-

ANTI-INFECTIVE AGENTS

149

lowing both regimens. When ganciclovir capsules were given with a meal containing 602 calories and 46.5% fat at a dose of 1000 mg every 8 hours to 20 HIV-positive subjects, the steady-state AUC increased 22% (range, 6% to 68%) and there was a significant prolongation of time to peak serum concentrations (T_{max}) from 1.8 to 3 hours and a higher C_{max} (0.85 vs 0.96 mcg/mL).

Adverse Reactions:

AIDS patients:

Selected Adverse Reactions Reported in 5% of Subjects: Oral vs IV Ganciclovir Maintenance Treatment		
Adverse reaction	Oral (3000 mg/day) (n = 326)	IV (5 mg/kg/day) (n = 179)
CNS		
Neuropathy	8%	9%
Paresthesia	6%	10%
GI		
Diarrhea	41%	44%
Nausea	26%	25%
Anorexia	15%	14%
Vomiting	13%	13%
Flatulence	6%	3%
Hemic/Lymphatic		
Leukopenia	29%	41%
Anemia	19%	25%
Thrombocytopenia	6%	6%
Miscellaneous		
Fever	38%	48%
Abdominal pain	17%	19%
Rash	15%	10%
Sweating	11%	12%
Infection	9%	13%
Chills	7%	10%
Pneumonia	6%	8%
Pruritus	6%	5%
Vitreous disorder	6%	4%
Sepsis	4%	15%
Catheter-related		
Total catheter events	6%	22%
Catheter infection	4%	9%
Catheter sepsis	1%	8%
Neutropenia (ANC/mm³)	(n = 320)	(n = 175)
< 500	18	25
500 to < 750	17	14
750 to < 1000	19	26
Total ANC ≤ 1000	54	66
Anemia hemoglobin (g/dL)	(n = 320)	(n = 175)
< 6.5	2	5
6.5 to < 8	10	16
8 to < 9.5	25	26
Total Hb < 9.5	36	46

Overall, subjects treated with IV ganciclovir experienced lower minimum acid-neutralizing capacities (ANCs) and hemoglobin levels, more consistent with neutropenia and anemia, compared with those who received oral ganciclovir.

For the majority of subjects, maximum serum creatinine levels were < 1.5 mg/dL and no difference was noted between IV and oral ganciclovir for the occurrence of renal impairment. Serum creatinine elevations > 2.5 mg/dL occurred in < 2% of all subjects

OPHTHALMIC DRUG FACTS

and no significant differences were noted in the time from the start of maintenance to the occurrence of elevations in serum creatinine values.

Transplant recipients –

Granulocytopenia/Thrombocytopenia with IV Ganciclovir				
	Heart allograft[1]		Bone marrow allograft[2]	
Hematologic effect	Ganciclovir (n = 76)	Placebo (n = 73)	Ganciclovir IV (n = 57)	Control (n = 55)
Neutropenia				
Minimum ANC < 500/mm^3	4%	3%	12%	6%
Minimum ANC 500 - 1000/mm^3	3%	8%	29%	17%
Total ANC ≤ 1000/mm^3	7%	11%	41%	23%
Thrombocytopenia				
Platelet count < 25,000/mm^3	3%	1%	32%	28%
Platelet count 25,000 - 50,000/mm^3	5%	3%	25%	37%
Total Platelet 50,000/mm^3	8%	4%	57%	65%

[1] Mean duration of treatment = 28 days.
[2] Mean duration of treatment = 45 days.

Elevated Serum Creatinine with IV Ganciclovir						
	Heart allograft		Bone marrow allograft			
Maximum serum creatinine levels	Ganciclovir IV (n = 76)	Placebo (n = 73)	Ganciclovir IV (n = 20)	Control (n = 20)	Ganciclovir IV (n = 37)	Placebo (n = 35)
Serum creatinine ≥ 2.5 mg/dL	18%	4%	20%	0%	0%	0%
Serum creatinine ≥ 1.5 - < 2.5 mg/dL	58%	69%	50%	35%	43%	44%

Cardiovascular: Arrhythmia, deep thrombophlebitis, hypertension, hypotension, vasodilatation (≤ 1%).

CNS: Abnormal dreams, abnormal gait, abnormal thinking, agitation, amnesia, anxiety, ataxia, coma, confusion, depression, dizziness, dry mouth, euphoria, hypertonia, hypesthesia, insomnia, libido decreased, manic reaction, nervousness, psychosis, seizures, somnolence, tremor, trismus (≈ 5%).

Dermatologic: Acne, alopecia, dry skin, fixed eruption, herpes simplex, maculopapular rash, skin discoloration, urticaria, vesiculobullous rash (≤ 1%).

GI: Abnormal liver function test, dyspepsia, nausea, vomiting (2%); constipation, dysphagia, eructation, fecal incontinence, hemorrhage, hepatitis, melena, mouth ulceration, tongue disorder (≤ 1%).

GU: Breast pain, creatinine clearance decreased/increased, hematuria, increased BUN, kidney failure, kidney function abnormal, urinary frequency, urinary tract infection.

Hematologic: Eosinophilia, hypochromic anemia, marrow depression, pancytopenia (≤ 1%).

Metabolic/Nutritional: Increased alkaline phosphatase, creatine phosphokinase, lactic dehydrogenase, AST, ALT (≤ 1%); hypokalemia, pancreatitis, decreased blood sugar (≤ 1%).

Musculoskeletal: Myalgia, myasthenia (≤ 1%).

Respiratory: Cough increased, dyspnea (≤ 1%).

ANTI-INFECTIVE AGENTS

Special senses: Abnormal vision, amblyopia, blindness, conjunctivitis, deafness, eye pain, glaucoma, retinitis, photophobia, taste perversion, tinnitus (≤ 1%).

Miscellaneous: Asthenia (6%); headache (4%); injection site inflammation, pain, phlebitis (2%); enlarged abdomen, abscess, back pain, cellulitis, chest pain, chills, fever, drug level increased (ganciclovir), edema, face edema, injection site abscess/edema/hemorrhage/pain, lab test abnormality, malaise, migraine, photosensitivity reaction, neck pain/rigidity (≤ 1%).

The following adverse reactions may be fatal: pancreatitis, sepsis, and multiple organ failure.

Adverse reactions reported in postmarket surveillance –

Reported on ≥ 2 occasions: Acidosis, anaphylactic reaction, cardiac arrest, cataracts, cholestasis, cholangitis, congenital anomaly, encephalopathy, hyponatremia, impotence, infertility, intracranial hypertension, leukemia, lymphoma, myocardial infarction, pericarditis, Stevens-Johnson syndrome, stroke, transverse myelitis, unexplained death.

Reported once: Allograft rejection, arthritis, asthma, bleeding disorder, cachexia, corneal erosion, cyanosis, diplopia, dry eyes, dysethesia, ear infection, elevated triglyceride levels, endocarditis, exfoliative dermatitis, exacerbation of psoriasis, facial palsy, gangrene, gingival hypertrophy, Guillain-Barre syndrome, hemolytic-uremic syndrome, hypernatremia, hypomagnesemia, icterus, inappropriate serum ADH, increased sweating, irritability, loss of memory, loss of sense of smell, multiple organ failure, myelopathy, myocarditis, nephritis, ophthalmoplegia, parathyroid disorder, Parkinsonism-like reaction, pneumothorax, peripheral ischemia, perforated intestine, pneumonia, proteinuria, pseudotumor cerebri, pulmonary fibrosis, pulmonary embolism, respiratory distress syndrome, rhabdomyolysis, sperm production abnormal, testicular hypotrophy, thyroid disorder, Wolff-Parkinson-White syndrome.

Overdosage:

IV: Overdosage with IV ganciclovir has been reported in 17 patients (13 adults and 4 children < 2 years of age). Five patients experienced no adverse events following overdosage at the following doses: 7 doses of 11 mg/kg over a 3 day period (adult), single dose of 3500 mg (adult), single dose of 500 mg (72.5 mg/kg) followed by 48 hours of peritoneal dialysis (4-month-old), single dose of ≈ 60 mg/kg followed by exchange transfusion (18-month-old), 2 doses of 500 mg instead of 31 mg (21-month-old).

Irreversible pancytopenia developed in 1 adult with AIDS and CMV colitis after receiving 3000 mg IV ganciclovir on each of 2 consecutive days. He experienced worsening GI symptoms and acute renal failure which required short-term dialysis. Pancytopenia developed and persisted until his death from a malignancy several months later. Other adverse events reported following overdosage include the following: Persistent bone marrow suppression (1 adult with neutropenia and thrombocytopenia after a single dose of 6000 mg), reversible neutropenia or granulocytopenia (4 adults, overdoses ranging from 8 mg/kg daily for 4 days to a single dose of 25 mg/kg), hepatitis (1 adult receiving 10 mg/kg daily, and one 2 kg infant after a single 40 mg dose), renal toxicity (1 adult with transient worsening of hematuria after a single 500 mg dose, and 1 adult with elevated creatinine [5.2 mg/dL] after a single 5000 to 7000 mg dose) and seizure (1 adult with known seizure disorder after 3 days of 9 mg/kg). In addition, 1 adult received 0.4 mL (instead of 0.1 mL) by intravitreal injection, and experienced temporary loss of vision and central retinal artery occlusion secondary to increased intraocular pressure related to the injected fluid volume.

152 OPHTHALMIC DRUG FACTS

Oral: There have been no reports of overdosage with oral ganciclovir. Doses ≤ 6000 mg/day did not result in overt toxicity other than transient neutropenia.

Treatment: Dialysis may be useful in reducing serum concentrations. Maintain adequate hydration. Consider the use of hematopoietic growth factors.

Patient Information:

Ganciclovir is not a cure for CMV retinitis, and immunocompromised patients may continue to experience progression of retinitis during or following treatment. Advise patients to have regular ophthalmologic examinations at a minimum of every 6 weeks while being treated.

The major toxicities of ganciclovir are granulocytopenia and thrombocytopenia. Dose modifications may be required, including possible discontinuation. Emphasize the importance of close monitoring of blood counts while on therapy.

Patients with AIDS may be receiving zidovudine. Treatment with zidovudine and ganciclovir will not be tolerated by many patients and may result in severe granulocytopenia.

Advise patients that ganciclovir may cause infertility. Advise women of childbearing potential that ganciclovir should not be used during pregnancy; use effective contraception during ganciclovir treatment. Similarly, advise men to practice barrier contraception during and for ≥ 90 days following ganciclovir treatment.

Although there is no information, consider ganciclovir a potential carcinogen.

Transplant recipients: Counsel transplant recipients regarding the high frequency of impaired renal function, particularly in patients receiving coadministration of nephrotoxic agents such as cyclosporine and amphotericin B.

Administration and Dosage:

IV: Do not administer by rapid or bolus IV injection. The toxicity may be increased as a result of excessive plasma levels. Do not exceed the recommended infusion rate. IM or SC injection of reconstituted ganciclovir may result in severe tissue irritation due to high pH.

CMV retinitis (normal renal function):

> *Induction –* The recommended initial dose is 5 mg/kg (given IV at a constant rate > 1 hour) every 12 hours for 14 to 21 days. Do not use oral ganciclovir for induction treatment.

> *Maintenance –*

> *IV –* Following induction treatment, the recommended maintenance dose is 5 mg/kg given as a constant rate IV infusion > 1 hour once daily 7 days per week, or 6 mg/kg once daily 5 days per week.

> *Oral –* Following induction treatment, the recommended maintenance dose of oral ganciclovir is 1000 mg 3 times daily with food. Alternatively, the dosing regimen of 500 mg 6 times daily every 3 hours with food, during waking hours, may be used.

ANTI-INFECTIVE AGENTS

For patients who experience progression of CMV retinitis while receiving maintenance treatment with either formulation of ganciclovir, reinduction treatment is recommended.

Prevention of CMV disease in transplant recipients: The recommended initial dose of IV ganciclovir for patients with normal renal function is 5 mg/kg (given IV at a constant rate > 1 hour) every 12 hours for 7 to 14 days, followed by 5 mg/kg once daily 7 days per week or 6 mg/kg once daily 5 days per week.

The duration of treatment with IV ganciclovir in transplant recipients is dependent on the duration and degree of immunosuppression. In controlled clinical trials in bone marrow allograft recipients, treatment was continued until day 100 to 120 post-transplantation. CMV disease occurred in several patients who discontinued treatment with ganciclovir prematurely. In heart allograft recipients, the onset of newly diagnosed CMV disease occurred after treatment with ganciclovir was stopped at day 28 post-transplant, suggesting that continued dosing may be necessary to prevent late occurrence of CMV disease in this patient population.

Renal impairment:

IV – Refer to the following table for recommended doses and adjust the dosing interval as indicated.

IV Ganciclovir Dose in Renal Impairment				
Creatinine clearance (mL/min)	Ganciclovir induction dose (mg/kg)	Dosing interval (hours)	Ganciclovir maintenance dose (mg/kg)	Dosing interval (hours)
≥ 70)	5	12	5	24
50 to 69	2.5	12	2.5	24
25 to 49	2.5	24	1.25	24
10 to 24	1.25	24	0.625	24
< 10	1.25	3 times per week following hemodialysis	0.625	3 times per week following hemodialysis

Hemodialysis: Dosing for patients undergoing hemodialysis should not exceed 1.25 mg/kg 3 times per week, following each hemodialysis session. Give shortly after completion of the hemodialysis session, since hemodialysis reduces plasma levels by ≈ 50%.

Oral – In patients with renal impairment, modify the dose of oral ganciclovir as follows:

Oral Ganciclovir Dose in Renal Impairment	
Creatinine clearance (mL/min)	Ganciclovir doses
≥ 70	1000 mg TID or 500 mg q3h, 6x/day
50 to 69	1500 mg QID or 500 mg TID
25 to 49	1000 mg QID or 500 mg BID
10 to 24	500 mg QID
< 10	500 mg 3 times per week, following hemodialysis

Ccr can be related to serum creatinine by the following formula:

Males: $$\frac{Weight\ (kg) \times (140 - age)}{72 \times serum\ creatinine\ (mg/dL)} = Ccr$$

Females: $0.85 \times$ above value

OPHTHALMIC DRUG FACTS

Patient monitoring: Due to the frequency of granulocytopenia and thrombocytopenia, it is recommended that neutrophil counts and platelet counts be performed frequently, especially in patients in whom ganciclovir or other nucleoside analogs have previously resulted in leukopenia, or in whom neutrophil counts are < 1000/mm^3 at the beginning of treatment. Because dosing with ganciclovir must be modified in patients with renal impairment, and because of the incidence of increased serum creatinine levels that has been observed in transplant recipients treated with IV ganciclovir, patients should have serum creatinine or Ccr values followed carefully.

Reduction of dose: Dose reductions are required for patients with renal impairment and for those with neutropenia or thrombocytopenia. Therefore, perform frequent white blood cell counts. Severe neutropenia (ANC < 500/mm^3) or severe thrombocytopenia (platelets < 25,000/mm^3) require a dose interruption until evidence of marrow recovery is observed (ANC > 750/mm^3).

Preparation of IV solution: Each 10 mL clear glass vial contains ganciclovir sodium equivalent to 500 mg of the free base form of ganciclovir and 46 mg of sodium. Prepare the contents of the vial for administration in the following manner:

Reconstituted solution –

1. Reconstitute lyophilized ganciclovir by injecting 10 mL of Sterile Water for Injection, USP, into the vial. Do not use bacteriostatic water for injection containing parabens; it is incompatible with ganciclovir and may cause precipitation.

2. Shake the vial to dissolve the drug.

3. Visually inspect the reconstituted solution for particulate matter and discoloration prior to proceeding with infusion solution. Discard the vial if particulate matter or discoloration is observed.

4. Reconstituted solution in the vial is stable at room temperature for 12 hours. Do not refrigerate.

Infusion solution – Based on patient weight, remove the appropriate volume of the reconstituted solution (ganciclovir concentration 50 mg/mL) from the vial and add to an acceptable (see below) infusion fluid (typically 100 mL) for delivery over the course of 1 hour. Infusion concentrations > 10 mg/mL are not recommended. The following infusion fluids have been determined to be chemically and physically compatible with ganciclovir IV solution: 0.9% Sodium Chloride, 5% Dextrose, Ringer's Injection, and Lactated Ringer's Injection, USP.

Handling and disposal: Exercise caution in the handling and preparation of ganciclovir. Solutions of IV ganciclovir are alkaline (pH 11). Avoid direct contact with the skin or mucous membranes of the powder contained in ganciclovir capsules or of ganciclovir IV solutions. If such contact occurs, wash thoroughly with soap and water; rinse eyes thoroughly with plain water. Do not open or crush ganciclovir capsules.

Because ganciclovir shares some of the properties of antitumor agents (ie, carcinogenicity and mutagenicity), give consideration to handling and disposal according to guidelines issued for antineoplastic drugs.

Storage/Stability: Reconstituted solution in the vial is stable at room temperature for 12 hours. Do not refrigerate. Because nonbacteriostatic infusion fluid must be used with ganciclovir IV solution, the infusion solution must be used within 24 hours of dilution to reduce the risk of bacterial contamination. Refrigerate the infusion solution. Freezing is not recommended.

ANTI-INFECTIVE AGENTS

155

Rx **Cytovene** (Roche)	**Capsules:** 250 mg	In 180s.
	Capsules: 500 mg	In 180s.
	Powder for injection, lyophilized: 500 mg/vial ganciclovir (as sodium)	In 10 mL vials.

GANCICLOVIR INTRAVITREAL IMPLANT

Actions:

Pharmacology: Ganciclovir is a synthetic nucleoside analog of 2'-deoxyguanosine that inhibits replication of herpes viruses both in vitro and in vivo. Sensitive human viruses include cytomegalovirus (CMV), herpes simplex virus-1 and -2 (HSV-1, HSV-2), Epstein-Barr virus (EBV), and varicella-zoster virus (VZV).

The median concentration of ganciclovir that effectively inhibits the replication of human CMV (ED_{50}) has ranged from 0.2 to 3 mcg/mL. The relationship of in vitro sensitivity of CMV to ganciclovir and clinical response has not been established. Ganciclovir inhibits mammalian cell proliferation in vitro at higher concentrations: ID_{50} values range from 10 to 60 mcg/mL, with the exception of bone marrow-derived colony-forming cells, which are more sensitive with ID_{50} values > 10 mcg/mL of the cell types tested.

In vitro sensitivity testing of CMV isolates from patients receiving intravenous ganciclovir has shown emergence of viral resistance. Because the prevalence of resistant isolates is unknown, there is a possibility that some patients may be infected with strains of CMV resistant to ganciclovir. Consequently, consider the possibility of viral resistance in patients showing poor clinical response.

Pharmacokinetics: In one clinical trial, 26 patients (30 eyes treated) received a total of 39 primary implants and 12 exchange implants (performed 32 weeks after the implant was inserted or earlier if progression of CMV retinitis occurred). Precise in vivo release rates of the ganciclovir implant could not be calculated because most of the exchanged implants were empty upon removal. It was unknown at what time the implant ran out of the drug. However, approximate in vivo release rates ranged from 1 mcg/hr to > 1.62 mcg/hr for the exchanged implants.

In another study, in 14 implants (3 exchanged, 11 autopsy) in which the in vivo release rate could be accurately calculated, the mean release rate was 1.4 mcg/hr, with a range of 0.5 to 2.88 mcg/hr. The mean vitreous drug levels in 8 eyes (4 collected at time of reginal detachment surgery; 2 collected from autopsy eyes within 6 hours of death and prior to fixation; 2 collected from implant exchange) was 4.1 mcg/mL.

Clinical Trials: Ganciclovir implant (*Vitrasert*) and intravenous (*Cytovene*) were compared in a randomized, controlled parallel group trial conducted between May 1993 and December 1994 in 188 patients with AIDS and newly diagnosed CMV retinitis. Patients in the intravenous treatment group received an induction dose of 5 mg/kg twice daily for 14 days followed by a maintenance dose of 5 mg/kg once daily. The median time to progression was $\approx$ 210 days for the implant (*Vitrasert*) treatment group, compared with $\approx$ 120 days for the intravenous (*Cytovene*) ganciclovir treatment group.

156 OPHTHALMIC DRUG FACTS

Indications:

For the treatment of CMV retinitis in patients with acquired immunodeficiency syndrome (AIDS). The implant is for intravitreal implantation only.

Contraindications:

Hypersensitivity to ganciclovir or acyclovir. Patients contraindicated for intraocular surgery (eg, external infection, severe thrombocytopenia).

Warnings:

Diagnosis of CMV retinitis: Diagnosis is ophthalmologic and should be made by indirect ophthalmoscopy. Other conditions in the differential diagnosis of CMV retinitis include candidiasis, toxoplasmosis, histoplasmosis, retinal scars, and cotton wool spots, any of which may produce a retinal appearance similar to CMV.

CMV retinitis: CMV retinitis may be associated with CMV disease elsewhere in the body. The implant provides localized therapy limited to the implanted eye. The implant does not provide treatment for systemic CMV disease. Monitor patients for extraocular CMV disease.

Surgical procedures: Surgical procedures involve risk. The following complications may occur with intraocular surgery to place the implant into the vitreous cavity: Vitreous loss, vitreous hemorrhage, cataract formation, retinal detachment, uveitis, endophthalmitis, and decrease in visual acuity.

Loss of visual acuity: Loss of visual acuity may occur immediately in the implanted eye of almost all patients postoperatively. This decrease is temporary and lasts for ≈ 2 to 4 weeks after implantation. This decrease in visual acuity is probably a result of the surgical implant procedure.

The Vitrasert implant: The *Virasert* implant is sterilized by an ethylene oxide-freon mixture, a substance which harms public health and the environment by destroying ozone in the upper atmosphere.

Carcinogenesis/Mutagenesis/Fertility Impairment: In mice, daily oral doses of 1000 mg/kg may have caused an increased incidence of tumors in the preputial gland of males, nonglandular mucosa of the stomach of males and females, and reproductive tissues (eg, ovaries, uterus, mammary gland, clitoral gland, vagina) and liver in females. A slightly increased incidence of tumors occurred in the preputial and harderian glands (males), forestomach in males and females, and liver in females in mice given 20 mg/kg/day. Except for histiocytic sarcoma of the liver, ganciclovir-induced tumors were generally of epithelial or vascular origin. Consider ganciclovir a potential carcinogen in humans.

Ganciclovir caused mutations in lymphoma cells in mice and DNA damage in human lymphocytes in vitro at concentrations of 50 to 500 mcg/mL and 250 to 2000 mcg/mL, respectively. In the mouse micronucleus assay, ganciclovir was clastogenic at doses of 150 and 500 mg/kg (2.8% to 10% human exposure based on AUC), but not 50 mg/kg (exposure approximately comparable to the human, based on AUC). Ganciclovir was not mutagenic in the Ames Salmonella assay at concentrations of 500 to 5000 mcg/mL.

Ganciclovir caused decreased mating behavior, decreased fertility, and an increased incidence of embryolethality in female mice following intravenous doses of 90 mg/

ANTI-INFECTIVE AGENTS

kg/day. Decreased fertility in male mice and hypospermatogenesis in mice and dogs occurred following daily oral or intravenous administration of ganciclovir ranging from 0.2 to 10 mg/kg.

Pregnancy: Category C. Ganciclovir is embryotoxic in rabbits and mice following IV administration and teratogenic in rabbits. Fetal resorptions were present in ≥ 85% of rabbits and mice administered 60 mg/kg/day and 108 mg/kg/day, respectively. Effects observed in rabbits included the following: Fetal growth retardation, embryolethality, teratogenicity, and maternal toxicity. Teratogenic changes included cleft palate, anophthalmia/microphthalmia, aplastic organs (kidney and pancreas), hydrocephaly, and brachygnathia. In mice, effects observed were maternal/fetal toxicity and embryolethality.

Daily IV doses of 90/mg/kg administered to female mice prior to mating, during gestation and during lactation, caused hypoplasia of the test and seminal vesicles in the month-old male offspring, as well as pathologic changes in the nonglandular region of the stomach.

There are no adequate and well-controlled studies in pregnant women. Use during pregnancy only if the potential benefits to the mother justify the potential risk to the fetus.

Lactation: It is not known whether ganciclovir is excreted in breast milk. However, because carcinogenic and teratogenic effects occurred in animals treated with ganciclovir, the possibility of serious adverse reactions from ganciclovir in nursing infants is considered likely. Instruct mothers to discontinue nursing if they have a ganciclovir implant.

Children: Safety and effectiveness in children < 9 years of age have not been established.

Precautions:

As with all intraocular surgery, rigorously maintain sterility of the surgical field and the ganciclovir implant. The implant should be handled only by the suture tab in order to avoid damaging the polymer coatings since this could affect release rate of ganciclovir inside the eye. Do not resterilize the implant by any method.

A high level of surgical skill is required for implantation. A surgeon should have observed or assisted in surgical implantation of the ganciclovir implant prior to attempting the procedure.

Drug Interactions:

No drug interactions have been observed with the ganciclovir implant. There is limited experience with the use of retinal tamponades in conjunction with the ganciclovir implant.

Adverse Reactions:

The most frequent adverse reactions reported involved the eye.

During first 2 months following implantation: Visual acuity loss of ≥ 3 lines, vitreous hemorrhage, and retinal detachments (≈ 10% to 20%).

Local: Cataract formation/lens opacities, macular abnormalities, intraocular pressure spikes, optic disk/nerve changes, hyphemas, uveitis (≈ 1% to 5%). Retinopathy,

158 OPHTHALMIC DRUG FACTS

anterior chamber cell and flare, synechia, hemorrhage (other than vitreous), cotton wool spots, keratophalthy, astigmatism, endophthalmitis, microangiopathy, sclerosis, choroiditis, chemosis, phthisis bulbi, angle-closure glaucoma with anterior chamber shallowing, vitreous detachment, vitreous traction, hypotony, severe postoperative inflammation, retinal tear, retinal hole, corneal dellen, choroidal folds, pellet extrusion from scleral wound, gliosis (< 1%).

Patient Information:

The ganciclovir implant is not a cure for CMV retinitis and immunocompromised patients may continue to experience progression of retinitis with the implant. Advise patients to have regular ophthalmic examinations on both eyes at appropriate intervals following implantation.

As with any surgical procedure, risk is involved. Potential complications accompanying implantation may include intraocular infection or inflammation, retinal detachment, or cataract formation in the natural crystalline lens.

Immediate and temporary decrease in visual acuity in the implanted eye(s) are experienced by almost all patients following implantation. This lasts ≈ 2 to 4 weeks postoperatively and is probably a result of the surgical implant procedure.

Administration and Dosage:

Each implant contains a minimum of 4.5 mg of ganciclovir, and is designed to release the drug over a 5- to 8-month period. Following depletion of ganciclovir from the implant, as evidenced by progression of retinitis, the implant may be removed and replaced.

Handling and disposal: Exercise caution in handling the implant in order to avoid damage to the polymer coating on the implant, which may result in an increased rate of drug release from the implant. Handle the implant by the suture tab only. Maintain aseptic technique at all times prior to and during the surgical implantation procedure.

Because the implant contains ganciclovir, which shares some of the properties of antitumor agents (ie, carcinogenicity, mutogenicity), give consideration to handling and disposal of the implant according to guidelines issued for antineoplastic drugs.

Storage/Stability: Store at room temperature 15° to 30°C (59° to 86°F). Do not freeze. Keep away from excessive heat and light.

Rx	**Vitrasert** (Bausch & Lomb Surgical)	**Implant:** Minimum 4.5 mg	In individual unit boxes in a sterile Tyvek package.

FOMIVIRSEN SODIUM

Actions:

Pharmacology: Fomivirsen is a phosphorothioate oligonucleotide that inhibits human cytomegalovirus (CMV) replication through an antisense mechanism. The nucleotide sequence of fomivirsen is complementary to a sequence in mRNA transcripts of the major immediate early region 2 (IE2) of CMV. This region of mRNA encodes several proteins responsible for regulation of viral gene expression that are essential for

ANTI-INFECTIVE AGENTS

the production of infectious CMV. Binding of fomivirsen to the target mRNA results in the inhibition of IE2 protein synthesis, subsequently inhibiting replication.

Cross-resistance – The antisense mechanisms of action and molecular target of fomivirsen are different from that of other inhibitors of CMV replication, which function by inhibiting the viral DNA polymerase. Fomivirsen was equally potent against 21 independent clinical CMV isolates, including several that were resistant to ganciclovir, foscarnet, or cidofovir.

Pharmacokinetics:

Ocular kinetics – Fomivirsen is cleared from the vitreous in rabbits over the course of 7 to 10 days by a combination of tissue distribution and metabolism, with metabolism as the primary route of elimination from the eye. Fomivirsen is metabolized by exonucleases in a process yielding shortened oligonucleotides and mononucleotide metabolites. Mononucleotide metabolites are further catabolized similar to endogenous nucleotides and are excreted as low molecular weight metabolites. Animal studies indicate a small amount is eliminated in urine (16%) or feces (3%) as low molecular weight metabolites.

Fomivirsen ocular concentrations were greatest in the retina and iris. It was detectable in the retina within hours after injection and concentrations increased over 3 to 5 days.

Systemic exposure – Systemic exposure to fomivirsen following single or repeated intravitreal injections in animals was below limits of quantitation. However, there were isolated instances when fomivirsen's metabolites were detected in liver, kidney, and plasma.

Protein binding – In animal studies of vitreous samples, ≈ 40% of fomivirsen is bound to proteins.

Indications:

CMV retinitis: Local treatment of CMV retinitis in patients with acquired immunodificiency syndrome (AIDS) who are intolerant of, or have a contraindication to, other treatments for CMV retinitis or who were sufficently responsive to previous treatments.

Contraindications:

Hypersensitivity to any component of this preparation.

Warnings:

Route of administration: Fomivirsen is for intravitreal injection (ophthalmic) use only.

Previous CMV therapy: Fomivirsen is not recommended for use in patients who have recently (2 to 4 weeks) been treated with either IV or intravitreal cidofovir because of the risk of exaggerated ocular inflammation.

Systemic CMV disease: CMV retinitis may be associated with CMV disease elsewhere in the body. Fomivirsen intravitreal injection provides localized therapy limited to the treated eye and does not provide treatment for systemic CMV disease. Monitor patients for extraocular CMV disease or disease in the other eye.

OPHTHALMIC DRUG FACTS

CMV retinitis diagnosis: The diagnosis and evaluation of CMV retinitis is ophthalmo-logic and should be made by comprehensive retinal examination including indirect ophthalmoscopy. Consider other conditions in the differential diagnosis of CMV reti-nitis including indirect ophthalmoscopy. Consider other conditions in the differen-tial diagnosis of CMV retinitis including ocular infections caused by syphilis, candidiasis, toxoplasmosis, histoplasmosis, herpes simplex virus, and varicella-zos-ter virus, as well as retinal appearance similar to CMV (retinal scars, cotton wool spots).

Pregnancy: Category C. It is not known whether fomivirsen sodium can cause fetal harm when administered to a pregnant woman or can affect reproduction capacity. There are no adequate and well-controlled studies in pregnant women. Use dur-ing pregnancy only if the potential benefit to the mother justifies the potential risk to the fetus.

Lactation: It is not known whether fomivirsen sodium is excreted in breast milk. Because of the potential for serious adverse reactions in nursing infants from fomi-virsen, decide whether to discontinue nursing or to discontinue the drug, taking into account the importance of the drug to the mother.

Children: Safety and efficacy have not been established.

Precautions:

Monitoring: Patients receiving fomivirsen should have regular ophthalmogic follow-up examinations. CMV may exist as a systemic disease in addition to CMV retinitis. Therefore, monitor patients for extraocular CMV infections (eg, pneumonitis, colitis) and retinitis in the opposite eye, if only 1 eye is being treated.

Ocular inflammations: Uveitis including iritis and vitritis has been reported in ≈ 25% of patients. Inflammatory reactions are more common during induction dosing. Delaying additional treatments with fomivirsen and topical corticosteroids have been useful in the management of inflammatory changes; patients may be able to con-tinue to receive intravitreal injections of fomivirsen after inflammation has resolved.

Increased intraocular pressure (IOP): IOP is common and is usually transient; in most cases, pressure returns to the normal range without any treatment or with temporary use of topical medications. Monitor IOP at each visit and manage IOP elevations, if sustained, with medications to lower IOP.

Adverse Reactions:

The most observed adverse experience has been ocular inflammation (uveitis) includ-ing iritis and vitritis. (≈ 25% of patients; see Precauctions).

Ophthalmic: Abnormal vision, anterior chamber inflammation, blurred vision, cata-ract, conjunctival hemorrhage, decreased visual acuity, desaturation of color vision, eye pain, floaters, increased intraocular pressure, photophobia, retinal detachment, retinal edema, retinal hemmorhage, retinal pigment changes, uveitis, vitritis (5% to 20%); application site reaction, conjunctival hyperemia, conjunctivitis, corneal edema, decreased peripheral vision, eye irritation, hypotony, keratic precipitates, optic neu-ritis, photopsia, retinal vascular disease, visual field defect, vitreous hemorrhage, vit-reous opacity (2% to 5%).

Systemic: Abdominal pain, anemia, asthenia, diarrhea, fever, headache, infection, nau-sea, pneumonia, rash, sepsis, sinusitis, systemic CMV, vomiting (5% to 20%); abnor-

ANTI-INFECTIVE AGENTS

161

mal liver function, abnormal thinking, allergic reactions, anorexia, back pain, bronchitis, cachexia, catheter infection, chest pain, decreased weight, dehydration, depression, dizziness, dysphea, flu syndrome, increased cough, increased GGTP, kidney failure, lymphoma-like reaction, neuropathy, neutropenia, oral monilia, pain, pancreatitis, sweating, thrombocytopenia (2% to 5%).

Overdosage:

In a clinical trial, 1 patient with advanced CMV retinitis unresponsive to other antiviral to other antiviral treatments was accidentally dosed once bilaterally with 990 mcg per eye. Anterior chamber paracentesis was performed bilaterally and vision was retained.

Patient Information:

Fomivirsen intravitreal injection is not a cure for CMV retinitis, and some immunocompromised patients may continue to experience progression of retinitis during and following treatment. Advise patients receiving fomivirsen to have regular ophthalmologic follow-up examinations. Patients may also experience other manifestations of CMV disease despite fomivirsen therapy.

Fomivirsen treats only the eye(s) in which it has been injected. CMV may exist as a systemic disease, in addition to CMV retinitis. Therefore, monitor patients for extraocular CMV infections (eg, pneumonitis, colitis) and retinitis in the opposite eye, if only 1 eye is being treated.

HIV-infected patients should continue antiretroviral therapy as otherwise indicated.

Administration and Dosage:

Dosage: The recommended induction dose is 330 mcg (0.05 mL) as a single intravitreal injection every other week for 2 doses followed by maintenance doses of 330 mcg (0.05 mL) once every 4 weeks. For patients whose disease progresses on fomivirsen during maintenance, an attempt at reinduction at the same dose may result in resumed disease control.

For unacceptable inflammation in the face of controlled CMV retinitis, it is worthwhile to interrupt therapy until inflammation decreases and therapy can resume.

Intravitreal injection instructions: Fomivirsen is administered by intravitreal injection (0.05 mL/eye) into the affected eye following application of standard topical or local anesthetics and antimicrobials using 30-gauge needle on a low-volume (eg, tuberculin) syringe. The following steps should be used:

- Disinfect rubber stopper with 70% ethyl alcohol.
- Attach a 5-micron filter needle to the injection syringe for solution withdrawal (to further guard against the introduction of stopper particulate), and withdraw ≈ 0.15 mL through the filter needle.
- Remove filter needle and attach a 30-gauge needle to syringe containing fomivirsen.
- Eject excess volume and air from syringe.
- Stabalize globe with cotton tip applicator and insert needle fully through an area 3.5 to 4 mm posterior to the limbus (avoiding the horizontal meridian) aiming toward the center of the globe, keeping fingers off the plunger until the needle has been completely inserted.
- Deliver the injection volume (0.05 mL) by injecting slowly. Roll cotton

tip applicator over injection site as needle is withdrawn to reduce the loss of eye fluid.

Post-injection monitoring instructions: Monitor light perception and optic nerve head perfusion. If not completely perfused by 7 to 10 minutes, perform anterior chamber paracentesis with a 30-gauge needle on a plungerless tuberculin syringe at the slit lamp.

Storage/Stability: Store between 2° to 25°C (35° to 77°F). Protect from excessive heat and light.

Rx	Vitravene (Novartis)	Injection (as sodium): 6.6 mg/mL	Preservative free. In 0.25 mL single use vials.[1]

[1] With sodium bicarbonate, NaCl, sodium carbonate.

FOSCARNET SODIUM (Phosphonoformic acid)

Warning:

Renal impairment, the major toxicity, occurs to some degree in most patients. Continual assessment of a patient's risk and frequent monitoring of serum creatinine with dose adjustment for changes in renal function are imperative.

Foscarnet causes alterations in plasma minerals and electrolytes that have led to seizures. Monitor patients frequently for such changes and their potential sequelae.

Actions:

Pharmacology: Foscarnet is an organic analog of inorganic pyrophosphate that inhibits replication of all known herpes viruses in vitro including cytomegalovirus (CMV), herpes simplex virus types 1 and 2 (HSV-1, HSV-2), human herpes virus 6 (HHV-6), Epstein-Barr virus (EBV), and varicella-zoster virus (VZV).

Foscarnet exerts its antiviral activity by a selective inhibition at the pyrophosphate binding site on virus-specific DNA polymerases and reverse transcriptases at concentrations that do not affect cellular DNA polymerases. Foscarnet does not require activation (phosphorylation) by thymidine kinase or other kinases, and therefore is active in vitro against HSV mutants deficient in thymidine kinase. CMV strains resistant to ganciclovir may be sensitive to foscarnet.

The quantitative relationship between the in vitro susceptibility of human CMV to foscarnet and clinical response to therapy has not been clearly established and virus sensitivity testing has not been standardized. If no clinical response to foscarnet is observed, test viral isolates for sensitivity to foscarnet; naturally resistant mutants may emerge under selective pressure both in vitro and in vivo. The latent state of any of the human herpes viruses is not known to be sensitive to foscarnet and viral reactivation of CMV occurs after foscarnet therapy is terminated.

Pharmacokinetics: Foscarnet is 14% to 17% bound to plasma protein at plasma drug concentrations of 1 to 1000 mcM. Plasma foscarnet concentrations in 2 studies are summarized in the following table:

ANTI-INFECTIVE AGENTS

Foscarnet Plasma Concentrations			
Mean dose (Infusion time)	Day of sampling	Mean plasma concentration (mcM)	
		C_{max} (range)	C_{min} (range)
57 ± 6 mg/kg q 8 hr (1 hour)	1	573 (213 to 1305)[1]	78 (< 33 to 139)[3]
47 ± 12 mg/kg q 8 hr (1 hour)	14 or 15	579 (246 to 922)[2]	110 (< 33 to 148)[4]
55 ± 6 mg/kg q 8 hr (hours)	3	445 (306 to 720)[1]	88 (< 33 to 162)[3]
57 ± 7 mg/kg q 8 hr (2 hours)	14 or 15	517 (348 to 789)[2]	105 (43 to 205)[4]

[1] Observed 0.9 to 2.4 hours after start of infusion.
[2] Observed 0.8 to 2.6 hours after start of infusion.
[3] Observed 4 to 8.1 hours after start of infusion.
[4] Observed 6.3 to 8.7 hours after start of infusion.

Mean plasma clearances were 130 ± 44 and 178 ± 48 mL/min/1.73 m² in 2 studies in which foscarnet was given by intermittent infusion and 152 ± 59 and 214 ± 25 mL/min/1.73 m² in 2 studies using continuous infusion. Approximately 80% to 90% of IV foscarnet is excreted unchanged in the urine of patients with normal renal function. Both tubular secretion and glomerular filtration account for urinary elimination of foscarnet. In one study, plasma clearance was less than creatinine clearance (Ccr), suggesting that foscarnet may also undergo tubular reabsorption. In 3 studies, decreases in plasma clearance of foscarnet were proportional to decreases in Ccr.

Two studies in patients with initially normal renal function who were treated with intermittent infusions showed average drug plasma half-lives of ≈ 3 hours determined on days 1 or 3 of therapy. This may be an underestimate of the effective half-life due to the limited observation period. Plasma half-life increases with the severity of renal impairment. Half-lives of 2 to 8 hours occurred in patients having estimated or measured 24 hour Ccr of 44 to 90 mL/min. Careful monitoring of renal function and dose adjustment is imperative (see Warnings and Administration and Dosage).

Following continuous foscarnet infusion for 72 hours in 6 HIV-positive patients, plasma half-lives of 0.45 ± 0.32 and 3.3 ± 1.3 hours were determined. A terminal half-life of 18 ± 2.8 hours was estimated from foscarnet urinary excretion over 48 hours after stopping infusion. When foscarnet was given as a continuous infusion to 13 patients with HIV infection for 8 to 21 days, plasma half-lives of 1.4 ± 0.6 and 6.8 ± 5 hours were determined. A terminal half-life of 87.5 ± 41.8 hours was estimated from foscarnet urinary excretion over 6 days after the last infusion; however, renal function at the time of discontinuing the infusion was not known.

Measurements of urinary excretion are required to detect the longer terminal half-life assumed to represent release of foscarnet from bone. In animal studies (mice), 40% of an IV dose is deposited in bone in young animals and 7% in adults. Evidence indicates that foscarnet accumulates in human bone; however, the extent to which this occurs has not been determined. Mean volumes of distribution at steady state range from 0.3 to 0.6 L/kg.

Variable penetration into cerebrospinal fluid (CSF) has been observed. Intermittent infusion of 50 mg/kg every 8 hours for 28 days in 9 patients produced CSF levels of 150 to 260 mcM 3 hours after the end of infusion or 39% to 103% of the plasma levels. In another 4 patients, CSF concentrations were 35% to 69% of the plasma drug level after a dose of 230 mg/kg/day by continuous infusion for 2 to 13 days. However, the CSF:plasma ratio was only 13% in one patient receiving a continuous infusion at a rate of 274 mg/kg/day. Disease-related defects in the blood-brain barrier may be responsible for the variations seen.

Clinical Trials: In most clinical studies, treatment for CMV retinitis began with an induction dosage of 60 mg/kg every 8 hours for the first 2 to 3 weeks, followed by a once-daily maintenance at doses ranging from 60 to 120 mg/kg.

OPHTHALMIC DRUG FACTS

A prospective, randomized, masked, controlled clinical trial was conducted in 24 patients with acquired immunodeficiency syndrome (AIDS) and CMV retinitis. Patients received induction treatment of 60 mg/kg every 8 hours for 3 weeks, followed by maintenance treatment with 90 mg/kg/day until retinitis progression (appearance of a new lesion or advancement of the border of a posterior lesion > 750 microns in diameter). The 13 patients randomized to treatment with foscarnet had a significant delay in progression of CMV retinitis compared to untreated controls. Median times to retinitis progression from study entry were 93 days (range, 21 to > 364) and 22 days (range, 7 to 42), respectively.

In another prospective clinical trial of CMV retinitis in AIDS patients, 33 were treated with 2 to 3 weeks of foscarnet induction (60 mg/kg 3 times a day) and then randomized to 2 maintenance dose groups, 90 and 120 mg/kg/day. Median times from study entry to retinitis progression were 96 days (range, 14 to > 176) and 140 days (range, 16 to > 233), respectively. This was not statistically significant.

Indications:

Treatment of CMV retinitis in patients with AIDS.

Contraindications:

Hypersensitivity to foscarnet.

Warnings:

Mineral and electrolyte imbalances: Foscarnet has been associated with changes in serum electrolytes including hypocalcemia (15%), hypophosphatemia (8%), hyperphosphatemia (6%), hypomagnesemia (15%), and hypokalemia (16%). Foscarnet is associated with a transient, dose-related decrease in ionized serum calcium, which may not be reflected in total serum calcium. This effect most likely is related to foscarnet's chelation of divalent metal ions such as calcium. Therefore, advise patients to report symptoms of low ionized calcium such as perioral tingling, numbness in the extremities, and paresthesias. Be prepared to treat these as well as severe manifestations of electrolyte abnormalities, such as tetany and seizures. The rate of infusion may affect the transient decrease in ionized calcium; slowing the rate may decrease or prevent symptoms.

Transient changes in calcium or other electrolytes (including magnesium, potassium, or phosphate) may also contribute to a patient's risk for cardiac disturbances and seizures (see Neurotoxicity and Seizures). Therefore, use particular caution in patients with altered calcium or other electrolyte levels before treatment, especially those with neurologic or cardiac abnormalities and those on other drugs known to influence minerals and electrolytes (see Monitoring and Drug Interactions).

Neurotoxicity and seizures: Foscarnet was associated with seizures in 18/189 (10%) of AIDS patients in 5 controlled studies. Three patients were not taking foscarnet at the time of seizure. In most cases (15/18), the patients had an active CNS condition (eg, toxoplasmosis, HIV encephalopathy) or a history of CNS diseases. The rate of seizures did not increase with duration of treatment. Three cases were associated with overdoses of foscarnet (see Overdosage).

Statistically significant risk factors associated with seizures were low baseline absolute neutrophil count (ANC), impaired baseline renal function, and low total serum calcium. Several cases of seizures were associated with death. However, seizures did not always necessitate drug discontinuation. Ten of 15 patients with seizures while on

ANTI-INFECTIVE AGENTS

the drug continued or resumed foscarnet following treatment of their underlying disease, electrolyte disturbances, or dose decreases. If factors predisposing to seizures are present, carefully monitor electrolytes, including calcium and magnesium (see Monitoring).

Other CMV infections: Safety and efficacy have not been established for the treatment of other CMV infections (eg, pneumonitis, gastroenteritis); congenital or neonatal CMV disease; or nonimmunocompromised individuals.

Renal function impairment: The major toxicity of foscarnet is renal impairment, which occurs to some degree in most patients. Approximately 33% of 189 patients with AIDS and CMV retinitis who received IV foscarnet in clinical studies developed significant impairment of renal function, manifested by a rise in serum creatinine concentration to $\geq$ 2 mg/dL. Therefore, use foscarnet with caution in all patients, especially those with a history of renal function impairment. Patients vary in their sensitivity to foscarnet-induced nephrotoxicity, and initial renal function may not be predictive of the potential for drug-induced renal impairment.

Renal impairment is most likely to become clinically evident as assessed by increasing serum creatinine during the second week of induction therapy at 60 mg/kg 3 times a day. However, renal impairment may occur at any time in any patient during treatment; therefore, monitor renal function carefully (see Monitoring).

Elevations in serum creatinine are usually, but not uniformly, reversible following discontinuation or dose adjustment. Recovery of renal function after foscarnet-induced impairment usually occurs within 1 week of drug discontinuation. However, of 35 patients who experienced grade II renal impairment (serum creatinine 2 to 3 times the upper limit of normal), 2 died with renal failure within 4 weeks of stopping foscarnet and 3 others died with renal insufficiency still present < 4 weeks after drug cessation.

Because of foscarnet's potential to cause renal impairment, dose adjustment for decreased baseline renal function and any change in renal function during treatment is necessary. In addition, it may be beneficial for adequate hydration to be established (eg, by inducing diuresis) prior to and during administration.

Mutagenesis: Foscarnet showed genotoxic effects in an in vitro transformation assay at concentrations > 0.5 mcg/mL and an increased frequency of chromosome aberrations in the sister chromatid exchange assay at 1000 mcg/mL. A high dose of foscarnet (350 mg/kg) caused an increase in micronucleated polychromatic erythrocytes in mice at doses that produced exposures comparable to that anticipated clinically.

Elderly: Since these individuals frequently have reduced glomerular filtration, pay particular attention to assessing renal function before and during administration (see Administration and Dosage).

Pregnancy: Category C. Daily SC doses up to 75 mg/kg administered to female rats prior to and during mating, during gestation, and 21 days postpartum caused a slight increase (< 5%) in the number of skeletal anomalies compared with the control group. Daily SC doses up to 75 mg/kg (one-third the maximal daily human exposure) administered to rabbits and 150 mg/kg (one-eighth the maximal daily human exposure) administered to rats during gestation caused an increase in the frequency of skeletal anomalies/variations. These studies are inadequate to define the potential teratogenicity at levels to which women will be exposed. There are no adequate and well-controlled studies in pregnant women. Use during pregnancy only if clearly needed.

OPHTHALMIC DRUG FACTS

Lactation: It is not known whether foscarnet is excreted in breast milk; however, in lactating rats administered 75 mg/kg, foscarnet was excreted in maternal milk at concentrations 3 times higher than peak maternal blood concentrations. Exercise caution if foscarnet is administered to a nursing woman.

Children: The safety and efficacy of foscarnet in children have not been studied. Foscarnet is deposited in teeth and bone, and deposition is greater in young and growing animals. Foscarnet adversely affects development of tooth enamel in mice and rats. The effects of this deposition on skeletal development have not been studied. Since deposition in human bone also occurs, it is likely that it does so to a greater degree in developing bone in children. Administer to children only after careful evaluation and only if the potential benefits for treatment outweigh the risks.

Precautions:

Monitoring: The majority of patients will experience some decrease in renal function due to foscarnet administration. Therefore it is recommended that Ccr, either measured or estimated using the modified Cockcroft and Gault equation based on serum creatinine, be determined at baseline, 2 to 3 times per week during induction therapy and at least once every 1 to 2 weeks during maintenance therapy, with foscarnet dose adjusted accordingly (see Dose Adjustment). More frequent monitoring may be required for some patients. It is also recommended that a 24-hour Ccr be determined at baseline and periodically thereafter to ensure correct dosing. Discontinue foscarnet if Ccr drops to < 0.4 mL/min/kg.

Due to foscarnet's propensity to chelate divalent metal ions and alter levels of serum electrolytes, closely monitor patients for such changes. It is recommended that a schedule similar to that recommended for serum creatinine (see above) be used to monitor serum calcium, magnesium, potassium, and phosphorus. Particular caution is advised in patients with decreased total serum calcium or other electrolyte levels before treatment, as well as in patients with neurologic or cardiac abnormalities, and in patients receiving other drugs known to influence serum calcium levels. Correct any clinically significant metabolic changes. Also, patients who experience mild (eg, perioral numbness or paresthesias) or severe symptoms (eg, seizures) of electrolyte abnormalities should have serum electrolyte and mineral levels assessed as close in time to the event as possible.

Careful monitoring and appropriate management of electrolytes, calcium, magnesium, and creatinine are of particular importance in patients with conditions that may predispose them to seizures (see Warnings).

Diagnosis of CMV retinitis: Determine diagnosis by indirect ophthalmoscopy. Other conditions in the differential diagnosis of CMV retinitis include candidiasis, toxoplasmosis, and other diseases producing a similar retinal pattern, any of which may produce a retinal appearance similar to CMV. For this reason it is essential that the diagnosis of CMV retinitis be established by an ophthalmologist familiar with the retinal presentation of these conditions. The diagnosis of CMV retinitis may be supported by culture of CMV from urine, blood, throat, or other sites, but a negative CMV culture does not rule out CMV retinitis.

Toxicity/Local irritation: In controlled clinical studies, the maximum single-dose administered was 120 mg/kg by IV infusion over 2 hours. It is likely that larger doses, or more rapid infusions, would result in increased toxicity. Take care to infuse solutions containing foscarnet only into veins with adequate blood flow to permit rapid dilution and distribution, and avoid local irritation (see Administration and Dosage). Local irritation and ulcerations of penile epithelium have occurred in male patients receiving foscarnet, possibly related to the presence of drug in urine. One case of vulvo-

ANTI-INFECTIVE AGENTS

vaginal ulceration in a female has occurred. Adequate hydration with close attention to personal hygiene may minimize the occurrence of such events.

Anemia: Anemia occurred in 33% of patients. This anemia was usually manageable with transfusions and required discontinuation of foscarnet in < 1% (1/189) of patients in the studies. Granulocytopenia occurred in 17% of patients; however, only 1% (2/189) were terminated from these studies because of neutropenia.

Drug Interactions:

Nephrotoxic drugs: The elimination of foscarnet may be impaired by drugs that inhibit renal tubular secretion. Because of foscarnet's tendency to cause renal impairment, avoid the use of foscarnet in combination with potentially nephrotoxic drugs such as aminoglycosides, amphotericin B, and IV pentamidine unless the potential benefits outweigh the risks to the patient.

Pentamidine: Concomitant treatment of 4 patients with foscarnet and IV pentamidine may have caused hypocalcemia; 1 patient died with severe hypocalcemia. Toxicity associated with concomitant use of aerosolized pentamidine has not been reported.

Zidovudine: Foscarnet was used concomitantly with zidovudine in approximately one-third of patients in the US studies. Although the combination was generally well tolerated, additive effects on anemia may have occurred. However, no evidence of increased myelosuppression was seen.

Foscarnet decreases serum levels of ionized calcium. Exercise particular caution when other drugs known to influence serum calcium levels are used concurrently.

Adverse Reactions:

The most frequently reported events were the following: fever (65%); nausea (47%); anemia (33%); diarrhea (30%); abnormal renal function including acute renal failure, decreased Ccr, and increased serum creatinine (27%); vomiting, headache (26%); seizure (10%) (see Warnings and Precautions).

Adverse events categorized as "severe" were the following: death (14%); abnormal renal function (14%); marrow suppression (10%); anemia (9%); seizures (7%). Although death was specifically attributed to foscarnet in only 1 case, other complications of foscarnet (ie, renal impairment, electrolyte abnormalities, seizures) may have contributed to patient deaths (see Warnings and Precautions).

Cardiovascular: Hypertension, palpitations, ECG abnormalities including sinus tachycardia, first-degree AV block and non-specific ST-T segment changes, hypotension, flushing, cerebrovascular disorder (see Warnings) (1% to 5%); cardiomyopathy, cardiac failure/arrest, bradycardia, extrasystole, arrhythmias, atrial arrhythmias/fibrillation, phlebitis, superficial thrombophlebitis of arm, mesenteric vein thrombophlebitis (< 1%).

CNS: Headache, paresthesia, dizziness, involuntary muscle contractions, hypoesthesia, neuropathy, seizures (including grand mal; see Warnings) (≥ 5%); tremor, ataxia, dementia, stupor, generalized spasms, sensory disturbances, meningitis, aphasia, abnormal coordination, leg cramps, EEG abnormalities (see Warnings) (1% to 5%); vertigo, coma, encephalopathy, abnormal gait, hyperesthesia, hypertonia, visual field defects, dyskinesia, extrapyramidal disorders, hemiparesis, hyperkinesia, vocal cord paralysis, paralysis, paraplegia, speech disorders, tetany, hyporeflexia, hyperreflexia, neuralgia, neuritis, peripheral neuropathy, cerebral edema, nystagmus (< 1%).

Dermatologic: Rash, increased sweating (≥ 5%); pruritus, skin ulceration, seborrhea, erythematous rash, maculopapular rash, skin discoloration, facial edema (1% to 5%); acne, alopecia, dermatitis, anal pruritus, genital pruritus, aggravated psoriasis, psoriaform rash, skin disorders, dry skin, urticaria, verruca (< 1%).

Endocrine: Antidiuretic hormone disorders, decreased gonadotropins, gynecomastia (< 1%).

GI: Anorexia, nausea, diarrhea, vomiting, abdominal pain (≥ 5%); constipation, dysphagia, dyspepsia, rectal hemorrhage, dry mouth, melena, flatulence, ulcerative stomatitis, pancreatitis (1% to 5%); enteritis, enterocolitis, glossitis, proctitis, stomatitis, tenesmus, increased amylase, pseudomembranous colitis, gastroenteritis, oral leukoplakia, oral hemorrhage, rectal disorders, colitis, duodenal ulcer, hematemesis, paralytic ileus, esophageal ulceration, ulcerative proctitis, tongue ulceration (< 1%).

GU: Alterations in renal function, including serum creatinine, decreased Ccr and abnormal renal function (see Warnings) (≥ 5%); albuminuria, dysuria, polyuria, urethral disorder, urinary retention, urinary tract infections, acute renal failure, nocturia (1% to 5%); hematuria, glomerulonephritis, micturition disorders/frequency, toxic nephropathy, nephrosis, urinary incontinence, renal tubular disorders, pyelonephritis, urethral irritation, uremia (< 1%). Perineal pain in women, penile inflammation (< 1%).

Hematologic/Lymphatic: Anemia, granulocytopenia, leukopenia (see Precautions) (≥ 5%); thrombocytopenia, platelet abnormalities, thrombosis, WBC abnormalities, lymphadenopathy (1% to 5%); pulmonary embolism, coagulation disorders, decreased coagulation factors, epistaxis, decreased prothrombin, hypochromic anemia, pancytopenia, hemolysis, leukocytosis, cervical lymphadenopathy, lymphopenia (< 1%).

Lymphoma-like disorder, sarcoma (1% to 5%); malignant lymphoma, skin hypertrophy (< 1%).

Hepatic: Abnormal A-G ratio, abnormal hepatic function, increased AST and ALT (1% to 5%); cholecystitis, cholelithiasis, hepatitis, cholestatic hepatitis, hepatosplenomegaly, jaundice (< 1%).

Local: Injection site pain or inflammation (1% to 5%).

Metabolic/Nutritional: Mineral/electrolyte imbalances (see Warnings), including hypokalemia, hypocalcemia, hypomagnesemia, hypo- or hyperphosphatemia (≥ 5%); hyponatremia, decreased weight, increased alkaline phosphatase, LDH and BUN, acidosis, cachexia, thirst, hypercalcemia (1% to 5%); dehydration, glycosuria, increased creatine phosphokinase, diabetes mellitus, abnormal glucose tolerance, hypervolemia, hypochloremia, periorbital edema, hypoproteinemia (< 1%).

Musculoskeletal: Arthralgia, myalgia (1% to 5%); arthrosis, synovitis, torticollis (< 1%).

Psychiatric: Depression, confusion, anxiety (≥ 5%); insomnia, somnolence, nervousness, amnesia, agitation, aggressive reaction, hallucination (1% to 5%); impaired concentration, emotional lability, psychosis, suicide attempt, delirium, personality disorders, sleep disorders (< 1%).

Respiratory: Coughing, dyspnea (≥ 5%); pneumonia, sinusitis, pharyngitis, rhinitis, respiratory disorders or insufficiency, pulmonary infiltration, stridor, pneumothorax, hemoptysis, bronchospasm (1% to 5%); bronchitis, laryngitis, respiratory depression, abnormal chest x-ray, pleural effusion, pulmonary hemorrhage, pneumonitis (< 1%).

ANTI-INFECTIVE AGENTS

Special senses: Vision abnormalities (≥ 5%); taste perversions, eye abnormalities, eye pain, conjunctivitis (1% to 5%); diplopia, blindness, retinal detachment, mydriasis, photophobia, deafness, earache, tinnitus, otitis (< 1%).

Miscellaneous: Fever, fatigue, rigors, asthenia, malaise, pain, infection, sepsis, death (≥ 5%); back/chest pain, edema, influenza-like symptoms, bacterial/fungal infections, moniliasis, abscess (1% to 5%); hypothermia, leg edema, peripheral edema, syncope, ascites, substernal chest pain, abnormal crying, malignant hyperpyrexia, herpes simplex, viral infection, toxoplasmosis (< 1%).

Overdosage:

Symptoms: In controlled clinical trials, overdosage was reported in 10 patients. All 10 patients experienced adverse events and all except 1 made a complete recovery. One patient died after receiving a total daily dose of > 12.5 for 3 days instead of the intended 10.9 g. The patient suffered a grand mal seizure and became comatose. Three days later the patient died with the cause of death listed as respiratory/cardiac arrest. The other 9 patients received doses ranging from 1.14 times to 8 times their recommended doses with an average of 4 times their recommended doses. Overall, 3 patients had seizures, 3 patients had renal function impairment, 4 patients had paresthesias either in limbs or periorally, and 5 patients had documented electrolyte disturbances primarily involving calcium and phosphate.

Treatment: There is no specific antidote. Hemodialysis and hydration may be of benefit in reducing drug plasma levels in patients who receive an overdosage, but these have not been evaluated in a clinical trial setting. Observe the patient for signs and symptoms of renal impairment and electrolyte imbalance. Institute medical treatment if clinically warranted.

Patient Information:

Foscarnet is not a cure for CMV retinitis; patients may continue to experience progression of retinitis during or following treatment.

Regular ophthalmologic examinations are necessary. The major toxicities of foscarnet are renal impairment, electrolyte disturbances, and seizures; dose modifications and possibly discontinuation may be required.

Close monitoring while on therapy is essential. Advise patients of the importance of perioral tingling, numbness in the extremities, or paresthesias during or after infusion as possible symptoms of electrolyte abnormalities. Should such symptoms occur, stop the infusion, obtain appropriate laboratory samples for assessment of electrolyte concentrations, and consult physician before resuming treatment. The rate of infusion must be ≤ 1 mg/kg/min.

The potential for renal impairment may be minimized by accompanying administration with hydration adequate to establish and maintain diuresis during dosing.

Administration and Dosage:

Caution: Do not administer by rapid or bolus IV injection. Toxicity may be increased as a result of excessive plasma levels. Take care to avoid unintentional overdose by carefully controlling the rate of infusion. Therefore, an infusion pump must be used. In spite of the use of an infusion pump, overdoses have occurred.

170 OPHTHALMIC DRUG FACTS

Administer by controlled IV infusion, either by using a central venous line or by using a peripheral vein. The standard 24 mg/mL solution may be used without dilution when using a central venous catheter for infusion. When a peripheral vein catheter is used, dilute the 24 mg/mL solution to 12 mg/mL with 5% Dextrose in Water or with a normal saline solution prior to administration to avoid local irritation of peripheral veins. Since the dose is calculated on the basis of body weight, it may be desirable to remove and discard any unneeded quantity from the bottle before starting with the infusion to avoid overdosage. Use solutions thus prepared within 24 hours of first entry into a sealed bottle.

Do not exceed the recommended dosage, frequency, or infusion rates. All doses must be individualized for patient's renal function.

Induction treatment: The recommended initial dose for patients with normal renal function is 60 mg/kg, adjusted for individual patient's renal function, given IV at a constant rate over a minimum of 1 hour every 8 hours for 2 to 3 weeks depending on clinical response. An infusion pump must be used to control the rate of infusion. Adequate hydration is recommended to establish diuresis, both prior to and during treatment to minimize renal toxicity (see Warnings), provided there are no clinical contraindications.

Maintenance treatment: 90 to 120 mg/kg/day (individualized for renal function) given as an IV infusion over 2 hours. Because the superiority of the 120 mg/kg/day has not been established in controlled trials, and given the likely relationship of higher plasma foscarnet levels to toxicity, it is recommended that most patients be started on maintenance treatment with a dose of 90 mg/kg/day. Escalation to 120 mg/kg/day may be considered should early reinduction be required because of retinitis progression. Some patients who show excellent tolerance to foscarnet may benefit from initiation of maintenance treatment at 120 mg/kg/day earlier in their treatment. An infusion pump must be used to control the rate of infusion with all doses. Again, hydration to establish diuresis both prior to and during treatment is recommended to minimize renal toxicity.

Patients who experience progression of retinitis while receiving maintenance therapy may be retreated with the induction and maintenance regimens given above.

Renal function abnormalities: Use with caution in patients with abnormal renal function because reduced plasma clearance of foscarnet will result in elevated plasma levels. In addition, foscarnet has the potential to further impair renal function (see Warnings). Foscarnet has not been specifically studied in patients with Ccr < 50 mL/min or serum creatinine > 2.8 mg/dL. Carefully monitor renal function at baseline and during induction and maintenance therapy with appropriate dose adjustments. If Ccr falls below the limits of the dosing nomograms (0.4 mL/min/kg) during therapy, discontinue foscarnet and monitor the patient daily until resolution of renal impairment is ensured.

Dose adjustment in renal impairment: Individualize foscarnet dosing according to the patient's renal function status. Refer to the table below for recommended doses and adjust the dose as indicated.

To use this dosing guide, actual 24 hour Ccr (mL/min) must be divided by body weight (kg) or the estimated Ccr in mL/min/kg can be calculated from serum creatinine (mg/dL) using the following formula (modified Cockcroft and Gault equation).

$$\text{Males:} \quad \frac{\text{Weight (kg)} \times (140 - \text{age})}{72 \times \text{serum creatinine (mg/dL)}} = \text{Ccr}$$

Females: 0.85 × above value

ANTI-INFECTIVE AGENTS

Foscarnet Dosing Guide Based on Ccr	
Induction	
Ccr (mL/min/kg)	Equivalent to 60 mg/kg dose every 8 hours
≥ 1.6	60
1.5	57
1.4	53
1.3	49
1.2	46
1.1	42
1	39
0.9	35
0.8	32
0.7	28
0.6	25
0.5	21
0.4	18

Foscarnet Dosing Guide Based on Ccr		
Maintenance		
Ccr (mL/min/kg)	Equivalent to 90 mg/kg dose every 24 hours	Equivalent to 120 mg/kg dose every 24 hours
≥ 1.4	90	120
1.2-1.4	78	104
1-1.2	75	100
0.8-1	71	94
0.6-0.8	63	84
0.4-0.6	57	76

IV incompatibility: Other drugs and supplements can be administered to a patient receiving foscarnet. However, take care to ensure that foscarnet is only administered with normal saline or Dextrose Solution 5% and that no other drug or supplement is administered concurrently via the same catheter. Foscarnet is chemically incompatible with dextrose 30%, amphotericin B, and solutions containing calcium such as Ringer's Lactate and TPN. Physical incompatibility with other IV drugs includes: Acyclovir sodium, ganciclovir, trimetrexate, pentamidine, vancomycin, trimethoprim/ sulfamethoxazole, diazepam, midazolam, digoxin, phenytoin, leucovorin, and prochlorperazine. Because of foscarnet's chelating properties, a precipitate can potentially occur when divalent cations are administered concurrently in the same catheter.

Rx **Foscavir** (Astra)   **Injection:** 24 mg/mL   In 250 and 500 mL bottles.

CIDOFOVIR

Warning:

Renal impairment is the major toxicity of cidofovir. To minimize possible nephrotoxicity, IV prehydration with Normal Saline and administration of probenecid must be used with each cidofovir infusion. Monitor renal function (serum creatinine and urine protein) within 48 hours prior to each dose of cidofovir and modify the dose for changes in renal function as appropriate.

Granulocytopenia has been observed in association with cidofovir treatment. Monitor neutrophil counts during cidofovir therapy.

OPHTHALMIC DRUG FACTS

Actions:

Pharmacology: Cidofovir is a nucleotide analog. Cidofovir suppresses cytomegalovirus (CMV) replication by selective inhibition of viral DNA synthesis. Biochemical data support selective inhibition of CMV DNA polymerase by cidofovir diphosphate, the active intracellular metabolite of cidofovir. Cidofovir diphosphate inhibits herpes virus polymerases at concentrations that are 8- to 600-fold lower than those needed to inhibit human cellular DNA polymerases alpha, beta and gamma. Incorporation of cidofovir into the growing viral DNA results in reductions in the rate of viral DNA synthesis.

Resistance – CMV isolates with reduced susceptibility to cidofovir have been selected in vitro in the presence of high concentration of cidofovir. IC_{50} values for selected resistant isolates ranged from 7 to 15 mcg.

Cross-resistance – Cidofovir-resistant isolates selected in vitro following exposure to increasing concentrations of cidofovir were assessed for susceptibility to ganciclovir and foscarnet. All were cross-resistant to ganciclovir, but remained susceptible to foscarnet. Ganciclovir or ganciclovir/foscarnet-resistant isolates that are cross-resistant to cidofovir have been obtained from drug-naive patients and from patients following ganciclovir or ganciclovir/foscarnet therapy. To date, the majority of ganciclovir-resistant isolates are UL97 gene product (phosphokinase) mutants and remain susceptible to cidofovir. However, reduced susceptibility to cidofovir has been reported for DNA polymerase mutants of CMV that are resistant to ganciclovir. To date, all clinical isolates that exhibit high level resistance to ganciclovir, because of mutations in the DNA polymerase gene, have been shown to be cross-resistant to cidofovir. Cidofovir is active against some, but not all, CMV isolates that are resistant to foscarnet. The incidence of foscarnet-resistant isolates that are resistant to cidofovir is not known.

A few triple-drug resistant isolates have been described. Genotypic analysis of 2 of these triple-resistant isolates revealed several point mutations in the CMV DNA polymerase gene.

Pharmacokinetics: Cidofovir must be administered with probenecid. Renal tubular secretion contributes to the elimination of cidofovir.

Cidofovir Pharmacokinetic Parameters Following 3 and 5 mg/kg Infusions With and Without Probenecid				
	Cidofovir administered without probenecid		Cidofovir administered with probenecid	
Parameters	3 mg/kg	5 mg/kg	3 mg/kg	5 mg/kg
AUC (mcg•hr/mL)	20	28.3	25.7	40.8
C_{max} (end of infusion) (mcg/mL)	7.3	11.5	9.8	19.6
Vdss (mL/kg)	537		410	
Clearance (mL/min/1.73 m^2)	179		148	
Renal Clearance (mL/min/1.73 m^2)	150		98.6	

In vitro, cidofovir was < 6% bound to plasma or serum proteins over the cidofovir concentration range 0.25 to 25 mcg/mL. CSF concentrations of cidofovir following IV infusion of cidofovir 5 mg/kg with concomitant probenecid and IV hydration were undetectable (< 0.1 mcg/mL, assay detection threshold) at 15 minutes after the end of a 1 hour infusion in 1 patient whose corresponding serum concentration was 8.7 mcg/mL.

ANTI-INFECTIVE AGENTS

173

Clinical Trials:

Delayed vs immediate therapy – In an open-label trial, previously untreated patients with peripheral CMV retinitis were randomized to either immediate treatment with cidofovir (5 mg/kg once a week for 2 weeks, then 5 mg/kg every other week), or delayed cidofovir treatment until progression of CMV retinitis occurred. Of 25 and 23 patients in the immediate and delayed groups respectively, 23 and 21 were evaluable for retinitis progression as determined by retinal photography. Based on masked readings of retinal photographs, the median (95% confidence internal [CI]) times to retinitis progression were 120 days (40, 134) and 22 days (10, 27) for the immediate and delayed therapy groups, respectively. This difference was statistically significant. Median (95% CI) times to the alternative endpoint of retinitis progression or study drug discontinuation (including adverse events, withdrawn consent, and systemic CMV disease) were 52 days (37, 85) and 22 days (13, 27) for the immediate and delayed therapy groups, respectively. This difference was statistically significant.

Indications:

CMV retinitis: For the treatment of CMV retinitis in patients with acquired immunodeficiency syndrome (AIDS).

The safety and efficacy of cidofovir have not been established for treatment of other CMV infections (such as pneumonitis or gastroenteritis), congenital or neonatal CMV disease, or CMV disease in non-HIV-infected individuals.

Contraindications:

Hypersensitivity to cidofovir; a history of clinically severe hypersensitivity to probenecid or other sulfa-containing medications; direct intraocular injection. It also is contraindicated in patients receiving other nephrotoxic agents.

Warnings:

Direct intraocular injection: Direct intraocular injection may be associated with significant decreases in intraocular pressure and impairment of vision.

Nephrotoxicity: Dose-dependent nephrotoxicity is the major dose-limiting toxicity related to cidofovir administration. Dose adjustment or discontinuation is required for changes in renal function while on therapy. Proteinuria may be an early indicator of cidofovir-related nephrotoxicity. Continued administration of cidofovir may lead to additional proximal tubular cell injury that may result in glycosuria; decreases in serum phosphate, uric acid, and bicarbonate; and elevations in serum creatinine. Patients with these adverse events occurring concurrently and meeting a criteria of Fanconi's syndrome have been reported. Renal function may not return to baseline after drug discontinuation.

Hematological toxicity: Neutropenia may occur during cidofovir therapy. Monitor neutrophil count while receiving cidofovir therapy.

Metabolic acidosis: Fanconi syndrome and decreases in serum bicarbonate associated with evidence of renal tubular damage have been reported. Serious metabolic acidosis, in association with liver failure, pancreatitis, mucormycosis, aspergillus, disseminated mycobacterial infection, and progression to death occurred in 1 patient.

174 OPHTHALMIC DRUG FACTS

Ocular hypotony: Among the subset of patients monitored for intraocular pressure changes, ocular hypotony (≥ 50% change from baseline) was reported in 5 patients. Hypotony was reported in 1 patient with concomitant diabetes mellitus. Risk of ocular hypotony may be increased in patients with preexisting diabetes.

Renal function impairment: It is recommended that cidofovir not be initiated in patients with baseline serum creatinine > 1.5 mg/dL or creatinine clearances ≤ 55 mL/min. In these patients, use cidofovir when the potential benefits exceed the potential risks.

Carcinogenesis: Mammary adenocarcinomas have occurred in rats and mice, and Zymbal's gland carcinomas have occurred in rats. Studies showed inhibition of spermatogenesis in rats and monkeys. However, no adverse effects on fertility or reproduction were seen following once weekly IV injections of cidofovir in male rats for 13 consecutive weeks.

Elderly: No studies of the safety and efficacy of cidofovir in patients > 60 years of age have been conducted. Because elderly individuals frequently have reduced glomerular filtration, pay particular attention to assessing renal function before and during cidofovir administration.

Pregnancy: Category C. Cidofovir was embryotoxic (reduced fetal body weights) in rats and in rabbits. An increased incidence of fetal external, soft tissue, and skeletal anomalies (eg, meningocele, short snout, short maxillary bones) occurred in rabbits. There are no adequate and well-controlled studies in pregnant women. Use cidofovir during pregnancy only if potential benefit to the mother justifies the potential risk to the fetus.

Lactation: It is not known whether cidofovir is excreted in breast milk. Since many drugs are excreted in breast milk and because of the potential for adverse reactions as well as the potential for tumorigenicity shown for cidofovir in animal studies, do not administer cidofovir to nursing women. The US Public Health Service Centers for Disease Control and Prevention advises HIV-infected women not to breastfeed and to avoid postnatal transmission of HIV to a child who may not yet be infected.

Children: Safety and effectiveness in children have not been studied. The use of cidofovir in children with AIDS warrants extreme caution due to the risk of long-term carcinogenicity and reproductive toxicity. Administer cidofovir to children only after careful evaluation and only if the potential benefits of treatment outweigh the risks.

Precautions:

Monitoring: Monitor serum creatinine, urine protein and white blood cell counts with differential prior to each dose. In patients with proteinuria, administer IV hydration and repeat the test. Periodically monitor intraocular pressure, visual acuity, and ocular symptoms.

Drug Interactions:

Nephrotoxic agents: Avoid concomitant administration of cidofovir and agents with nephrotoxic potential (eg, amphotericin B, aminoglycosides, foscarnet, IV pentamidine).

Adverse Reactions:

Cardiovascular: Hypotension; postural hypotension; pallor; syncope; tachycardia.

ANTI-INFECTIVE AGENTS

CNS: Headache (27%); asthenia (46%); amnesia; anxiety; confusion; convulsion; depression; dizziness; abnormal gait; hallucinations; insomnia; neuropathy; paresthesia; somnolence; vasodilation.

Dermatologic: Alopecia (25%); rash (30%); acne; skin discoloration; dry skin; herpes simplex; pruritus; rash; sweating; urticaria.

GI: Nausea, vomiting (65%); diarrhea (27%); anorexia (22%); abdominal pain (17%); colitis; constipation; tongue discoloration; dyspepsia; dysphagia; flatulence; gastritis; hepatomegaly; abnormal liver function tests; melena; oral candidiasis; rectal disorder; stomatitis; aphthous stomatitis; mouth ulceration; dry mouth.

GU: Decreased creatinine clearance; glycosuria; hematuria; urinary incontinence; urinary tract infection.

Hematologic/Lymphatic: Thrombocytopenia; neutropenia (< 750/mm^3; 31%); anemia (20%).

Metabolic/Nutritional: Edema; dehydration; hyperglycemia; hyperlipemia; hypocalcemia; hypokalemia; increased alkaline phosphatase; increased SGOT; increased SGPT; weight loss.

Musculoskeletal: Arthralgia; myasthenia; myalgia.

Renal: Renal toxicity (53%); proteinuria (80%); serum creatinine elevations (29%) (see Warnings).

Respiratory: Asthma; bronchitis; coughing; dyspnea (22%); hiccough; increased sputum; lung disorder; pharyngitis; pneumonia (9%); rhinitis; sinusitis.

Special senses: Amblyopia; conjunctivitis; eye disorder; hypotony (12%) (see Warnings); iritis; retinal detachment; taste perversion; uveitis; abnormal vision.

Miscellaneous: Fever (57%); infections (24%); chills (24%); allergic reaction; face edema; malaise; back, chest, neck pain; sarcoma; sepsis.

Overdosage:

Overdosage with cidofovir has not been reported; however, hemodialysis and hydration may reduce drug plasma concentrations in patients who receive an overdosage of cidofovir. Probenecid may reduce the potential for nephrotoxicity in patients who receive an overdose of cidofovir through reduction of active tubular secretion.

Patient Information:

Advise patients that cidofovir is not a cure for CMV retinitis, and that they may continue to experience progression of retinitis during and following treatment. Advise patients receiving cidofovir to have regular follow-up ophthalmologic examinations. Patients may also experience other manifestations of CMV disease despite cidofovir therapy.

HIV-infected patients may continue taking antiretroviral therapy. However, because probenecid reduces metabolic clearance of zidovudine, advise those taking zidovudine to temporarily discontinue zidovudine administration or decrease their zidovudine dose by 50% on days of cidofovir administration only.

176 OPHTHALMIC DRUG FACTS

Inform patients of the major toxicity of cidofovir, namely renal impairment, and that dose modification, including reduction, interruption, and possibly discontinuation, may be required. Emphasize close monitoring of renal function (routine urinalysis and serum creatinine) while on therapy.

Emphasize the importance of completing a full course of probenecid with each cidofovir dose. Warn patients of potential adverse events caused by probenecid (eg, headache, nausea, vomiting, hypersensitivity reactions). Hypersensitivity/allergic reactions may include rash, fever, chills and anaphylaxis. Administration of probenecid after a meal or use of antiemetics may decrease the nausea. Prophylactic or therapeutic antihistamines or acetaminophen may be used to ameliorate hypersensitivity reactions.

Cidofovir caused reduced testes weight and hypospermia in animals. Such changes may occur in humans and cause infertility. Advise women of childbearing potential that cidofovir is embryotoxic in animals and not to use the drug during pregnancy. Women of childbearing potential should use effective contraception during and for 1 month following treatment. Men should practice barrier contraceptive methods during and for 3 months following treatment.

Administration and Dosage:

Do not administer by intraocular injection.

Dosage: The recommended dosage, frequency, or infusion rate must not be exceeded. Cidofovir must be diluted in 0.9% Saline Solution 100 mL prior to administration. To minimize potential nephrotoxicity, probenecid and IV saline prehydration must be administered with each cidofovir infusion.

Induction treatment: The recommended dose of cidofovir is 5 mg/kg body weight (given as an IV infusion at a constant rate over 1 hour) administered once weekly for 2 consecutive weeks.

Maintenance treatment: The recommended maintenance dose of cidofovir is 5 mg/kg body weight (given as an IV infusion at a constant rate over 1 hour) administered once every 2 weeks.

Probenecid: Probenecid must be administered orally with each cidofovir dose. Two grams must be administered 3 hours prior to the cidofovir dose, and > 1 g administered at 2 hours and again at 8 hours after completion of the 1 hour cidofovir infusion (for a total of 4 g).

Ingestion of food prior to each dose of probenecid may reduce drug-related nausea and vomiting. Administration of an antiemetic may reduce the potential for nausea associated with probenecid ingestion. In patients who develop allergic or hypersensitivity symptoms to probenecid, consider the use of an appropriate prophylactic or therapeutic antihistamine or acetaminophen.

Hydration: Patients should receive a total of 1 L of 0.9% Saline Solution IV with each infusion of cidofovir. Infuse the saline solution over a 1- to 2-hour period immediately before the cidofovir infusion. Patients who can tolerate the additional fluid load should receive a second liter. If administered, initiate the second liter of saline at the start of the cidofovir infusion or immediately afterwards, and infuse over a 1- to 3-hour period.

Nephrotoxicity: For increases in serum creatinine (0.3 to 0.4 mg/dL), reduce the cidofovir dose from 5 mg/kg to 3 mg/kg. Discontinue cidofovir therapy for an increase in serum creatinine of ≥ 0.5 mg/dL or development of ≥ 3+ proteinuria.

ANTI-INFECTIVE AGENTS 177

Renal function impairment:

Dosing of Cidofovir with Renal Function Impairment		
Creatinine Clearance (mL/min)	Induction (once weekly for 2 weeks)	Maintenance (once every 2 weeks)
41 - 55	2 mg/kg	2 mg/kg
30 - 40	1.5 mg/kg	1.5 mg/kg
20-29	1 mg/kg	1 mg/kg
≤ 19	0.5 mg/kg	0.5 mg/kg

Storage/Stability: Store at controlled room temperature 20° to 25°C (68° to 77°F).

Admixtures may be stored under refrigeration (2° to 8°C; 36° to 46°F) for ≤ 24 hours. Allow refrigerated admixtures to equilibrate to room temperature prior to use.

Rx	**Vistide** (Gilead Sciences)	**Injection:** 75 mg/mL	In 5 mL amps.

AGENTS FOR GLAUCOMA

Glaucoma is a condition of the eye in which there is often an elevation of the intraocular pressure (IOP) that leads to progressive cupping and atrophy of the optic nerve head, deterioration of the visual fields, and ultimately to blindness. *Primary open-angle glaucoma* is the most common type of glaucoma. *Angle-closure glaucoma* and *congenital glaucoma* are treated primarily by surgical methods, although short-term drug therapy is used to decrease IOP prior to surgery.

Drugs used in the therapy of primary open-angle glaucoma include a variety of agents with different mechanisms of action. The therapeutic goal in treating glaucoma is reducing the IOP, a major risk factor in the pathogenesis of glaucomatous visual field loss. The higher the level of IOP, the greater the likelihood of optic nerve damage and glaucomatous visual field loss. Reduction of IOP may be accomplished by: 1) decreasing the rate of production of aqueous humor or 2) increasing the rate of outflow (drainage) of aqueous humor from the eye.

The seven groups of agents used in the therapy of primary open-angle glaucoma are listed in Table 1: Agents for Glaucoma, which summarizes their mechanism of decreasing IOP, effects on pupil size and ciliary muscle, and duration of action.

EPINEPHRINES

Epinephrine (eg, *Epifrin*) and dipivefrin (*Propine*) have both α and β activity. They lower IOP mainly by increasing aqueous outflow. Epinephrine, usually used as an adjunct to miotic or beta blocker therapy, may also be used as primary therapy. The combination of a miotic and a sympathomimetic (eg, epinephrine) will have additive effects in lowering IOP.

Dipivefrin HCl is a prodrug metabolized to epinephrine in vivo. The IOP-lowering and intraocular effects are qualitatively and quantitatively similar to epinephrine; however, dipivefrin may be better tolerated and have a lower incidence of adverse effects because of its lower concentration.

OPHTHALMIC DRUG FACTS

Table 1: Agents for Glaucoma						
Drug	Strength	Duration (hrs)	Decrease aqueous production	Increase aqueous outflow	Effect on pupil	Effect on ciliary muscle
Epinephrines						
Epinephrine	0.1%-2%	12	+	++	mydriasis	NR
Dipivefrin	0.1%	12	+	++	mydriasis	NR
Alpha-2 Adrenergic Agonists						
Apraclonidine	0.5%-1%	7-12	+++	NR	NR	NR
Brimonidine	0.2%	6-8	++	++	NR	NR
Beta Blockers						
Betaxolol	0.25%-0.5%	12	+++	NR	NR	NR
Carteolol	1%	12	+++	nd	NR	NR
Levobunolol	0.25%-0.5%	12-24	+++	NR	NR	NR
Metipranolol	0.3%	12-24	+++	NR	NR	NR
Timolol	0.25%-0.5%	12-24	+++	NR	NR	NR
Miotics, Direct-Acting						
Carbachol[1]	0.75%-3%	6-8	NR	+++	miosis	accommodation
Pilocarpine[2]	0.25%-10%	4-8	NR	+++	miosis	accommodation
Miotics, Cholinesterase Inhibitors						
Physostigmine	0.25%-0.5%	12-36	NR	+++	miosis	accommodation
Demecarium	0.125%-0.25%	days/wks	NR	+++	miosis	accommodation
Echothiophate	0.03%-0.25%	days/wks	NR	+++	miosis	accommodation
Carbonic Anhydrase Inhibitors						
Acetazolamide[3]	125-500 mg	8-12	+++	NR	NR	NR
Brinzolamide [4]	1%	≈ 8	+++	NR	NR	NR
Dichlorphenamide[3]	50 mg	6-12	+++	NR	NR	NR
Dorzolamide[4]	2%	≈ 8	+++	NR	NR	NR
Methazolamide[3]	25-50 mg	10-18	+++	NR	NR	NR
Prostaglandins and Prostamide						
Latanoprost	0.005%	24	NR	+++	NR	NR
Bimatoprost	0.03%	24	NR	+++	NR	N
Travoprost	0.004%	24	NR	+++	NR	N

+++ = Significant activity.
++ = Moderate activity.
+ = Some activity.
NR = No activity reported.
nd = No data available.
[1] Available as intraocular administration during surgery; carbachol also available as a topical agent.
[2] Also available as a gel and an insert; the duration of these doseforms is longer (18 to 24 hours and 1 week, respectively) than the solution.
[3] Systemic agents.
[4] Topical ophthalmic agent.

ALPHA-2 ADRENERGIC AGONISTS

Alpha-2 adrenergic agonists (apraclonidine [*Iopidine*] and brimonidine [*Alphagan*]) are relatively new to the treatment of glaucoma. Apraclonidine is used primarily before or after laser surgery to control or prevent postsurgical elevations of IOP and as short-term adjunctive therapy for patients requiring additional IOP reduction. Approximately 30% of patients on apraclonidine developed an allergic response. Also, the drug loses its effectiveness in ≈ 40% of patients after 2 to 3 months of chronic use. Brimonidine, the newer alpha-2 agonist, seems to have a much lower allergic response associated with it and is much more successful as chronic therapy for most patients.

AGENTS FOR GLAUCOMA

BETA-ADRENERGIC BLOCKING AGENTS

Beta-adrenergic blocking agents (eg, betaxolol [*Betoptic*], carteolol [*Ocupress*], levo-bunolol [eg, *Betagan Liquifilm*], metipranolol [*OptiPranolol*], timolol [eg, *Betimol, Timoptic*]) may be used alone or in conjunction with other agents. They may be more effective than either pilocarpine or epinephrine alone and have the advantage of not affecting either pupil size or accommodation. They lower IOP by decreasing the rate of aqueous production.

DIRECT-ACTING MIOTICS

Direct-acting miotics, (eg, carbachol [eg, *Isopto Carbachol*], pilocarpine [eg, *Isopto Carpine*]) were considered the first step in glaucoma therapy. They have now yielded to the β-blockers and other ocular hypotensive agents. They are useful adjunctive agents that are additive to either the β-blockers, carbonic anhydrase inhibitors, or the sympathomimetics. Dosage and frequency of administration must be individualized. Study data indicate pilocarpine 2% and carbachol 1.5% every 12 hours with naso-lacrimal occlusion (NLO) provide maximum effect. Increasing the concentration and dosage intervals may correct an inadequate response. Concentrations greater than pilocarpine 4% or carbachol 3% are occasionally required in patients with darkly pigmented irides.

CHOLINESTERASE INHIBITOR MIOTICS

Cholinesterase inhibitor miotics include both reversible/short-acting (physostigmine, demecarium [*Humorsol*]), and irreversible/long-acting (echothiophate [*Phospholine Iodide*]) agents, which enhance the effects of endogenous acetylcholine by inactivation of the enzyme acetylcholinesterase. These agents are more potent and longer acting than the direct-acting cholinergic agents. Side effects and systemic toxicity are more common and of greater significance. Using a direct-acting cholinergic and a cholinesterase inhibitor provides no improvement in response.

CARBONIC ANHYDRASE INHIBITORS

Carbonic anhydrase inhibitors (eg, acetazolamide [eg, *Diamox*], dichlorphenamide [*Daranide*], methazolamide [eg, *Neptazane*]) are administered systemically. Dorzol-amide (*Trusopt*) and brinzolamide (*Azopt*) are administered topically. IOP is lowered by a direct action on the ciliary epithelium to suppress the secretion of aqueous humor (inflow). Carbonic anhydrase inhibitors are often used as adjunctive therapy.

HYPEROSMOTIC AGENTS

Hyperosmotic agents (eg, mannitol [eg, *Osmitrol*]), urea [*Ureaphil*], glycerin [*Osmo-glyn*], isosorbide [*Ismotic*]) are useful in lowering IOP in acute situations (see the Hyperosmotic Agents chapter). These agents lower IOP by creating an osmotic gradient between the ocular fluids and plasma. These agents are not for chronic use.

PROSTAGLANDINS AND PROSTAMIDES

Although it has been long recognized that prostaglandins have IOP-lowering effects, side effects such as ocular redness, stinging, and burning discouraged use of this drug class as chronic treatment for glaucoma. The prostaglandin analog latanoprost (*Xalatan*) appears to be fairly well tolerated with a similar side effect profile of timo-lol in regard to ocular redness, stinging, and burning. However, latanoprost does

OPHTHALMIC DRUG FACTS

change the iris color in some patients after chronic use. Yellow-blue, yellow-green, and blue-gray irises appear to be most susceptible to color change.

Consequently, this drug is approved only as adjunctive therapy. It is as effective or more effective than the beta blockers for lowering IOP and appears to be an acceptable additive with most ocular hypotensive agents. Travoprost has similar effects as latanoprost. Bimatoprost works on aqueous humor outflow through the uveoscleral and trabecular meshwork pathways.

Thom J. Zimmerman, MD, PhD
University of Louisville

For More Information

Bartlett JD, Jaanus SD, eds. *Clinical Ocular Pharmacology*, ed. 3. Boston: Butterworth-Heinemann, 1995.

Becker B, Shaffer RN. *Diagnosis and Therapy of the Glaucomas*, ed. 4. St. Louis: C.V. Mosby Co., 1987.

Chandler PA, Grant WM. *Lectures on Glaucoma*. Philadelphia: Lea & Febiger, 1965.

Duane TD, ed. *Clinical Ophthalmology*. Philadelphia: Lippincott-Raven, 1997.

Zimmerman TJ, ed. *Textbook of Ocular Pharmacology*. Philadelphia: Lippincott-Raven, 1997.

AGENTS FOR GLAUCOMA

EPINEPHRINES

Actions:

Pharmacology: Epinephrine, a direct-acting sympathomimetic agent, acts on α and β receptors. Topical application, therefore, causes conjunctival decongestion (vasoconstriction), transient mydriasis (pupillary dilation), and reduction in intraocular pressure (IOP). It is believed IOP reduction is primarily caused by increased aqueous outflow. The duration of decrease in IOP is 12 to 24 hours.

Epinephrine is available as the bitartrate hydrochloride and borate salts. These preparations are therapeutically equal when given in equivalent doses of epinephrine base.

Indications:

Glaucoma: Management of open-angle (chronic simple) glaucoma; may be used in combination with miotics, beta blockers (not usually additive), hyperosmotic agents, or carbonic anhydrase inhibitors.

Contraindications:

Hypersensitivity to epinephrine or any component of the formulation; narrow- or angle-closure glaucoma; aphakia; patients with a narrow angle but no glaucoma; if the nature of the glaucoma is not clearly established. Do not use while wearing soft contact lenses; discoloration of lenses may occur.

Warnings:

For ophthalmic use only: Not for injection or intraocular use.

Gonioscopy: Because pupil dilation may precipitate an acute attack of angle-closure glaucoma, evaluate anterior chamber angle by gonioscopy prior to beginning therapy.

Anesthesia: Discontinue use prior to general anesthesia with anesthetics that sensitize the myocardium to sympathomimetics (eg, cyclopropane, halothane).

Aphakic patients: Maculopathy with associated decrease in visual acuity may occur in the aphakic eye; if this occurs, promptly discontinue use.

Elderly: Use with caution.

Pregnancy: Category C. Safety for use during pregnancy has not been established. Use only when clearly needed.

Lactation: It is not known whether this drug is excreted in breast milk. Exercise caution when administering to a nursing woman.

Children: Safety and efficacy for use in children have not been established.

Precautions:

Instillation discomfort: Epinephrine is relatively uncomfortable upon instillation. Discomfort lessens as concentration of epinephrine decreases.

184 OPHTHALMIC DRUG FACTS

Special risk patients: Use with caution in the presence of or history of hypertension, diabetes, hyperthyroidism, heart disease, cerebral arteriosclerosis, or bronchial asthma.

Hazardous tasks: Epinephrine may cause temporarily blurred or unstable vision after instillation; observe caution while driving, operating machinery, or performing other tasks requiring coordination or physical dexterity.

Sulfite sensitivity: Some of these products contain sulfites which may cause allergic-type reactions (eg, hives, itching, wheezing, anaphylaxis) in certain susceptible persons. Although the overall prevalence of sulfite sensitivity in the general population is probably low, it is seen more frequently in asthmatics or atopic nonasthmatics.

Drug Interactions:

Beta-adrenergic blockers, nonselective: Nonselective beta-adrenergic blockers administered concomitantly with epinephrine may block the ocular hypotensive effects of epinephrine.

Bretylium: Bretylium may potentiate the action of vasopressors on adrenergic receptors, possibly resulting in arrhythmias.

Guanethidine: Guanethidine may increase the pressor response of the direct-acting vasopressors, possibly resulting in severe hypertension.

Halogenated hydrocarbon anesthetics: Halogenated hydrocarbon anesthetics may sensitize the myocardium to the effects of catecholamines. Use of vasopressors may lead to serious arrhythmias; use with extreme caution.

Oxytocic drugs: In obstetrics, if vasopressor drugs are used to correct hypotension or added to the local anesthetic solution, some oxytocic drugs may cause severe persistent hypertension.

Tricyclic antidepressants: The pressor response of the direct-acting vasopressors may be potentiated by these agents; use with caution.

Drug/Lab test interactions: After prolonged use or epinephrine overdosage, elevated serum lactic acid levels with severe metabolic acidosis may occur. Transient elevations of blood glucose may be associated with epinephrine administration.

Adverse Reactions:

Local: Transient stinging and burning; eye pain/ache; browache; headache; allergic lid reaction; conjunctival hyperemia; conjunctival or corneal pigmentation; ocular irritation (hypersensitivity); localized adrenochrome deposits in conjunctiva and cornea (prolonged use); cystoid macular edema may result from use in aphakic patients.

Systemic: Headache; palpitations; tachycardia; extrasystoles; cardiac arrhythmia; hypertension; faintness.

Overdosage:

If ocular overdosage occurs, flush eye(s) with water or normal saline.

AGENTS FOR GLAUCOMA

Patient Information:

To avoid contamination, do not touch tip of container to any surface. Replace cap after using.

Do not use if solution is brown or contains a precipitate.

Do not use while wearing soft contact lenses.

Transitory stinging may occur upon initial instillation. Headache or browache may occur.

Patients should immediately report any decrease in visual acuity.

Refer to the Dosage Forms and Routes of Administration chapter for more complete information.

Administration and Dosage:

Instill 1 drop into affected eye(s) twice daily.

More frequent instillation than 1 drop twice daily does not usually elicit any further improvement in therapeutic response.

When used in conjunction with miotics, instill the miotic last.

Storage: Store at 2° to 24°C (36° to 75°F). Keep container tightly sealed. Protect solution from light; store in cool place. Do not freeze. Discard if solution becomes discolored or contains a precipitate.

EPINEPHRINE HYDROCHLORIDE

Rx	Epifrin (Allergan)	Solution: 0.5% (as base)	In 15 mL dropper bottles.[1]
Rx	Epifrin (Allergan)	Solution: 1% (as base)	In 15 mL dropper bottles.[1]
Rx	Glaucon (Alcon)	Solution: 1%	In 10 mL Drop-Tainers.[2]
Rx	Epifrin (Allergan)	Solution: 2% (as base)	In 15 mL dropper bottles.[1]
Rx	Glaucon (Alcon)	Solution: 2%	In 10 mL Drop-Tainers.[2]

[1] With benzalkonium chloride, sodium metabisulfite, EDTA, hydrochloric acid.
[2] With 0.01% benzalkonium chloride, sodium metabisulfite, EDTA, sodium chloride, hydrochloric acid, sodium hydroxide.

EPINEPHRYL BORATE

Rx	Epinal (Alcon)	Solution: 0.5%	In 7.5 mL.[1]
		1%	In 7.5 mL.[1]

[1] With 0.01% benzalkonium chloride, ascorbic acid, acetylcysteine, boric acid, sodium carbonate.

DIPIVEFRIN HYDROCHLORIDE (Dipivalyl epinephrine)

Refer to the Agents for Glaucoma introduction for a general discussion of these products.

OPHTHALMIC DRUG FACTS

Actions:

Pharmacology: Dipivefrin is a prodrug of epinephrine formed by diesterification of epinephrine and pivalic acid, enhancing its lipophilic character and, consequently, penetrating the anterior chamber. Corneal penetration is ≈ 17 times that of epinephrine. Dipivefrin, converted to epinephrine in the eye by enzymatic hydrolysis, appears to act by enhancing outflow facility. It has the same therapeutic effects as epinephrine with fewer local and systemic side effects.

Dipivefrin does not produce the miosis or accommodative spasm that cholinergic agents produce. The blurred vision and night blindness often associated with miotic agents do not occur with dipivefrin. In patients with cataracts, the inability to see around lenticular opacities caused by constricted pupil is avoided.

Pharmacokinetics: The onset of action with 1 drop occurs ≈ 30 minutes after treatment, with maximum effect seen at ≈ 1 hour.

Clinical Trials: In patients with a history of epinephrine intolerance, only 3% of dipivefrin-treated patients exhibited intolerance, while 55% treated with epinephrine again developed an intolerance. Response to dipivefrin twice daily is less than that to 2% epinephrine twice daily and comparable to 2% pilocarpine 4 times daily. Patients using dipivefrin twice daily had mean IOP reductions ranging from 20% to 24%.

Indications:

Glaucoma: Initial therapy or as an adjunct with other antiglaucoma agents for the control of IOP in chronic open-angle glaucoma.

Contraindications:

Hypersensitivity to dipivefrin or any formulation component; narrow-angles (any dilation of pupil may predispose patient to an attack of angle-closure glaucoma).

Warnings:

Pregnancy: Category B. There are no adequate and well-controlled studies in pregnant women. Use only when clearly needed.

Lactation: It is not known whether this drug is excreted in breast milk. Use caution in nursing mothers.

Children: Safety and efficacy for use in children have not been established.

Precautions:

Aphakic patients: Macular edema occurs in up to 30% of aphakic patients treated with epinephrine. Discontinuation generally results in reversal of the maculopathy.

Adverse Reactions:

Cardiovascular: Tachycardia; arrhythmias; hypertension (reported with epinephrine).

AGENTS FOR GLAUCOMA

Local: Burning and stinging (6%); conjunctival injection (6.5%); follicular conjunctivitis; mydriasis; allergic reactions (infrequent). Epinephrine therapy can lead to adrenochrome deposits in the conjunctiva and cornea.

Dipivefrin 0.1% is less irritating than 1% epinephrine HCl. Only 1.8% of dipivefrin patients reported discomfort from photophobia, glare, or light sensitivity.

Patient Information:

Slight stinging or burning on initial instillation may occur.

Do not try to "catch up" on missed doses by applying > 1 dose at a time.

Administration and Dosage:

Initial glaucoma therapy: Instill 1 drop into the eye(s) every 12 hours.

Concomitant therapy: When patients receiving other antiglaucoma agents require additional therapy, add 1 drop of dipivefrin every 12 hours.

Rx	**Dipivefrin HCl** (Falcon)	**Solution:** 0.1%	In 5, 10, and 15 mL.
Rx	**Propine** (Allergan)		In 5, 10, and 15 mL C Cap Compliance Cap B.I.D.[1]

[1] With 0.005% benzalkonium chloride, sodium chloride, EDTA, hydrochloric acid.

ALPHA$_2$-ADRENERGIC AGONISTS

APRACLONIDINE HYDROCHLORIDE

Actions:

Pharmacology: Apraclonidine has the action of reducing elevated, as well as normal, intraocular pressure (IOP) whether accompanied by glaucoma or not. Apraclonidine is a relatively selective α_2-adrenergic agonist that does not have significant membrane stabilizing (local anesthetic) activity. Topical application of apraclonidine reduces IOP and has minimal effect on cardiovascular parameters.

Optic nerve head damage and visual field loss may result from an acute elevation in IOP that can occur after argon laser surgical procedures. The higher the peak or spike of IOP, the greater the likelihood of visual field loss and optic nerve damage, especially in patients with previously compromised optic nerves. The onset of action is usually within 1 hour and the maximum IOP reduction occurs 3 to 5 hours after application of a single dose. Apraclonidine's mechanism of action is not completely established, although its predominant action may be related to a reduction of aqueous formation via stimulation of the alpha-adrenergic system.

Pharmacokinetics: Topical use of apraclonidine 0.5% leads to systemic absorption. Studies of apraclonidine ophthalmic solution 1 drop 3 times daily in both eyes for 10 days in healthy volunteers yielded mean peak and trough concentrations of 0.9 and 0.5 ng/mL, respectively. The half-life of apraclonidine 0.5% was calculated to be 8 hours.

188 OPHTHALMIC DRUG FACTS

Clinical Trials: The clinical utility of apraclonidine 0.5% is most apparent for those glaucoma patients on maximally tolerated medical therapy (ie, patients using combinations of a topical beta blocker, sympathomimetics, parasympathomimetics, oral carbonic anhydrase inhibitors). Patients with advanced glaucoma and uncontrolled IOP scheduled to undergo laser trabeculoplasty or trabeculectomy surgery were enrolled in a study to determine whether apraclonidine dosed 3 times daily could delay the need for surgery for ≤ 3 months. Apraclonidine treatment resulted in a significantly greater percentage of treatment successes compared with patients treated with placebo.

Indications:

1%: To control or prevent postsurgical elevations in IOP that occur in patients after argon laser trabeculoplasty or iridotomy.

0.5%: Short-term adjunctive therapy in patients on tolerated maximal medical therapy who require additional IOP reduction.

Contraindications:

Hypersensitivity to any component of this medication or to clonidine; concurrent monoamine oxidase inhibitor therapy (see Drug Interactions).

Warnings:

Concomitant therapy: The addition of apraclonidine 0.5% to patients already using 2 aqueous-suppressing drugs (eg, beta blocker plus carbonic anhydrase inhibitor) as part of their medical therapy may not provide additional benefit. This is because apraclonidine is an aqueous-suppressing drug and the addition of a third aqueous suppressant may not significantly reduce IOP.

Tachyphylaxis: The IOP-lowering efficacy of apraclonidine 0.5% diminishes over time in some patients. This loss of effect, or tachyphylaxis, appears to be an individual occurrence with a variable time of onset and should be closely monitored. The benefit for most patients is < 3 months.

Hypersensitivity: Apraclonidine can lead to an allergic-like reaction characterized wholly or in part by the symptoms of hyperemia, pruritus, discomfort, tearing, foreign body sensation, and edema of the lids and conjunctiva. If ocular allergic-like symptoms occur, discontinue therapy.

Renal/Hepatic function impairment: Although the topical use of apraclonidine has not been studied in renal failure patients, structurally related clonidine undergoes a significant increase in half-life in patients with severe renal impairment. Close monitoring of cardiovascular parameters in patients with impaired renal function is advised if they are candidates for topical apraclonidine therapy. Close monitoring of cardiovascular parameters in patients with impaired liver function is also advised as the systemic dosage form of clonidine is partly metabolized in the liver.

Pregnancy: Category C. Apraclonidine has an embryocidal effect in rabbits when given in an oral dose of 3 mg/kg (60 times the maximum recommended human dose). There are no adequate and well controlled studies in pregnant women. Use during pregnancy only if the potential benefit to the mother justifies the potential risk to the fetus.

AGENTS FOR GLAUCOMA

Lactation: It is not known if topically applied apraclonidine is excreted in breast milk. Exercise caution when apraclonidine is administered to a nursing woman. Consider discontinuing nursing for the day(s) on which apraclonidine is used.

Children: Safety and efficacy for use in children have not been established.

Precautions:

Monitoring: Glaucoma patients on tolerated maximal medical therapy who are treated with apraclonidine 0.5% to delay surgery should have their visual fields monitored periodically. Discontinue treatment if IOP rises significantly or is not lowered.

IOP reduction: Apraclonidine is a potent depressor of IOP. An unpredictable decrease of IOP effect in some patients and incidence of ocular allergic responses and systemic side effects may limit the utility of apraclonidine 0.5%. However, patients on tolerated maximal medical therapy may still benefit from the additional IOP reduction provided by the short-term use of apraclonidine 0.5%.

Cardiovascular disease: Acute administration of apraclonidine has had minimal effect on heart rate or blood pressure; however, observe caution in treating patients with severe cardiovascular disease.

Use apraclonidine 0.5% with caution in patients with coronary insufficiency, recent myocardial infarction, cerebrovascular disease, chronic renal failure, Raynaud's disease, or thromboangiitis obliterans.

Depression: Caution and monitor depressed patients; apraclonidine has been infrequently associated with causing depression or worsening existing depression.

Vasovagal attack: Consider the possibility of a vasovagal attack occurring during laser surgery; use caution in patients with a history of such episodes.

Corneal changes: Topical ocular administration of apraclonidine 1.5% to rabbits 3 times daily for 1 month resulted in sporadic and transient instances of minimal corneal cloudiness. No corneal changes were observed in humans given ≥ 1 dose of apraclonidine 1%.

Drug Interactions:

Apraclonidine Drug Interactions			
Precipitant drug	Object drug*		Description
Apraclonidine	Cardiovascular agents	↓	Because apraclonidine may reduce pulse and blood pressure, caution in using cardiovascular drugs is advised. Patients using cardiovascular drugs concurrently with apraclonidine 0.5% should have pulse and blood pressures frequently monitored.
Apraclonidine	MAO inhibitors	↑	Apraclonidine should not be used in patients receiving MAO inhibitors (see Contraindications).

* ↑ = Object drug increased. ↓ = Object drug decreased.

Adverse Reactions:

In clinical studies, the overall discontinuation rate related to apraclonidine was 15%. The most commonly reported events leading to discontinuation included (in decreasing order of frequency): Hyperemia; pruritus; tearing; discomfort; lid edema; dry mouth; foreign body sensation.

190   OPHTHALMIC DRUG FACTS

The following adverse effects were reported with the use of apraclonidine in laser surgery: Upper lid elevation (1.3%); conjunctival blanching (0.4%); mydriasis (0.4%).

The following additional adverse effects were reported (listed by solution strength):

Cardiovascular:

1% – Bradycardia; vasovagal attack; palpitations; orthostatic episode.

0.5% – Asthenia (< 3%); peripheral edema, arrhythmia (< 1%). Although there are no reports of bradycardia, consider the possibility.

CNS:

1% – Insomnia; dream disturbances; irritability; decreased libido; headache; paresthesia.

0.5% – Headache (< 3%); somnolence, dizziness, nervousness, depression, insomnia, paresthesia (< 1%).

Hypersensitivity: Use can lead to an allergic-like reaction (see Warnings).

GI:

1% – Abdominal pain; diarrhea; stomach discomfort; emesis; dry mouth.

0.5% – Dry mouth (2%); constipation, nausea (< 1%).

Ophthalmic:

1% – Conjunctival blanching; upper lid elevation; mydriasis; burning; discomfort; foreign body sensation; dryness; itching; hypotony; blurred or dimmed vision; allergic response; conjunctival microhemorrhage.

0.5% – Hyperemia (13%); pruritus (10%); discomfort (6%); tearing (4%); lid edema, blurred vision, foreign body sensation, dry eye, conjunctivitis, discharge, blanching (< 3%); lid margin crusting, conjunctival follicles, conjunctival edema, edema, abnormal vision, pain, lid disorder, keratitis, blepharitis, photophobia, corneal staining, lid erythema, blepharoconjunctivitis, irritation, corneal erosion, corneal infiltrate, keratopathy, lid scales, lid retraction (< 1%).

Respiratory:

0.5% – Dry nose (2%); rhinitis, dyspnea, pharyngitis, asthma (< 1%).

Miscellaneous:

1% – Taste abnormalities; nasal burning or dryness; head cold sensation; chest heaviness or burning; clammy or sweaty palms; body heat sensation; shortness of breath; increased pharyngeal secretion; extremity pain or numbness; fatigue; pruritus not associated with rash.

0.5% – Taste perversion (3%); contact dermatitis, dermatitis, chest pain, abnormal coordination, malaise, facial edema (< 1%); myalgia, parosmia (0.2%).

Patient Information:

Do not touch dropper tip to any surface as this may contaminate the contents.

AGENTS FOR GLAUCOMA

Apraclonidine can cause dizziness and somnolence. Patients who engage in hazardous activities requiring mental alertness should be warned of the potential for a decrease in mental alertness, physical dexterity, or coordination while using apraclonidine.

Administration and Dosage:

0.5%: Instill 1 to 2 drops in the affected eye(s) 3 times daily. Because apraclonidine 0.5% will be used with other ocular glaucoma therapies, use an approximate 5 minute interval between instillation of each medication to prevent washout of the previous dose. Not for injection into the eye.

1%: Instill 1 drop in scheduled operative eye 1 hour before initiating anterior segment laser surgery. Instill second drop into same eye immediately upon completion of surgery.

Storage: Store at room temperature. Protect from light and freezing (0.5%).

Rx **Iopidine** (Alcon)	**Solution:** 0.5%	In 5 mL and 10 mL Drop-Tainers.[1]
	Solution: 1%	In 0.1 mL (2s).[1]

[1] With 0.01% benzalkonium chloride.

BRIMONIDINE TARTRATE

Actions:

Pharmacology: Brimonidine tartrate is a relatively selective alpha-2 adrenergic agonist for ophthalmic use. It has a peak ocular hypotensive effect occurring at 2 hours post-dosing. Fluorophotometric studies in animals and humans suggest that brimonidine tartrate has a dual mechanism of action by reducing aqueous humor production and increasing uveoscleral outflow.

Pharmacokinetics: After ocular administration of a 0.2% solution, plasma concentration peaked within 1 to 4 hours and declined with a systemic half-life of ≈ 3 hours. In humans it is systemically metabolized by the liver primarily, with urinary excretion as the major route of elimination of the drug and its metabolites.

Clinical Trials: Elevated IOP presents a major risk factor in glaucomatous field loss. The higher the level of IOP, the greater the likelihood of optic nerve damage and visual field loss. Brimonidine tartrate has the action of lowering IOP with minimal effect on cardiovascular and pulmonary parameters.

Indications:

To lower intraocular pressure in patients with open-angle glaucoma or ocular hypertension. The ability to lower IOP diminishes over time in some patients. This loss of effect appears with a variable time of onset in each patient, and should be closely monitored.

Contraindications:

Hypersensitivity to brimonidine tartrate or any component of this medication. It also is contraindicated in patients receiving monoamine oxidase (MAO) inhibitor therapy.

OPHTHALMIC DRUG FACTS

Warnings:

Pregnancy: Category B. Reproduction studies performed in rats revealed no evidence of impaired fertility or harm to the fetus due to brimonidine tartrate. There are no studies of brimonidine tartrate in pregnant women; however, in animal studies, brimonidine crossed the placenta and entered into the fetal circulation to a limited extent. Brimonidine tartrate should be used during pregnancy only if the potential benefit to the mother justifies the potential risk to the fetus.

Lactation: It is not known whether brimonidine tartrate is excreted in human milk, although in animal studies brimonidine tartrate has been shown to be excreted in breast milk. A decision should be made whether to discontinue nursing or to discontinue the drug, taking into account the importance of the drug to the mother.

Children: Safety and efficacy in children have not been established. Agitation, apnea, bradycardia, convulsions, cyanosis, depression, dyspnea, emotional instability, hypotension, hypothermia, hypotonia, hypoventilation, irritability, lethargy, somnolence, and stupor have been reported in pediatric patients receiving brimondine tartrate 0.2%.

Precautions:

Cardiovascular disease: Although in clinical studies, brimonidine tartrate had minimal effect on blood pressure, exercise caution in treating patients with severe cardiovascular disease.

Renal/Hepatic function impairment: Brimonidine tartrate has not been studied in patients with hepatic or renal impairment; use caution in treating such patients.

Depression: Use caution in patients with depression, cerebral or coronary insufficiency, Raynaud's phenomenon, orthostatic hypotension, or thromboangiitis obliterans.

Hazardous tasks: Brimonidine tartrate may cause fatigue and drowsiness in some patients. Observe caution while driving, operating machinery, or performing other tasks requiring coordination or physical dexterity.

Drug Interactions:

CNS depressants: Consider the possibility of an additive or potentiating effect with CNS depressants (eg, alcohol, barbiturates, opiates, sedatives, anesthetics).

Concomitant therapy: Brimonidine tartrate did not have significant effects on pulse and blood pressure in clinical studies. However, caution is advised in using concomitant drugs such as beta blockers (ophthalmic or systemic), antihypertensives, or cardiac glycosides.

Tricyclic antidepressants: Tricyclic antidepressants have been reported to blunt the hypotensive effect of systemic clonidine. It is not known whether the concurrent use of these agents with brimonidine tartrate can lead to an interference in IOP-lowering effect. No data on the level of circulating catecholamines after brimonidine tartrate is instilled are available. Caution is advised in patients taking tricyclic antidepressants, which can affect the metabolism and uptake of circulating amines.

AGENTS FOR GLAUCOMA

Adverse Reactions:

The most commonly reported adverse events included oral dryness, ocular hyperemia, burning and stinging, headache, blurring, foreign body sensation, fatigue/drowsiness, conjunctival follicles, ocular allergic reactions, ocular pruritus, corneal staining/erosion, photophobia, eyelid erythema, ocular ache/pain, ocular dryness, tearing, upper respiratory symptoms, eyelid edema, conjunctival edema, dizziness, blepharitis, ocular irritation, gastrointestinal symptoms, asthenia, conjunctival blanching, abnormal vision, muscular pain, lid crusting, conjunctival hemorrhage, abnormal taste, insomnia, conjunctival discharge, depression, hypertension, anxiety, palpitations, nasal dryness, and syncope.

Patient Information:

Do not touch dropper tip to any surface as this may contaminate the contents.

The preservative in brimonidine tartrate, benzalkonium chloride, may be absorbed by soft contact lenses. Patients wearing soft contact lenses should be instructed to wait ≥ 15 minutes after instilling brimonidine tartrate to insert soft contact lenses.

Brimonidine tartrate may cause fatigue and drowsiness in some patients. Caution patients who engage in hazardous activities of the potential for a decrease in mental alertness.

Administration and Dosage:

Instill 1 drop of brimonidine tartrate in the affected eye(s) 3 times daily, ≈ 8 hours apart. Brimonidine is often dosed 2 times daily in clinical practice based upon clinical study data.

Storage: Store at ≤ 25°C (77°F).

Rx	**Alphagan** (Allergan)	**Solution:** 0.2%	In 5, 10, and 15 mL dropper bottles.[1]
Rx	**Alphagan P** (Allergan)	**Solution:** 0.15%	In 5, 10, and 15 mL dropper bottles.[2]

[1] Polyvinyl alcohol, NaCl, 0.05 mg benzalkonium chloride per mL.
[2] Sodium borate, boric acid, NaCl, KCl.

BETA-ADRENERGIC BLOCKING AGENTS

Actions:

Pharmacology: Timolol, levobunolol, carteolol, and metipranolol are noncardioselective (β_1 and β_2) β-blockers; betaxolol is a cardioselective (β_1) β-blocker. Topical β-blockers generally do not have significant membrane-stabilizing (local anesthetic) actions or intrinsic sympathomimetic activity (ISA) except for carteolol, which does have ISA.

The exact mechanism of ocular hypotensive action is not established, but it appears to be a reduction of aqueous production. Some studies show a slight increase in outflow facility with timolol and metipranolol.

These agents reduce IOP with little or no effect on pupil size or accommodation. Blurred vision and night blindness often associated with miotics are not associated with these agents. In addition, in patients with cataracts, the inability to see around

OPHTHALMIC DRUG FACTS

lenticular opacities when the pupil is constricted, is avoided. These agents, as well as all topically applied ocular agents, may be absorbed systemically (see Warnings).

Pharmacokinetics:

Pharmacokinetics of Ophthalmic β-Adrenergic Blocking Agents				
Drug	β-receptor selectivity	Onset (min)	Maximum effect (hr)	Duration (hr)
Carteolol)	β_1 and β_2	nd	nd	12
Betaxolol	β_1	30	2	12
Levobunolol	β_1 and β_2	< 60	2 to 6	12 to 24
Metipranolol	β_1 and β_2	≤ 30	≈ 2	12 to 24
Timolol	β_1 and β_2	30	1 to 2	12 to 24

nd = No data

Clinical Trials:

Timolol – In controlled studies of untreated IOP of ≥ 22 mm Hg, timolol 0.25% or 0.5% twice daily caused greater IOP reduction than 4% pilocarpine solution 4 times daily or 2% epinephrine HCl solution twice daily. In comparative studies, mean IOP reduction was 31% to 33% with timolol, 22% with pilocarpine, and 28% with epinephrine.

In ocular hypertension, effects of timolol and acetazolamide are additive. Timolol, generally well tolerated, produces fewer and less severe side effects than pilocarpine or epinephrine. Timolol has been well tolerated in patients wearing conventional (PMMA) hard contact lenses.

Betaxolol – Betaxolol ophthalmic was compared with ophthalmic timolol and placebo in patients with reactive airway disease. Betaxolol had no significant effect on pulmonary function as measured by Forced Expiratory Volume (FEV$_1$), Forced Vital Capacity (FVC), and FEV$_1$/VC. Also, action of isoproterenol was not inhibited. Timolol significantly decreased these pulmonary functions. No evidence of cardiovascular β-blockade during exercise was observed with betaxolol. Mean arterial blood pressure was not affected by any treatment; however, timolol significantly decreased mean heart rate. Betaxolol reduces mean IOP 25% from baseline. In controlled studies, the magnitude and duration of the ocular hypotensive effects of betaxolol and timolol were clinically similar. Clinical observation of glaucoma patients treated with betaxolol solution for up to 3 years shows that the IOP-lowering effect is well maintained.

Betaxolol has been successfully used in glaucoma patients who have undergone laser trabeculoplasty and have needed long-term hypotensive therapy. The drug is well tolerated in glaucoma patients with hard or soft contact lenses and in aphakic patients.

Levobunolol – Levobunolol effectively reduced IOP in controlled clinical studies from 3 months to > 1 year when given topically twice daily; IOP was well maintained. The mean IOP decrease is clinically similar to timolol.

Metipranolol – Metipranolol reduced the average intraocular pressure ≈ 20% to 26% in controlled studies of patients with IOP > 24 mm Hg at baseline. Clinical studies in patients with glaucoma treated ≤ 2 years indicate that an intraocular pressure lowering effect is maintained.

Carteolol – Carteolol produced a median percent IOP reduction of 22% to 25% when given twice daily in clinical trials ranging from 1.5 to 3 months.

AGENTS FOR GLAUCOMA

Indications:

Glaucoma: Lowering IOP in patients with chronic open-angle glaucoma.

For specific approved indications, refer to individual drug monographs.

Contraindications:

Bronchial asthma, a history of bronchial asthma, or severe chronic obstructive pulmonary disease; sinus bradycardia; second-degree and third-degree AV block; overt cardiac failure; cardiogenic shock; hypersensitivity to any component of the products.

Warnings:

Systemic absorption: These agents may be absorbed systemically. The same adverse reactions found with systemic β-blockers may occur with topical use. For example, severe respiratory reactions and cardiac reactions, including death due to bronchospasm in asthmatics, and rarely, death associated with cardiac failure, have been reported with topical β-blockers. These agents may decrease heart rate and blood pressure, and betaxolol has had adverse effects on pulmonary and cardiovascular parameters. Exercise caution with all of these agents.

Cardiovascular: Timolol can decrease resting and maximal exercise heart rate even in healthy subjects.

> *Cardiac failure* – Sympathetic stimulation may be essential for circulation support in diminished myocardial contractility; its inhibition by β-receptor blockade may precipitate more severe failure.

> *In patients without history of cardiac failure* – Continued depression of myocardium with β-blockers may lead to cardiac failure. Discontinue at the first sign or symptom of cardiac failure.

Non-allergic bronchospasm: Patients with a history of chronic bronchitis, emphysema, etc, should receive β-blockers with caution; they may block bronchodilation produced by catecholamine stimulation of β_2-receptors.

Major surgery: Withdrawing β-blockers before major surgery is controversial. Beta-receptor blockade impairs the heart's ability to respond to β-adrenergically mediated reflex stimuli. This may augment the risk of general anesthesia. Some patients on β-blockers have had protracted severe hypotension during anesthesia. Difficulty restarting and maintaining heartbeat has been reported. In elective surgery, gradual withdrawal of β-blockers may be appropriate.

The effects of β-blocking agents may be reversed by β-agonists such as isoproterenol, dopamine, dobutamine, or norepinephrine.

Diabetes mellitus: Administer with caution to patients subject to spontaneous hypoglycemia or to diabetic patients (especially labile diabetics). Beta-blocking agents may mask signs and symptoms of acute hypoglycemia.

Thyroid: Beta-adrenergic blocking agents may mask clinical signs of hyperthyroidism (eg, tachycardia). Manage patients suspected of developing thyrotoxicosis carefully to avoid abrupt withdrawal of β-blockers, which might precipitate thyroid storm.

196 OPHTHALMIC DRUG FACTS

Cerebrovascular insufficiency: Because of potential effects of β-blockers on blood pressure and pulse, use with caution in patients with cerebrovascular insufficiency. If signs or symptoms suggesting reduced cerebral blood flow develop, consider alternative therapy.

Carcinogenesis: In female mice receiving oral metipranolol doses of 5, 50, and 100 mg/kg/day, the low dose had an increased number of pulmonary adenomas.

Pregnancy: Category C. There have been no adequate and well controlled studies in pregnant women. Use during pregnancy only if the potential benefits to the mother outweigh potential hazards to the fetus.

Carteolol – Increased resorptions and decreased fetal weights occurred in rabbits and rats at maternal doses ≈ 1052 and 5264 times the maximum human dose, respectively. A dose-related increase in wavy ribs was noted in the developing rat fetus when pregnant rats received doses ≈ 212 times the maximum human dose.

Betaxolol – In oral studies with rats and rabbits, evidence of post-implantation loss was seen at dose levels above 12 mg/kg and 128 mg/kg, respectively. Betaxolol was not teratogenic; however, there were no other adverse effects on reproduction at subtoxic dose levels.

Levobetaxolol – There was evidence of drug-related post-implantation loss in rabbits with levobetaxolol at 12 mg/kg/day and sternebrae malformations at 4 mg/kg/day. No other adverse effects on reproduction were noted at subtoxic dose levels.

Levobunolol – Fetotoxicity was observed in rabbits at doses 200 and 700 times the glaucoma dose.

Metipranolol – Increased fetal resorption, fetal death, and delayed development occurred in rabbits receiving 50 mg/kg orally during organogenesis.

Timolol – Doses 1000 times the maximum recommended human oral dose were maternotoxic in mice and resulted in increased fetal resorptions. Increased fetal resorptions were also seen in rabbits at 100 times the maximum recommended human oral dose.

Lactation: It is not known whether *betaxolol, levobunolol,* or *metipranolol* are excreted in breast milk. Systemic β-blockers and topical *timolol maleate* are excreted in milk. *Carteolol* is excreted in breast milk of animals. Exercise caution when administering to a nursing mother.

Because of the potential for serious adverse reactions from *timolol* in nursing infants, decide whether to discontinue nursing or discontinue the drug taking into account the importance of the drug to the mother.

Children: Safety and efficacy for use in children have not been established.

Precautions:

Angle-closure glaucoma: The immediate objective is to reopen the angle, requiring constriction of the pupil with a miotic. These agents have little or no effect on the pupil. When they are used to reduce elevated IOP in angle-closure glaucoma, use with a miotic.

AGENTS FOR GLAUCOMA

Muscle weakness: Beta-blockade may potentiate muscle weakness consistent with certain myasthenic symptoms (eg, diplopia, ptosis, generalized weakness). *Timolol* has increased muscle weakness in some patients with myasthenic symptoms.

Long-term therapy: Diminished responsiveness to *betaxolol* and *timolol* after prolonged therapy has occurred. However, in long-term studies (2 and 3 years), no significant differences in mean IOP were observed after initial stabilization.

Sulfite sensitivity: Some of these products contain sulfites, which may cause allergic-type reactions (eg, hives, itching, wheezing, anaphylaxis) in certain susceptible patients. Although the overall prevalence of sulfite sensitivity in the general population is probably low, it is seen more frequently in asthmatics or atopic nonasthmatics.

Drug Interactions:

Ophthalmic Beta Blocker Drug Interactions			
Precipitant drug	Object drug*		Description
Beta blockers, ophthalmic	Beta blockers, oral	↑	Use topical beta blockers with caution because of the potential for additive effects on systemic and ophthalmic beta-blockade.
Beta blockers, ophthalmic	Calcium antagonists	↑	Possible cases of hypotension, left ventricular failure, and atrioventricular conduction disturbances may occur from coadministration of timolol maleate and calcium antagonists. Avoid use in patients with imparied cardiac function.
Beta blockers, ophthalmic	Catechol-amine-depleting drugs (eg, reserpine)	↑	Use of reserpine with ophthalmic beta blockers can cause additive effects and the production of hypotension or marked bradycardia, which may result in syncope, vertigo, or postural hypotension. Close observation is recommended.
Catecholamine-depleting drugs (eg, reserpine)	Beta blockers, ophthalmic		
Beta blockers, ophthalmic	Digitalis	↑	Coadministration of ophthalmic beta blockers with digitalis and calcium antagonists may have additive effects in prolonging atrioventricular condution time.
Digitalis	Beta blockers, ophthalmic		
Quinidine	Beta blockers, ophthalmic	↑	Decreased heart rate has been reported during combined treatment with timolol maleate and quinidine, possibly because quinidine inhibits the metabolism of timolol maleate via the P450 enzyme, CYP2D6.
Beta Blockers	Phenothiazine compounds	↑	Potential additive hypotensive effects due to mutual inhibition of metabolism.

* ↑ = Object drug increased. ↔ = Undetermined effect.

Other drugs that may interact with systemic β-adrenergic blocking agents may also interact with ophthalmic agents. These agents are listed below.

Antithyroid agents	Insulin	Phenothiazines
Calcium channel blockers	Lidocaine	Prazosin
Cimetidine	Morphine	Rifampin
Clonidine	Neuromuscular blockers,	Salicylates
Contraceptives, oral	nondepolarizing	Smoking
Digoxin	Nicotine	Sympathomimetics
Disopyramide	NSAIDs	Theophylline
Haloperidol	Phenobarbital	Thyroid hormones
Hydralazine		

Adverse Reactions:

The following have occurred with ophthalmic β_1 and β_2 (nonselective) blockers:

Cardiovascular: Arrhythmia; syncope; heart block; cerebral vascular accident; cerebral ischemia; congestive heart failure; palpitation.

CNS: Headache; depression.

Dermatologic: Hypersensitivity, including localized and generalized rash.

Endocrine: Masked symptoms of hypoglycemia in insulin-dependent diabetics (see Warnings).

GI: Nausea.

Ophthalmic: Keratitis; blepharoptosis; visual disturbances including refractive changes (due to withdrawal of miotic therapy in some cases); diplopia; ptosis.

The following adverse reactions have occurred with the individual agent:

Respiratory: Bronchospasm (predominantly in patients with preexisting bronchospastic disease); respiratory failure.

Carteolol:

>*Ophthalmic* – Transient irritation, burning, tearing, conjunctival hyperemia, edema ($\approx$ 25%), blurred/cloudy vision; photophobia; decreased night vision; ptosis; blepharoconjunctivitis; abnormal corneal staining; corneal sensitivity.

>*Systemic* – Bradycardia; decreased blood pressure; arrhythmia; heart palpitation; dyspnea; asthenia; headache; dizziness; insomnia; sinusitis; taste perversion.

Betaxolol:

>*Ophthalmic* – Brief discomfort (> 25%); occasional tearing (5%), decreased corneal sensitivity, erythema, itching, corneal punctate staining, keratitis, anisocoria; photophobia (rare).

>*Systemic* – Insomnia; depressive neurosis (rare).

Levobetaxolol:

>*Cardiovascular* – Bradycardia; heart block; hypertension; hypotension; tachycardia; vascular anomaly (< 2%).

>*CNS* – Anxiety; dizziness; hypertonia; vertigo (< 2%).

>*Dermatologic* – Alopecia; dermatitis; psoriasis (< 2%).

>*Endocrine* – Diabetes; hypothyroidism (< 2%).

>*GI* – Constipation; dyspepsia (< 2%).

>*GU* – Breast abscess; cystitis (< 2%).

>*Metabolic/Nutritional* – Gout; hypercholesteremia; hyperlipidemia (< 2%).

>*Musculoskeletal* – Arthritis; tendonitis (< 2%).

AGENTS FOR GLAUCOMA

Ophthalmic – Transient ocular discomfort upon instillation (11%); transient blurred vision (≈ 2%); cataracts, vitreous disorders (< 2%).

Pulmonary – Pulmonary distress characterized by bronchitis, dyspnea, pharyngitis, pneumonia, rhinitis, and sinusitis (< 2%).

Special Senses – Ear pain; otitis media; taste perversion; tinnitus (< 2%).

Miscellaneous – Accidental injury; headache; infection (< 2%).

Levobunolol:

Cardiovascular – Effects may resemble those of timolol.

CNS – Ataxia, dizziness, lethargy (rare).

Dermatologic – Urticaria, pruritus (rare).

Ophthalmic – Transient burning/stinging (25%); blepharoconjunctivitis (5%); iridocyclitis (rare); decreased corneal sensitivity.

Metipranolol:

Ophthalmic – Transient local discomfort; conjunctivitis; eyelid dermatitis; blepharitis; blurred vision; tearing; browache; abnormal vision; photophobia; edema.

Systemic – Allergic reaction; headache; asthenia; hypertension; myocardial infarction; atrial fibrillation; angina; palpitation; bradycardia; nausea; rhinitis; dyspnea; epistaxis; bronchitis; coughing; dizziness; anxiety; depression; somnolence; nervousness; arthritis; myalgia; rash.

Timolol:

CNS – Dizziness; depression; fatigue; lethargy; hallucinations; confusion.

Cardiovascular – Bradycardia; arrhythmia; hypotension; syncope; heart block; cerebral vascular accident; cerebral ischemia; heart failure; palpitation; cardiac arrest. These generally occur in the elderly or in patients with preexisting cardiovascular problems.

Ophthalmic – Ocular irritation including conjunctivitis; blepharitis; keratitis; blepharoptosis; decreased corneal sensitivity; visual disturbances including refractive changes (in some cases, due to withdrawal of miotics); diplopia; ptosis.

Respiratory – Bronchospasm (mainly in patients with preexisting bronchospastic disease); respiratory failure; dyspnea.

Miscellaneous – Aggravation of myasthenia gravis; alopecia; nail pigmentary changes; nausea; hypersensitivity, including localized and generalized rash; urticaria; asthenia; sexual dysfunction, including impotence, decreased libido; decreased ejaculation; hyperkalemia; masked symptoms of hypoglycemia in insulin-dependent diabetics; diarrhea; paresthesia.

Causal relationship unknown: Hypertension; chest pain; dyspepsia; anorexia; dry mouth; behavioral changes (eg, anxiety, disorientation, nervousness, somnolence, psychic disturbance); aphakic cystoid macular edema; retroperitoneal fibrosis.

Systemic β-adrenergic blocker-associated reactions: Consider potential effects with ophthalmic use (see Warnings).

Overdosage:

If ocular overdosage occurs, flush eye(s) with water or normal saline. If accidentally ingested, efforts to decrease further absorption may be appropriate (gastric lavage).

The most common signs and symptoms of overdosage from systemic β-blockers are bradycardia, hypotension, bronchospasm, and acute cardiac failure. If these occur, discontinue therapy and initiate appropriate supportive therapy.

Patient Information:

Refer to the Dosage Forms and Routes of Administration chapter for more complete information.

Transient stinging/discomfort is relatively common; notify physician if severe.

Administration and Dosage:

Concomitant therapy: If IOP is not controlled with these agents, institute concomitant pilocarpine, other miotics, dipivefrin, or carbonic anhydrase inhibitors.

Use of epinephrine with topical β-blockers is controversial. Some reports indicate that initial effectiveness of the combination decreases over time (see Drug Interactions).

Monitoring: The IOP-lowering response to betaxolol and timolol may require a few weeks to stabilize. Determine the IOP during the first month of treatment. Thereafter, determine IOP on an individual basis.

Because of diurnal IOP variations in individual patients, satisfactory response to twice-a-day therapy is best determined by measuring IOP at different times during the day. Intraocular pressures ≤ 22 mm Hg may not be optimal to control glaucoma in each patient; therefore, individualize therapy.

Individual drug monographs are on the following pages.

AGENTS FOR GLAUCOMA

BETAXOLOL HYDROCHLORIDE

For complete prescribing information, refer to the Beta-adrenergic Blocking Agents group monograph.

Indications:

Treatment of ocular hypertension and chronic open-angle glaucoma. Betaxolol may be used alone or in combination with other antiglaucoma drugs.

Administration and Dosage:

Usual dose: Instill 1 drop twice daily.

Replacement therapy (single agent): Continue the agent already used and add 1 drop of betaxolol twice daily. The following day, discontinue the previous agent and continue betaxolol. Monitor with tonometry.

Replacement therapy (multiple agents): When transferring from several concomitant antiglaucoma agents, individualize dosage. Adjust 1 agent at a time at intervals of ≥ 1 week. One may continue the agents being used and add 1 drop betaxolol twice daily. The next day, discontinue another agent. Decrease or discontinue remaining antiglaucoma agents according to patient response.

Storage/Stability: Store at room temperature 15° to 30°C (59° to 86°F). Shake suspension well.

Rx	**Betoptic** (Alcon)	**Solution:** 5.6 mg (equiv. to 5 mg base) per mL (0.5%)	In 10 mL Drop-Tainer bottles.[1]
Rx	**Betoptic S** (Alcon)	**Suspension:** 2.8 mg (equiv. to 2.5 mg base) per mL (0.25%)	In 5, 10, and 15 mL Drop-Tainer bottles.[2]

[1] With 0.01% benzalkonium chloride, NaCl, hydrochloric acid or sodium hydroxide, EDTA.
[2] With 0.01% benzalkonium chloride, mannitol, poly sulfonic acid, carbomer 934P, hydrochloric acid or sodium hydroxide, EDTA.

CARTEOLOL HYDROCHLORIDE

For complete prescribing information, refer to the Beta-adrenergic Blocking Agents group monograph.

Indications:

Treatment of chronic open-angle glaucoma and ocular hypertension. It may be used alone or in combination with other IOP lowering drugs.

Administration and Dosage:

Usual dose: Instill 1 drop in affected eye(s) twice daily. If the patient's IOP is not at a satisfactory level on this regimen, concomitant therapy can be instituted.

Rx	**Ocupress** (Novartis)	**Solution:** 1%	In 5, 10, and 15 mL dropper bottles.[1]

[1] With 0.005% benzalkonium chloride, NaCl, sodium phosphate.

LEVOBETAXOLOL HYDROCHLORIDE

For complete prescribing information, refer to the Beta-adrenergic Blocking Agents group monograph.

Indications:

For lowering intraocular pressure in patients with chronic open-angle gluacoma or ocular hypertension.

Administration and Dosage:

Usual dose: Instill 1 drop twice daily.

Storage/Stability: Store upright 39° to 77°F (4° to 25°C). Protect from light. Shake well before using.

Rx	**Betaxon** (Alcon)	**Suspension, ophthalmic:** 0.5% as base (5.6 mg/mL)	In 5, 10, and 15 mL Drop-tainers.[1]

[1] 0.01% benzalkonium Cl, EDTA, hydrochloric acid, boric acid.

LEVOBUNOLOL HYDROCHLORIDE

For complete prescribing information, refer to the Beta-adrenergic Blocking Agents group monograph.

Indications:

Lower IOP in chronic open-angle glaucoma or ocular hypertension.

Administration and Dosage:

Usual dose: Instill 1 drop in the affected eye(s) once or twice daily.

Rx	**Levobunolol** (Various, eg, Bausch & Lomb)	**Solution:** 0.25%	In 5 and 10 mL.
Rx	**Betagan Liquifilm** (Allergan)		In 5 and 10 mL dropper bottles with BID *C Cap.*[1]
Rx	**Levobunolol** (Various, eg, Bausch & Lomb)	**Solution:** 0.5%	In 5, 10, and 15 mL.
Rx	**Betagan Liquifilm** (Allergan)		In 2, 5, 10 and 15 mL bottles with BID and QD*C Cap.*[1]

[1] With 1.4% polyvinyl alcohol, 0.004% benzalkonium chloride, sodium metabisulfite, EDTA.

METIPRANOLOL HYDROCHLORIDE

For complete prescribing information, refer to the Beta-adrenergic Blocking Agents group monograph.

AGENTS FOR GLAUCOMA

Indications:

Treatment of ocular conditions in which lowering IOP is likely to be of therapeutic benefit, including ocular hypertension and chronic open-angle glaucoma.

Administration and Dosage:

Usual dose: Instill 1 drop in the affected eye(s) twice a day. If the patient's IOP is not at a satisfactory level on this regimen, more frequent administration or a larger dose is of benefit. Concomitant therapy to lower IOP can be instituted.

Rx	**OptiPranolol** (Bausch & Lomb)	**Solution**: 0.3%	In 5 or 10 mL dropper bottles.[1]

[1] With 0.004% benzalkonium chloride, EDTA, NaCl.

TIMOLOL MALEATE

For complete prescribing information, refer to the Beta-adrenergic Blocking Agents group monograph.

Indications:

Treatment of elevated IOP in chronic open-angle glaucoma, ocular hypertension, aphakic glaucoma patients, some patients with secondary glaucoma, and patients with elevated IOP who need ocular pressure lowering.

Administration and Dosage:

Solution:

> *Initial therapy* – Instill 1 drop of 0.25% or 0.5% twice daily. Because the pressure-lowering response may require a few weeks to stabilize, evaluation should include a determination of IOP after $\approx$ 4 weeks of treatment.

Gel: Invert the closed container and shake once before each use; it is not necessary to shake it more than once. Administer other ophthalmics $\geq$ 10 minutes before the gel. Dose is 1 drop (0.25% or 0.5%) once daily. Consider concomitant therapy if IOP is not at a satisfactory level. When patients are switched from timolol solution twice daily to the gel once daily, the ocular hypotensive effect should remain constant.

Because the pressure-lowering response may require a few weeks to stabilize, determine IOP after $\approx$ 4 weeks of treatment.

Rx	**Timolol Maleate** (Various, eg, Akorn, Bausch & Lomb, Falcon, Fougera)	**Solution**: 0.25%	In 2.5, 5, 10, and 15 mL.
Rx	**Betimol**[1] (Novartis)		In 2.5, 5, 10, and 15 mL.[2]
Rx	**Timoptic**[3] (Merck)		Preservative free. In UD 60s Ocu-dose.[4]
Rx	**Timoptic**[3] (Merck)		In 2.5, 5, 10, and 15 mL Ocumeters[5]

204			OPHTHALMIC DRUG FACTS

Rx	**Timolol Maleate** (Various, eg, Akorn, Bausch & Lomb, Falcon, Fougera)	**Solution:** 0.5%	In 2.5, 5, 10, and 15 mL.
Rx	**Betimol**[1] (Novartis)		In 2.5, 5, 10, and 15 mL.[2]
Rx	**Timoptic**[3] (Merck)		Preservative free. In UD 60s Ocu-dose.[4]
Rx	**Timoptic**[3] (Merck)		In 2.5, 5, 10, and 15 mL Ocumeters[5]
Rx	**Timolol Maleate Ophthalmic** (Falcon)	**Solution, gel-forming:** 0.25%	In 2.5 and 5 mL.[5]
Rx	**Timoptic-XE**[3] (Merck)		In 2.5 and 5 mL Ocumeters.[6]
Rx	**Timolol Maleate Ophthalmic** (Falcon)	**Solution, gel-forming:** 0.5%	In 2.5 and 5 mL.[5]
Rx	**Timoptic-XE**[3] (Merck)		In 2.5 and 5 mL Ocumeters.[6]

[1] As hemihydrate.
[2] With 0.01% benzalkonium chloride and monosodium and disodium phosphate dihydrate.
[3] As maleate.
[4] Use immediately after opening; discard remaining contents. With monobasic and dibasic sodium phosphate and sodium hydroxide.
[5] With 0.01% benzalkonium chloride, sodium hydroxide, and monobasic and dibasic sodium phosphate.
[6] With 0.012% benzododecinium bromide.

MIOTICS, DIRECT-ACTING

Refer to the Agents for Glaucoma introduction for a general discussion of these products.

Actions:

Pharmacology: The direct-acting miotics are parasympathomimetic (cholinergic) drugs that duplicate the muscarinic effects of acetylcholine. When applied topically, these drugs produce pupillary constriction, stimulate the ciliary muscles, and increase aqueous humor outflow facility. Miosis, produced through contraction of the iris sphincter, causes increased tension on the scleral spur (reducing outflow resistance) and opening of the trabecular meshwork spaces facilitating outflow. With the increase in outflow facility, there is a decrease in intraocular pressure (IOP). Topical ophthalmic instillation of acetylcholine causes no discernible response as cholinesterase destroys the molecule more rapidly than it can penetrate the cornea; therefore, acetylcholine is used only intraocularly.

Miosis Induction of Direct-Acting Miotics			
Topical Miotic	Onset	Peak	Duration
Carbachol	10 to 20 min	—	4 to 8 hours
Pilocarpine	10 to 30 min	—	4 to 8 hours

Indications:

Carbachol, topical; pilocarpine: To decrease elevated IOP in glaucoma.

Acetylcholine; carbachol, intraocular: To induce miosis during surgery.

See individual monographs for specific indications.

AGENTS FOR GLAUCOMA

Contraindications:

Hypersensitivity to any component of the formulation; where constriction is undesirable (eg, acute iritis, acute or anterior uveitis, some forms of secondary glaucoma, pupillary block glaucoma, acute inflammatory disease of the anterior chamber).

Warnings:

Corneal abrasion: Use carbachol with caution in the presence of corneal abrasion to avoid excessive penetration.

Pregnancy: Category C (carbachol, pilocarpine). Safety for use during pregnancy has not been established. Use only when clearly needed.

Lactation: It is not known whether these drugs are excreted in breast milk; exercise caution when administering to a nursing woman.

Children: Safety and efficacy for use in children have not been established.

Precautions:

Systemic reactions: Caution is advised in patients with acute cardiac failure, bronchial asthma, peptic ulcer, hyperthyroidism, GI spasm, urinary tract obstruction, Parkinson's disease, recent MI, hypertension, or hypotension.

Retinal detachment: Retinal detachment has been caused by miotics in susceptible individuals, in individuals with preexisting retinal disease, or in those who are predisposed to retinal tears. Fundus examination is advised for all patients prior to initiation of therapy.

Miosis: Miosis usually causes difficulty in dark adaptation. Advise patients to use caution while night driving or performing hazardous tasks in poor light.

Angle-closure: Although withdrawal of the peripheral iris from the anterior chamber angle by miosis may reduce the tendency for angle-closure, miotics can occasionally precipitate angle closure by increasing resistance to aqueous flow from posterior to anterior chamber.

Pilocarpine ocular system (Ocusert): Carefully consider and evaluate patients with acute infectious conjunctivitis or keratitis prior to use.

Drug Interactions:

Nonsteroidal anti-inflammatory agents, topical: Although studies with acetylcholine chloride or carbachol revealed no interference, and there is no known pharmacological basis for an interaction, there have been reports that both of these drugs have been ineffective when used in patients treated with topical nonsteroidal anti-inflammatory agents.

Adverse Reactions:

Acetylcholine:

> *Ophthalmic* – Corneal edema; clouding; decompensation.

> *Systemic* – Bradycardia; hypotension; flushing; breathing difficulties; sweating.

Carbachol:

> *Ophthalmic* – Transient stinging and burning; corneal clouding; persistent bullous keratopathy; postoperative iritis following cataract extraction with intraocular use; retinal detachment; transient ciliary and conjunctival injection; ciliary spasm with resultant temporary decrease of visual acuity.

> *Systemic* – Headache; salivation; GI cramps; vomiting; diarrhea; asthma; syncope; cardiac arrhythmia; flushing; sweating; epigastric distress; tightness in bladder; hypotension; frequent urge to urinate.

Pilocarpine:

> *Ophthalmic* – Transient stinging and burning; tearing; ciliary spasm; conjunctival vascular congestion; temporal, peri- or supra-orbital headache; superficial keratitis; induced myopia (especially in younger individuals who have recently started administration); blurred vision; poor dark adaptation; reduced visual acuity in poor illumination in older individuals and in individuals with lens opacity. A subtle corneal granularity has occurred with pilocarpine gel. Lens opacity (prolonged use), retinal detachment (rare; see Precautions).

> *Systemic* – Hypertension; tachycardia; bronchiolar spasm; pulmonary edema; salivation; sweating; nausea; vomiting; diarrhea (rare).

Pilocarpine ocular system (Ocusert):

> *Ophthalmic* – Conjunctival irritation, including mild erythema with or without a slight increase in mucus secretion with first use. These symptoms tend to lessen or disappear after the first week of therapy. Ciliary spasm may occur with pilocarpine usage but is not a contraindication to continued therapy unless the induced myopia is debilitating to the patient. Rarely, a sudden increase in pilocarpine effects has been reported during use.

> Irritation from pilocarpine has been infrequently encountered and may require cessation of therapy. True allergic reactions are uncommon, but require discontinuation of therapy. Corneal abrasion and visual impairment have occurred.

Overdosage:

Should accidental overdosage in the eye(s) occur, flush with water.

Treatment: Treatment includes usual supportive measures. Observe patients for signs of toxicity (eg, salivation, lacrimation, sweating, nausea, vomiting, diarrhea). If these occur, therapy with anticholinergics (atropine) may be necessary. Bronchial constriction may be a problem in asthmatic patients.

Patient Information:

May sting upon instillation, especially first few doses.

AGENTS FOR GLAUCOMA 207

May cause headache, browache, and decreased night vision. Use caution while driving at night or performing hazardous tasks in poor light.

To avoid contamination, do not touch tip of container to any surface. Replace cap after using. Keep bottle tightly closed when not in use. Discard solution after expiration date. Wash hands immediately after use.

Individual drug monographs are on the following pages.

ACETYLCHOLINE CHLORIDE, INTRAOCULAR

For complete prescribing information, refer to the Miotics, Direct-Acting group monograph. The following section is included here for completeness to show all of the clinical uses of this class of drug.

Indications:

Miosis: To produce complete miosis rapidly in cataract surgery, penetrating keratoplasty, iridectomy, and other anterior segment surgery where rapid, complete miosis is desirable.

Administration and Dosage:

Solution: 0.5 to 2 mL produces satisfactory miosis. Solution need not be flushed from the chamber after miosis occurs. Because acetylcholine has a short duration of action, pilocarpine may be applied topically after the operation to maintain miosis.

Preparation of solution: The aqueous solution of acetylcholine chloride is unstable. Prepare solution immediately before use. Do not use solution that is not clear and colorless. Discard any solution that has not been used. Do not gas sterilize.

Storage/Stability: Store at room temperature 15° to 30°C (59° to 86°F). Do not freeze.

Rx	**Miochol-E** (Novartis)	**Solution**: 1:100 acetylcholine chloride when reconstituted	In 2 mL dual chamber univial (lower chamber 20 mg lyophilized acetylcholine chloride and 56 mg mannitol; upper chamber 2 mL electrolyte diluent[1] and sterile water for injection).

[1] Sodium chloride, potassium chloride, magnesium chloride hexahydrate, calcium chloride dihydrate.

CARBACHOL, INTRAOCULAR

For complete prescribing information, refer to the Miotics, Direct-Acting group monograph. The following section is included here for completeness to show all of the clinical uses of this class of drug.

Indications:

Miosis: Intraocular use for miosis during surgery.

Administration and Dosage:

For single-dose intraocular use only. Discard unused portion.

Open under aseptic conditions only.

Gently instill ≤ 0.5 mL into the anterior chamber before or after securing sutures. Miosis is usually maximal 2 to 5 minutes after application.

Storage/Stability: Store at room temperature 15° to 30°C (59° to 86°F).

AGENTS FOR GLAUCOMA

Rx	**Carbastat** (Novartis)	**Solution:** 0.01%	In 1.5 mL vials.[1]
Rx	**Miostat** (Alcon)		In 1.5 mL vials.[1]

[1] With 0.64% sodium chloride, 0.075% potassium chloride dihydrate, 0.048% calcium chloride dihydrate, 0.03% magnesium chloride hexahydrate, 0.39% sodium acetate trihydrate, 0.17% sodium citrate dihydrate, sodium hydroxide, hydrochloric acid.

CARBACHOL, TOPICAL

For complete prescribing information, refer to the Miotics, Direct-Acting group monograph.

Indications:

Glaucoma: For lowering intraocular pressure in the treatment of glaucoma.

Administration and Dosage:

Instill 1 drop into eye(s) up to 3 times daily.

Storage/Stability: Store at 8° to 27°C (46° to 80°F).

Rx	**Isopto Carbachol** (Alcon)	**Solution:** 0.75%	In 15 and 30 mL Drop-Tainers.[1]
		1.5%	In 15 and 30 mL Drop-Tainers.[1]
		2.25%	In 15 mL Drop-Tainers.[1]
Rx	**Isopto Carbachol** (Alcon)	3%	In 15 and 30 mL Drop-Tainers.[1]
Rx	**Carboptic** (Optopics)		In 15 mL.[2]

[1] With 0.005% benzalkonium chloride, 1% hydroxypropyl methylcellulose, sodium chloride, boric acid, sodium borate.
[2] With benzalkonium chloride, polyvinyl alcohol, sodium phosphate dibasic and monobasic.

PILOCARPINE HYDROCHLORIDE

For complete prescribing information, refer to the Miotics, Direct-Acting group monograph.

Indications:

To lower intraocular pressure (IOP) in glaucoma.

Chronic angle-closure glaucoma.

Acute (angle-closure) glaucoma: Alone, or in combination with β–adrenergic blocking agents, carbonic anhydrase inhibitors, apraclonidine, or hyperosmotic agents to decrease IOP and break the attack.

Pre- and postoperative elevated IOP.

210 OPHTHALMIC DRUG FACTS

Administration and Dosage:

Solution:

Initial – Instill 1 drop 3 to 4 times daily. The frequency of instillation and the concentration are determined by patient response. Individuals with heavily pigmented irides may require higher strengths.

Gel: Apply a 0.5-inch ribbon in the lower conjunctival sac of affected eye(s) once daily at bedtime. If other glaucoma medication is also used at bedtime, use drops ≥ 5 minutes before the gel.

Storage/Stability: Do not freeze. Store at room temperature; 2° to 26°C (36° to 80°F).

Rx	**Isopto Carpine** (PolyMedica)	**Solution**: 0.25%	In 15 mL.[1]
Rx	**Pilocarpine HCl** (Various, eg, Martec)	**Solution**: 0.5%	In 15 mL.
Rx	**Isopto Carpine** (PolyMedica)		In 15 and 30 mL.[1]
Rx	**Pilocar** (Novartis)		In 15 mL and twin-pack (2 × 15 mL).[2]
Rx	**Pilocarpine HCl** (Various, eg, Alcon)	**Solution**: 1%	In 2, 5, and 15 mL and 15 mL twin-pack (2 × 15 mL).
Rx	**Akarpine** (Akorn)		In 15 mL.
Rx	**Isopto Carpine** (Alcon)		In 15 and 30 mL.[1]
Rx	**Pilocar** (Novartis)		In 15 mL, twin-pack (2 × 15 mL) and 1 mL dropperettes.[2]
Rx	**Pilocarpine HCl** (Various, eg, Alcon)	**Solution**: 2%	In 2 and 15 mL and 15 mL twin-pack (2 × 15 mL)
Rx	**Akarpine** (Akorn)		In 15 mL dropper bottles.
Rx	**Isopto Carpine** (Alcon)		In 15 and 30 mL.[1]
Rx	**Pilocar** (Novartis)		In 15 mL, twin-pack (2 × 15 mL), and 1 mL dropperettes.[2]
Rx	**Pilostat** (Bausch & Lomb)		In 15 mL and twin-pack (2 × 15 mL).[4]
Rx	**Pilocarpine HCl** (Various, eg, Baush & Lomb)	**Solution**: 3%	In 15 mL.
Rx	**Isopto Carpine** (Alcon)		In 15 and 30 mL.[1]
Rx	**Pilocar** (Novartis)		In 15 mL and twin-pack (2 × 15 mL).[2]

AGENTS FOR GLAUCOMA

Rx	Pilocarpine HCl (Various, eg, Alcon)	Solution: 4%	In 2 and 15 mL.
Rx	Akarpine (Akorn)		In 15 mL dropper bottles.
Rx	Isopto Carpine (Alcon)		In 15 and 30 mL.[1]
Rx	Pilocar (Novartis)		In 15 mL, twin-pack (2 × 15 mL) and 1 mL dropperettes.[2]
Rx	Pilopto-Carpine (Lebeh Pharmacal)		In 15 mL.
Rx	Isopto Carpine (Alcon)	Solution: 5%	In 15 mL.[1]
Rx	Pilocarpine HCl (Various, eg, Alcon)	Solution: 6%	In 15 mL.
Rx	Isopto Carpine (Alcon)		In 15 and 30 mL.[1]
Rx	Pilocar (Ciba Vision)		In 15 mL and twin-pack (2 × 15 mL).[3]
Rx	Pilocarpine HCl (Alcon)	Solution: 8%	In 2 mL.
Rx	Isopto Carpine (Alcon)		In 15 mL.[1]
Rx	Isopto Carpine (PolyMedica)	Solution: 10%	In 15 mL.[1]
Rx	Pilopine HS (Alcon)	Gel: 4%	In 3.5 g.[5]

[1] With 0.5% hydroxypropyl methylcellulose, 0.01% benzalkonium chloride.
[2] With hydroxypropyl methylcellulose, benzalkonium chloride, EDTA.
[3] With polyvinyl alcohol, benzalkonium chloride, EDTA.
[4] With hydroxypropyl methylcellulose, 0.01% benzalkonium chloride, EDTA.
[5] With 0.008% benzalkonium chloride, carbopol 940, EDTA.

PILOCARPINE NITRATE

For complete prescribing information, refer to the Miotics, Direct-Acting group monograph.

Indications:

To control IOP in glaucoma.

For emergency relief of angle-closure glaucoma.

Administration and Dosage:

Glaucoma: Instill 1 drop 2 to 4 times daily. Patient response may vary.

Storage/Stability: Do not freeze. Keep out of reach of children.

Rx	Pilagan (Allergan)	Solution: 1%	In 15 mL.[1]
		2%	In 15 mL.[1]
		4%	In 15 mL.[1]

[1] With 1.4% polyvinyl alcohol, 0.5% chlorobutanol, menthol, camphor, phenol, eucalyptol.

212 OPHTHALMIC DRUG FACTS

PILOCARPINE OCULAR THERAPEUTIC SYSTEM

Refer to the general discussion in the Miotics, Direct-Acting group monograph.

Actions:

Pharmacology: An elliptical unit designed for continuous release of pilocarpine following placement in the cul-de-sac of the eye.

Pharmacokinetics: Ocusert initially releases the drug at 3 times the rated value in the first hours and declines to the rated value in ≈ 6 hours. A total of 0.3 to 0.7 mg pilocarpine is released during this initial 6-hour period (1 drop of 2% pilocarpine ophthalmic solution contains 1 mg pilocarpine). During the remainder of the 7-day period, the release rate is within ± 20% of the rated value.

Ocular hypotensive effect is fully developed within 1.5 to 2 hours after placement in the cul-de-sac. A satisfactory ocular hypotensive response is maintained around the clock. IOP reduction for the entire week is achieved with the system from either 3.4 or 6.7 mg pilocarpine (20 or 40 mcg/hr times 24 hrs/day times 7 days, respectively), vs 28 mg given as a 2% ophthalmic solution 4 times daily.

During the first several hours after insertion, induced myopia may occur. In contrast to fluctuating and high levels of induced myopia typical of pilocarpine eye drop use, the amount of induced myopia with *Ocusert* decreases after the first several hours to a low baseline level (≤ 0.5 diopters), which persists for the therapeutic life of the system. Pilocarpine-induced miosis approximately parallels induced myopia.

Indications:

IOP reduction: Control of elevated IOP in pilocarpine-responsive patients.

Patient Information:

Patient package insert is available with the product.

Wash hands with soap and water before touching or manipulating the system. If a displaced system contacts an unclean surface, rinse with cool tap water before replacing. Discard contaminated system and replace with a fresh unit.

Check for the presence of the system before retiring at night and upon awakening.

Administration and Dosage:

Damaged or deformed systems: Do not place or retain in the eye. Remove and replace systems believed to be associated with an unexpected increase in drug action.

Initiation of therapy: There is no direct correlation between the strength of *Ocusert* used and the strength of pilocarpine eyedrop solutions required to achieve a given level of pressure lowering. It has been estimated that *Ocusert* 20 mcg is roughly equal to 0.5% or 1% drops and 40 mcg is roughly equal to 2% or 3% drops. *Ocusert* reduces the amount of drug necessary to achieve adequate medical control; therefore, therapy may be started with the 20 mcg system, regardless of the strength of pilocarpine solution the patient previously required. Because of the patient's age, family history, and disease status or progression, therapy may be started with the 40 mcg system. The patient should return during the first week of therapy for evaluation of IOP and as often thereafter as deemed necessary.

AGENTS FOR GLAUCOMA

If pressure is satisfactorily reduced with the 20 mcg system, the patient should continue its use, replacing each unit every 7 days. If IOP reduction greater than that achieved by 20 mcg is needed, transfer the patient to the 40 mcg system. If necessary, concurrently use epinephrine, a β-blocker or carbonic anhydrase inhibitor; *Ocusert's* release rate is not influenced by other ophthalmic preparations.

Placement and removal of the system: The system is placed in and removed from the eye by the patient. Because pilocarpine-induced myopia may occur during the first several hours of therapy, place the system into the conjunctival cul-de-sac at bedtime. By morning, the myopia is at a stable level (≤ 0.5 diopters).

For those patients in whom retention is a problem, superior cul-de-sac placement is often more desirable. The unit can be manipulated from lower to upper conjunctival cul-de-sac by gentle digital massage through the eyelid. If possible, move the unit before sleep to the upper conjunctival cul-de-sac for best retention. Should the unit slip out during sleep, its ocular hypotensive effect after loss continues for a period comparable to that following instillation of eyedrops.

Ocusert has been used concomitantly with various ophthalmic medications.

Storage/Stability: Refrigerate at 2° to 8°C (36° to 46°F).

Rx	**Ocusert Pilo-20** (Akorn)	**Ocular Therapeutic System**: Releases 20 mcg pilocarpine per hour for 1 week	In packs of 8 individ. sterile systems.
Rx	**Ocusert Pilo-40** (Akorn)	**Ocular Therapeutic System**: Releases 40 mcg pilocarpine per hour for 1 week	In packs of 8 individ. sterile systems.

CHOLINESTERASE INHIBITORS

Actions:

Pharmacology: These indirect-acting agents inhibit the enzyme cholinesterase, potentiating the action of acetylcholine on the parasympathomimetic end organs. Topical application to the eye produces intense miosis and ciliary muscle contraction. Intraocular pressure (IOP) is reduced by a decreased resistance to aqueous outflow.

Cholinesterase inhibitors are subdivided into reversible and irreversible agents. Reversible agents (eg, physostigmine, demecarium) quickly combine with cholinesterase; the resulting complex is slowly hydrolyzed and the inhibited enzyme is regenerated. The demecarium-enzyme complex is hydrolyzed more slowly than the physostigmine complex; therefore, its duration of action is longer.

Irreversible agents (eg, echothiophate) also bind to cholinesterase; however, the resulting covalent bond is not hydrolyzed. Therefore, cholinesterase is not regenerated. More cholinesterase must be synthesized or supplied from depots elsewhere in the body before ophthalmic action dependent on cholinesterase returns. Echothiophate will depress both plasma and erythrocyte cholinesterase levels in most patients after a few weeks of eyedrop therapy.

These effects are accompanied by increased permeability of the blood-aqueous barrier and vasodilation. Myopia may be induced or, if present, may be augmented by the increased refractive power of the lens that results from the accommodative effect of the drug. Demecarium indirectly produces some of the muscarinic and nicotinic effects of acetylcholine as quantities of the latter accumulate.

Cholinesterase-Inhibiting Miotics					
	Miosis		IOP reduction		
Miotics	Onset (minutes)	Duration	Onset (hours)	Peak (hours)	Duration
Reversible					
Physostigmine	20 to 30	12 to 36 hrs	—	2 to 6	12 to 36 hrs
Demecarium	15 to 60	3 to 10 days	—	24	7 to 28 days
Irreversible					
Echothiophate	10 to 30	1 to 4 weeks	4 to 8	24	7 to 28 days

Indications:

Glaucoma: Therapy of open-angle glaucoma.

For other specific indications, refer to the individual monographs.

Contraindications:

Hypersensitivity to cholinesterase inhibitors or any component of the formulation; active uveal inflammation or any inflammatory disease of the iris or ciliary body; glaucoma associated with iridocyclitis.

Demecarium: Pregnancy.

Echothiophate: Most cases of angle-closure glaucoma (due to the possibility of increasing angle-block).

Warnings:

Myasthenia gravis: Because of possible additive adverse effects, only administer demecarium and echothiophate with extreme caution to patients with myasthenia gravis who are receiving systemic anticholinesterase therapy. Conversely, exercise extreme caution in the use of anticholinesterase drugs for the treatment of myasthenia gravis patients who are already undergoing topical therapy with cholinesterase inhibitors.

Surgery: In patients receiving cholinesterase inhibitors, administer succinylcholine with extreme caution before and during general anesthesia (see Drug Interactions). Stop these drugs 4 to 6 weeks prior to ophthalmic surgery to avoid a severe inflammatory response.

Pregnancy: Category X (demecarium). Contraindicated in women who are or who may become pregnant. If this drug is used during pregnancy, or if the patient becomes pregnant while taking this drug, apprise the patient of the potential hazard to the fetus.

Category C (physostigmine, echothiophate). Safety for use during pregnancy has not been established. Use only when clearly needed and when the potential benefits to the mother outweigh the potential hazards to the fetus.

Lactation: It is not known whether these drugs are excreted in breast milk. Exercise caution when administering to a nursing woman. Because of the potential for serious adverse reactions in nursing infants, decide whether to discontinue nursing or the drug, taking into account the importance of the drug to the mother.

AGENTS FOR GLAUCOMA

Children: The occurrence of iris cysts is more frequent in children (see Precautions). Exercise extreme caution in children receiving demecarium who may require general anesthesia. Safety and efficacy for use of physostigmine have not been established.

Precautions:

Concomitant therapy: Cholinesterase inhibitors may be used in combination with adrenergic agents, β-blockers, carbonic anhydrase inhibitors, or hyperosmotic agents.

Narrow angle glaucoma: Use with caution in patients with chronic angle-closure (narrow-angle) glaucoma or in patients with narrow angles, because of the possibility of producing pupillary block and increasing angle blockage.

Special risk patients: Use caution in patients with marked vagotonia, bronchial asthma, spastic GI disturbances, peptic ulcer, pronounced bradycardia/hypotension, recent MI, epilepsy, parkinsonism, and other disorders that may respond adversely to vagotonic effects. Temporarily discontinue if cardiac irregularities occur.

Ophthalmic ointments: Ophthalmic ointments may retard corneal healing.

Miosis: Miosis usually causes difficulty in dark adaptation. Use caution while driving at night or performing hazardous tasks in poor light.

Gonioscopy: Use only when shorter-acting miotics have proved inadequate. Gonioscopy is recommended prior to use of these medications. Routine examination (eg, slit-lamp) to detect lens opacities should accompany therapy.

Concomitant ocular conditions: When an intraocular inflammatory process is present, breakdown of the blood-aqueous barrier from anticholinesterase therapy requires abstention from, or cautious use of, these drugs. Use with great caution where there is a history of quiescent uveitis. After long-term use, blood vessel dilation and resultant greater permeability increase the possibility of hyphema or a severe inflammatory response during or after ophthalmic surgery. Discontinue 4 to 6 weeks before surgery.

Systemic effects: Repeated administration may cause depression of the concentration of cholinesterase in the serum and erythrocytes, with resultant systemic effects. Discontinue if salivation, urinary incontinence, diarrhea, profuse sweating, muscle weakness, respiratory difficulties, shock, or cardiac irregularities occur.

Although systemic effects are infrequent, use digital compression of the nasolacrimal ducts immediately before and for 2 minutes after instillation to minimize systemic absorption.

Iris cysts: Iris cysts may form, enlarge, and obscure vision (more frequent in children). The iris cyst usually shrinks upon discontinuation of the miotic, or following reduction in strength of the drops or frequency of instillation. Rarely, the cyst may rupture or break free into the aqueous humor. Frequent examination for this occurrence is advised.

Sulfite sensitivity: Some of these products contain sulfites, which may cause allergic-type reactions (eg, hives, itching, wheezing, anaphylaxis) in certain susceptible persons. Although the overall prevalence of sulfite sensitivity in the general population is probably low, it is seen more frequently in asthmatics or atopic nonasthmatics.

216 OPHTHALMIC DRUG FACTS

Drug Interactions:

Ophthalmic Cholinesterase Inhibitor Drug Interactions			
Precipitant drug	Object drug*		Description
Carbamate/ Organophosphate insecticides, pesticides	Cholinester- ase inhibitors	↑	Warn patients on cholinesterase inhibitors who are exposed to these substances (eg, gardeners, organo- phosphate plant or warehouse workers, farmers) of sys- temic effects possible from absorption through respiratory tract or skin. Advise use of respiratory masks, frequent washing, and clothing changes.
Succinylcholine	Cholinester- ase inhibitors	↑	Use extreme caution before or during general anesthe- sia in patients on cholinesterase inhibitors because of possible respiratory and cardiovascular collapse.
Anticholinester- ases, systemic	Cholinester- ase inhibitors	↑	Additive effects are possible; coadminister topical cho- linesterase inhibitors cautiously, regardless of which therapy is added (see Warnings).

* ↑ = Object drug increased

Adverse Reactions:

Ophthalmic: Iris cysts (see Precautions); burning; lacrimation; lid muscle twitching; conjunctival and ciliary redness; browache; headache; activation of latent iritis or uve- itis; induced myopia with visual blurring; retinal detatchment; lens opacities (see Pre- cautions); conjunctival thickening and destruction of nasolacrimal canals (prolonged use).

Paradoxical increase in IOP by pupillary block may follow instillation.

Systemic: Nausea; vomiting; abdominal cramps; diarrhea; urinary incontinence; faint- ing; sweating; salivation; difficulty in breathing; cardiac irregularities.

Overdosage:

Treatment: Systemic effects can be reversed with atropine sulfate.

Adults – 0.4 to 0.6 mg.

Infants and children up to 12 years – 0.01 mg/kg repeated every 2 hours as needed until the desired effect is obtained, or adverse effects of atropine preclude fur- ther usage. The maximum single dose should not exceed 0.4 mg.

Much larger atropine doses for anticholinesterase intoxication in adults have been used. Initially, 2 to 6 mg followed by 2 mg/hr or more often, as long as muscarinic effects continue. Consider the greater possibility of atropinization with large doses, particularly in sensitive individuals.

Pralidoxime chloride (see Antidotes) has been useful in treating systemic effects due to cholinesterase inhibitors. However, use in addition to, not as a substitute for, atro- pine.

A short-acting barbiturate is indicated for convulsions not relieved by atropine. Promptly treat marked weakness or paralysis of respiratory muscles by maintaining a clear airway and by artificial respiration.

AGENTS FOR GLAUCOMA

Patient Information:

Local irritation and headache may occur at initiation of therapy.

Notify physician if abdominal cramps, diarrhea, or excessive salivation occurs.

Wash hands immediately after administration.

Use caution while driving at night or performing hazardous tasks in poor light.

Refer to the Dosage Forms and Routes of Administration chapter for more complete information.

Individual drug monographs are on the following pages.

PHYSOSTIGMINE

For complete prescribing information, refer to the Miotics, Cholinesterase Inhibitors group monograph.

Indications:

Glaucoma: Reduction of IOP.

Administration and Dosage:

Ointment: Apply small quantity to lower fornix, up to 3 times daily.

Storage/Stability: Keep tightly closed. Protect from heat.

Rx	**Physostigmine Sulfate** (Fougera)	**Ointment**: 0.25% (as sulfate)	In 3.5 g.[1]

[1] Lanolin, white petrolatum, mineral oil.

DEMECARIUM BROMIDE

For complete prescribing information, refer to the Miotics, Cholinesterase Inhibitors group monograph. The following section is included here for completeness to show all of the clinical uses of this class of drug.

Indications:

Glaucoma: Treatment of open-angle glaucoma (use only when shorter-acting miotics have proved inadequate).

Aqueous outflow: Conditions affecting aqueous outflow (eg, synechial formation) that are amenable to miotic therapy.

Iridectomy: Following iridectomy procedure.

Accommodative esotropia: Treatment of accomodative esotripia (accomodative convergent strabismus).

Administration and Dosage:

Do not use more often than directed. Caution is necessary to avoid overdosage. Individualize dosage to use as little drug as possible to achieve the desired therapeutic effect.

Closely observe the patient during the initial period. If the response is not adequate within the first 24 hours, consider other measures. Keep frequency of use to a minimum in all patients, especially children, to reduce the chance of side effects.

Glaucoma:

> *Initial* – Instill 1 drop into eye(s). A decrease in IOP should occur within a few hours. During this period, keep patient under supervision and perform tonometric examinations at least hourly for 3 or 4 hours to make sure no immediate rise in pressure occurs.

AGENTS FOR GLAUCOMA

Usual dose – Instill 1 drop twice a week to 1 drop twice a day.

Accommodative esotropia: Essentially equal visual acuity of both eyes is a prerequisite to successful treatment.

Diagnosis – For initial evaluation, use as a diagnostic aid to determine if an accommodative factor exists. This is especially useful preoperatively in young children and in patients with normal hypermetropic refractive errors. Instill 1 drop/day for 2 weeks, then 1 drop every 2 days for 2 to 3 weeks. If the eyes become straighter, an accommodative factor is demonstrated. This technique may supplement or complement standard testing with atropine and trial with glasses for the accommodative factor.

Therapy – In esotropia uncomplicated by amblyopia or anisometropia, instill ≤ 1 drop at a time in both eyes every day for 2 to 3 weeks; too severe a degree of miosis may interfere with vision. Then reduce dosage to 1 drop every other day for 3 to 4 weeks and reevaluate the patient's status. Continue with a dosage of 1 drop every 2 days to 1 drop twice a week (the latter dosage may be maintained for several months). Evaluate the patient's condition every 4 to 12 weeks. If improvement continues, reduce to 1 drop once a week and eventually to a trial without medication. However, discontinue therapy after 4 months if control of the condition still requires 1 drop every 2 days.

Storage/Stability: Do not freeze. Protect from heat.

Rx	**Humorsol** (Merck)	**Solution:** 0.125%	In 5 mL Ocumeters.[1]
		0.25%	In 5 mL Ocumeters.[1]

[1] With 1:5000 benzalkonium chloride, sodium chloride.

ECHOTHIOPHATE IODIDE

For complete prescribing information, refer to the Miotics, Cholinesterase Inhibitors group monograph. The following section is included here for completeness to show all of the clinical uses of this class of drug.

Indications:

Glaucoma: Chronic open-angle glaucoma; if therapeutic goal is not achieved with direct-acting miotics, usually not useful in angle-closure glaucoma and most secondary glaucomas.

Accommodative esotropia: Concomitant esotropias with a significant accommodative component.

Administration and Dosage:

Tolerance may develop after prolonged use.

Glaucoma: 1 drop to eye(s) once or twice daily. Less frequent dosing can also produce the desired effect. Individualize dosage.

Concomitant therapy: May be coadministered with other glaucomal medication classes.

220 OPHTHALMIC DRUG FACTS

Accommodative esotropia:

Diagnosis – Instill 1 drop of 0.125% solution once a day into both eyes at bedtime for 2 or 3 weeks. If the esotropia is accommodative, a favorable response may begin within a few hours.

Treatment – Use the lowest concentration and frequency that gives satisfactory results. After initial period of treatment for diagnostic purposes, reduce schedule to 0.125% every other day or 0.06% every day. Dosages can often be gradually lowered as treatment progresses. The 0.03% strength has proven effective in some cases. The maximum recommended dose is 0.125% once a day, although more intensive therapy has been used for short periods.

Duration of treatment – In diagnosis, only a short period is required and little time will be lost in instituting other procedures if the esotropia proves to be unresponsive. In therapy, there is no definite limit if the drug is well tolerated. However, if the eyedrops, with or without eyeglasses, are gradually withdrawn after 1 to 2 years and deviation recurs, consider surgery.

Storage/Stability: Store at room temperature 15° to 30°C (59° to 86°F). After reconstitution, keep eyedrops in refrigerator to obtain maximum useful life of 6 months. Use within 1 month if stored at room temperature.

Rx	**Phospholine Iodide** (Wyeth)	**Powder for Reconstitution**: 1.5 mg to make 0.03%	With 5 mL diluent.[1]
		6.25 mg to make 0.125%	With 5 mL diluent.[1]

[1] With potassium acetate, 0.55% chlorobutanol, 1.2% mannitol.

PILOCARPINE AND EPINEPHRINE

Refer to the general discussion of Miotics, Cholinesterase Inhibitors for more information.

Indications:

Pilocarpine lowers IOP by a direct cholinergic action that improves outflow facility (see Agents for Glaucoma: Miotics, Direct-Acting).

Epinephrine reduces IOP by increasing outflow facility (see Agents for Glaucoma: Sympathomimetics).

The combination of pilocarpine and epinephrine provides additive effects in lowering IOP; opposing actions on the pupil may prevent marked miosis. These fixed combinations do not permit the flexibility necessary to adjust the dosage of each agent.

Administration and Dosage:

Instill 1 drop into the eye(s) 1 to 4 times daily. Determine concentration and frequency of instillation by patient response.

Storage/Stability: Store at 8° to 30°C (46° to 86°F). Keep tightly closed. Do not use solution if it is brown or contains a precipitate. Protect from light and heat.

AGENTS FOR GLAUCOMA

Rx	**E-Pilo-1** (Ciba Vision)	**Solution:** 1% pilocarpine HCl, 1% epinephrine bitartrate	In 10 mL dropper bottles.[1]
Rx	**P₁E₁** (Alcon)		In 15 mL Drop-Tainers.[2]
Rx	**E-Pilo-2** (Ciba Vision)	**Solution:** 2% pilocarpine HCl, 1% epinephrine bitartrate	In 10 mL dropper bottles.[1]
Rx	**P₂E₁** (Alcon)		In 15 mL Drop-Tainers.[2]
Rx	**E-Pilo-4** (Ciba Vision)	**Solution:** 4% pilocarpine HCl, 1% epinephrine bitartrate	In 10 mL dropper bottles.[1]
Rx	**P₄E₁** (Alcon)		In 15 mL Drop-Tainers.[2]
Rx	**E-Pilo-6** (Ciba Vision)	**Solution:** 6% pilocarpine HCl, 1% epinephrine bitartrate	In 10 mL dropper bottles.[1]
Rx	**P₆E₁** (Alcon)		In 15 mL Drop-Tainers.[2]

[1] With benzalkonium chloride, EDTA, mannitol, sodium bisulfite.
[2] With 0.01% benzalkonium chloride, methylcellulose, EDTA, chlorobutanol, polyethylene glycol, sodium bisulfite.

CARBONIC ANHYDRASE INHIBITORS

Actions:

Pharmacology: These agents are nonbacteriostatic sulfonamides that inhibit the enzyme carbonic anhydrase. This action reduces the rate of aqueous humor formation, resulting in decreased intraocular pressure (IOP).

Pharmacokinetics:

Pharmacokinetics of Oral Carbonic Anhydrase Inhibitors				
Carbonic anhydrase inhibitor	IOP Lowering Effects			Relative inhibitor potency
	Onset (hours)	Peak effect (hours)	Duration (hours)	
Dichlorphenamide	within 1	2 to 4	6 to 12	30
Acetazolamide				
Tablets	1 to 1.5	1 to 4	8 to 12	1
Capsules, sustained-release	2	3 to 6	18 to 24	
Injection (IV)	2 min	15 min	4 to 5	
Methazolamide	2 to 4	6 to 8	10 to 18	*

* Quantitative data not available; reported to be more active than acetazolamide.

Methazolamide – Peak plasma concentrations for the 25, 50, and 100 mg twice daily regimens were 2.5, 5.1, and 10.7 mcg/mL, respectively. Approximately 55% is bound to plasma proteins. The mean steady-state plasma elimination half-life is ≈ 14 hours. At steady state, ≈ 25% of the dose is recovered unchanged in the urine. Renal clearance accounts for 20% to 25% of the total clearance of drug. After repeated dosing, methazolamide accumulates to steady-state concentrations in 7 days.

Dorzolamide – When topically applied, dorzolamide reaches the systemic circulation. It binds moderately to plasma proteins (≈ 33%). The drug is primarily excreted unchanged in the urine, and the metabolite is also excreted in the urine.

After dosing is stopped, dorzolamide washes out of RBCs nonlinearly, resulting in a rapid decline of drug concentration initially, followed by a slower elimination phase with a half-life of ≈ 4 months.

OPHTHALMIC DRUG FACTS

Indications:

The following section is included here for completeness to show all of the clinical uses of this class of drug.

Oral: For adjunctive treatment of glaucoma.

Ophthalmic: Treatment of elevated IOP in patients with ocular hypertension or open-angle glaucoma.

Dorzolamide: Only indicated to decrease IOP in patients with ocular hypertension or open-angle glaucoma.

Contraindications:

Hypersensitivity to these agents; depressed sodium or potassium serum levels; marked kidney and liver disease or dysfunction; suprarenal gland failure; hyperchloremic acidosis; adrenocortical insufficiency; severe pulmonary obstruction with inability to increase alveolar ventilation because acidosis may be increased (dichlorphenamide); cirrhosis (acetazolamide, methazolamide).

Warnings:

Renal function impairment: Dorzolamide has not been studied in patients with severe renal impairment (Ccr < 30 mL/min). However, because dorzolamide and its metabolite are excreted predominantly by the kidney, dorzolamide is not recommended in such patients.

Hepatic function impairment: Use of methazolamide in this condition could precipitate hepatic coma. Dorzolamide has not been studied in patients with hepatic impairment and should be used with caution in such patients.

Carcinogenesis:

> *Dorzolamide* – In a 2-year study of dorzolamide administered orally to rats, urinary bladder papillomas were seen in male rats in the highest dosage group of 20 mg/kg/day (250 times the recommended human ophthalmic dose). The increased incidence of urinary bladder papillomas is a class effect of carbonic anhydrase inhibitors in rats.

Pregnancy: Category C. Animal studies with some of these drugs have demonstrated teratogenicity (skeletal anomalies). Do not use during pregnancy, especially during the first trimester, unless the potential benefits to the mother outweigh the potential hazards to the fetus.

Lactation: Safety for use in the nursing mother has not been established. It is not known whether all carbonic anhydrase inhibitors are excreted in breast milk. Acetazolamide appeared in breast milk of a patient taking 500 mg twice/day. However, the infant ingested only 0.06% of the dose, an amount unlikely to cause adverse effects.

Children: Safety and efficacy have not been established.

Precautions:

Monitoring: Monitor for hematologic reactions common to sulfonamides.

AGENTS FOR GLAUCOMA

Hypokalemia: During concomitant use of steroids or ACTH, and with interference with adequate oral electrolyte intake, hypokalemia may develop when severe cirrhosis is present. Hypokalemia can sensitize or exaggerate the response of the heart to the toxic effects of digitalis (eg, increased ventricular irritability). Hypokalemia may be avoided or treated with potassium supplements or foods with a high potassium content.

Pulmonary conditions: Use dichlorphenamide with caution in patients with severe degrees of respiratory acidosis. These drugs may precipitate or aggravate acidosis. Use with caution in patients with pulmonary obstruction or emphysema when alveolar ventilation may be impaired.

Cross-sensitivity: Cross-sensitivity between antibacterial sulfonamides and sulfonamide derivative diuretics, including acetazolamide and various thiazides, has occurred.

Corneal endothelium effects: The effect of continued administration of dorzolamide on the corneal endothelium has not been fully evaluated.

Ocular effects: Local ocular adverse effects, primarily conjunctivitis and lid reactions, occurred with chronic administration of dorzolamide. Many of these reactions had the clinical appearance and course of an allergic-type reaction that resolved upon discontinuation of drug therapy. If such reactions are observed, discontinue dorzolamide and evaluate the patient before considering restarting the drug.

Concomitant oral CA inhibitors: The concomitant administration of dorzolamide and oral CA inhibitors is not recommended.

Contact lenses: The preservative in dorzolamide solution, benzalkonium chloride, may be absorbed by soft contact lenses. Dorzolamide should be administered with this in mind.

Hazardous tasks: Carbonic anhydrase inhibitors may cause drowsiness in some patients. Observe caution while driving, operating machinery, or performing other tasks requiring coordination or physical dexterity.

Drug Interactions:

Carbonic Anhydrase Inhibitor (CAI) Drug Interactions			
Precipitant drug	Object drug*		Description
Acetazolamide	Cyclosporine	↑	Increased trough cyclosporine levels with possible nephrotoxicity and neurotoxicity may occur.
Acetazolamide	Primidone	↓	Primidone serum and urine concentrations may be decreased.
CAIs	Salicylates	↑	Concurrent use may result in accumulation and toxicity of the CAI, including CNS depression and metabolic acidosis. Also, CAI-induced acidosis may allow increased CNS penetration by salicylates.
Salicylates	CAIs	↑	
Diflunisal	CAIs	↑	Concurrent use may result in a significant decrease in intraocular pressure; the effect may be less pronounced with methazolamide. Increased side effects may also occur.

* ↑ = Object drug increased. ↓ = Object drug decreased

Adverse Reactions:

Sulfonamide-type adverse reactions may occur.

OPHTHALMIC DRUG FACTS

Dorzolamide:

Miscellaneous – Ocular burning, stinging, or discomfort immediately following administration (≈ 33%); bitter taste following administration (≈ 25%); superficial punctate keratitis (10% to 15%); signs and symptoms of ocular allergic reaction (≈ 10%); blurred vision, tearing, dryness, photophobia (≈ 1% to 5%); urolithiasis, iridocyclitis (rare).

CNS: Convulsions; weakness; malaise; fatigue; nervousness; drowsiness; depression; dizziness; disorientation; confusion; ataxia; tremor; tinnitus; headache; lassitude; flaccid paralysis; paresthesias of the extremities.

Dermatologic: Urticaria; pruritus; skin eruptions; rash (including erythema multiforme, Stevens-Johnson syndrome, toxic epidermal necrolysis); photosensitivity.

GI:: Melena; anorexia; nausea; vomiting; constipation; taste alteration; diarrhea.

Hematologic: Bone marrow depression; thrombocytopenia; thrombocytopenic purpura; hemolytic anemia; leukopenia; pancytopenia; agranulocytosis.

Renal: Hematuria; glycosuria; urinary frequency; renal colic; renal calculi; crystalluria; polyuria; phosphaturia.

Miscellaneous: Weight loss; fever; acidosis (usually corrected with bicarbonate); decreased/absent libido; impotence; electrolyte imbalance; hepatic insufficiency; transient myopia.

Overdosage:

Symptoms: Symptoms of overdosage or toxicity may include drowsiness, anorexia, nausea, vomiting, dizziness, paresthesias, ataxia, tremor, and tinnitus.

Treatment: In the event of overdosage, induce emesis or perform gastric lavage. The electrolyte disturbance most likely to be encountered from overdosage is hyperchloremic acidosis, which may respond to bicarbonate administration. Potassium supplementation may be required. Observe carefully; give supportive treatment.

Patient Information:

Oral: If GI upset occurs, take with food.

Avoid prolonged exposure to sunlight or sunlamps; may cause photosensitivity.

May cause drowsiness; observe caution while driving or performing other tasks requiring alertness, coordination, or physical dexterity.

Notify physician if sore throat, fever, unusual bleeding or bruising, tingling or tremors in the hands or feet, flank or loin pain, skin rash, or eye irritation occurs.

Bioavailability – Consult physician before switching brands of carbonic anhydrase inhibitors. Problems with bioavailability have been documented with products from different manufacturers.

Ophthalmic: To avoid contamination, do not touch tip of container to any surface. Replace cap after use.

AGENTS FOR GLAUCOMA

Advise patients that if they develop an intercurrent ocular condition (eg, trauma, ocular surgery, infection), they should immediately seek their physician's advice concerning the continued use of the present multidose container.

If more than one topical ophthalmic drug is being used, administer the drugs at least 10 minutes apart.

Dorzolamide should not be administered while wearing soft contact lenses.

Individual drug monographs are on the following pages.

ACETAZOLAMIDE

For complete prescribing information, see the Carbonic Anhydrase Inhibitors group monograph. The following section is included here for completeness to show all of the clinical uses of this class of drug.

Administration and Dosage:

To lower IOP:

Adults – 250 mg to 1 g/day, in divided doses every 6 to 12 hours. Dosage > 1 g/day does not usually increase the effect.

Secondary glaucoma and preoperative treatment of acute congestive (closed-angle) glaucoma:

Adults –

Short-term therapy: 250 mg every 4 hours or 250 mg twice daily.

Acute cases: 500 mg followed by 125 or 250 mg every 4 hours.

IV therapy may be used for rapid decreases of intraocular pressure. A complementary effect occurs when used with miotics or beta blockers.

Children:

Parenteral – 5 to 10 mg/kg/dose, IM or IV, every 6 hours.

Oral – 10 to 15 mg/kg/day in divided doses, every 6 to 8 hours.

Sustained release: 500 mg twice daily.

Parenteral: Direct IV administration is preferred; IM administration is painful because of the alkaline pH of the solution.

Preparation and storage of parenteral solution: Reconstitute each 500 mg vial with ≥ 5 mL of sterile water for injection. Reconstituted solutions retain potency for 1 week if refrigerated. However, because this product contains no preservative, use within 24 hours of reconstitution.

Oral liquid dose form: If required, acetazolamide tablets may be crushed and suspended in a cherry, chocolate, raspberry, or other sweet syrup. Do not use a vehicle with alcohol or glycerin. Alternatively, 1 tablet can be submerged in 10 mL of hot water and added to 10 mL of honey or syrup. When prepared in a 70% sorbitol solution with a pH of 4 to 5 and stored in amber glass bottles, the suspension is stable for ≥ 2 to 3 months at temperatures < 30°C (86°F).

Rx	**Acetazolamide** (Various, eg, Mutual, URL)	**Tablets**: 125 mg	In 50s, 100s, 250s, 500s, and 1000s.
Rx	**Diamox** (Wyeth)		In 100s.
Rx	**Acetazolamide** (Various, eg, Qualitest, Schein, URL)	**Tablets**: 250 mg	In 50s, 100s, 250s, 500s, 1000s, and UD 100s.
Rx	**Dazamide** (Major)		In 100s, 250s, 1000s, and UD 100s.

AGENTS FOR GLAUCOMA

Rx	**Diamox Sequels** (Wyeth)	**Capsules, sustained release:** 500 mg	In 100s.
Rx	**Acetazolamide** (Various, eg, Bedford Labs)	**Powder for injection, lyophilized:** 500 mg (as sodium)	In vials.
Rx	**Diamox** (Wyeth)		

DICHLORPHENAMIDE

For complete prescribing information, refer to the Carbonic Anhydrase Inhibitors group monograph.

Administration and Dosage:

Glaucoma: Use adjunctively. In acute angle-closure glaucoma, dichlorphenamide may be used with miotics and osmotic agents to rapidly reduce intraocular tension.

Adults: Individualize dosage, 25 to 50 mg 1 to 3 times daily.

Rx	**Daranide** (Merck)	**Tablets:** 50 mg	Lactose. In 100s.

METHAZOLAMIDE

For complete prescribing information, refer to the Carbonic Anhydrase Inhibitors group monograph.

Administration and Dosage:

Glaucoma: 25 to 100 mg 2 or 3 times daily. May be used with glaucoma agents from other classes.

Rx	**Methazolamide** (Various, eg, Teva)	**Tablets:** 25 mg	In 100s and 1000s.
Rx	**GlaucTabs** (Akorn)		In 100s.
Rx	**Neptazane** (Wyeth)		In 100s.
Rx	**Methazolamide** (Various, eg, Teva)	**Tablets:** 50 mg	In 100s and 1000s.
Rx	**GlaucTabs** (Akorn)		In 100s.
Rx	**Neptazane** (Wyeth)		In 100s.

DORZOLAMIDE HYDROCHLORIDE

Actions:

Pharmacology: Dorzolamide is a carbonic anhydrase inhibitor formulated for topical ophthalmic use. Carbonic anhydrase (CA) is an enzyme found in many tissues of the body, including the eye. It catalyzes the reversible reaction involving the hydration of carbon dioxide and the dehydration of carbonic acid. In humans, carbonic

228   OPHTHALMIC DRUG FACTS

anhydrase exists as a number of isoenzymes, the most active being carbonic anhydrase II (CA-II), found primarily in red blood cells (RBCs), but also in other tissues. Inhibition of CA in the ciliary processes of the eye decreases aqueous humor secretion, presumably by slowing the formation of bicarbonate ions with subsequent reduction in sodium and fluid transport. The result is a reduction in intraocular pressure (IOP). Dorzolamide, by inhibiting CA-II, reduces elevated IOP. Elevated IOP is a major risk factor in the pathogenesis of optic nerve damage and glaucomatous visual field loss.

Pharmacokinetics: When topically applied, dorzolamide reaches the systemic circulation. To assess the potential for systemic CA inhibition following topical administration, drug and metabolite concentrations in RBCs and plasma and CA inhibition in RBCs were measured. Dorzolamide accumulates in RBCs, during chronic dosing as a result of binding to CA-II. The parent drug forms a single N-desethyl metabolite that inhibits CA-II less potently than the parent drug but also inhibits CA-I. The metabolite also accumulates in RBCs, where it binds primarily to CA-I. Plasma concentrations of parent and metabolite are generally below the assay limit of quantitation. Dorzolamide binds moderately to plasma proteins ($\approx$ 33%). The drug is primarily excreted unchanged in the urine, and the metabolite is also excreted in urine. After dosing is stopped, dorzolamide washes out of RBCs nonlinearly, resulting in a rapid decline of drug concentration initially, followed by a slower elimination phase with a half-life of $\approx$ 4 months.

To simulate the systemic exposure after long-term topical ocular administration, dorzolamide was given orally to 8 healthy subjects for up to 20 weeks. The oral dose of 2 mg twice daily closely approximates the amount of drug delivered by topical ocular administration of 2% three times daily. Steady-state was reached within 8 weeks. The inhibition of CA-II and total CA activities was below the degree of inhibition anticipated to be necessary for a pharmacological effect on renal function and respiration in healthy individuals.

Clinical Trials: The efficacy of dorzolamide was demonstrated in clinical studies in the treatment of elevated IOP in patients with glaucoma or ocular hypertension (baseline IOP $\geq$ 23 mm Hg). The IOP-lowering effect of dorzolamide was $\approx$ 3 to 5 mm Hg throughout the day, and this was consistent in clinical studies with durations of up to 1 year.

Indications:

Elevated intraocular pressure (IOP): Treatment of elevated IOP in patients with ocular hypertension or open-angle glaucoma.

Contraindications:

Hypersensitivity to any component of this product.

Warnings:

Systemic effects: Dorzolamide is a sulfonamide and, although administered topically, is absorbed systemically. Therefore, the same types of adverse reactions attributable to sulfonamides may occur with topical administration of dorzolamide. Fatalities have occurred, although rarely, due to severe reactions to sulfonamides including Stevens-Johnson syndrome, toxic epidermal necrolysis, fulminant hepatic necrosis, agranulocytosis, aplastic anemia, and other blood dyscrasias. Sensitization may recur

AGENTS FOR GLAUCOMA

when a sulfonamide is readministered, regardless of the route of administration. If signs of serious reactions or hypersensitivity occur, discontinue the use of this preparation.

Renal/Hepatic function impairment: Dorzolamide has not been studied in patients with severe renal impairment (Ccr < 30 mL/min). However, because dorzolamide and its metabolite are excreted predominantly by the kidney, dorzolamide is not recommended in such patients.

Dorzolamide has not been studied in patients with hepatic impairment and should be used with caution in such patients.

Carcinogenesis: In a 2 year study of dorzolamide administered orally to male and female Sprague-Dawley rats, urinary bladder papillomas were seen in male rats in the highest dosage group of 20 mg/kg/day (250 times the recommended human ophthalmic dose); papillomas were not seen in rats given oral doses equivalent to $\approx$ 12 times the recommended dose. The increased incidence of urinary bladder papillomas is a class effect of CA inhibitors in rats.

Elderly: Of all the patients in clinical studies, 44% were $\geq$ 65 years of age and 10% were $\geq$ 75 years of age. No overall differences in efficacy or safety were observed between these patients and younger patients, but greater sensitivity of some older individuals to the product cannot be ruled out.

Pregnancy: Category C. Studies in rabbits at oral doses of $\geq$ 2.5 mg/kg/day (31 times the recommended human ophthalmic dose) revealed malformations of the vertebral bodies. These malformations occurred at doses that caused metabolic acidosis with decreased body weight gain in dams and decreased fetal weights. There are no adequate and well-controlled studies in pregnant women. Use during pregnancy only if the potential benefit to the mother justifies the risk to the fetus.

Lactation: In lactating rats, decreases in body weight gain of 5% to 7% were seen in offspring at an oral dose of 7.5 mg/kg/day (94 times the recommended human ophthalmic dose). A slight delay in postnatal development (incisor eruption, vaginal canalization, eye openings), secondary to lower fetal body weight, was noted.

It is not known whether this drug is excreted in breast milk. Because of the potential for serious adverse reactions in nursing infants, decide whether to discontinue nursing or to discontinue the drug, taking into account the importance of the drug to the mother.

Children: Safety and efficacy have not been established.

Precautions:

Corneal endothelium effects: The effect of continued administration of dorzolamide on the corneal endothelium has not been fully evaluated.

Ocular effects: Local ocular adverse effects, primarily conjunctivitis and lid reactions, were reported with chronic administration of dorzolamide. Many of these reactions had the clinical appearance and course of an allergic-type reaction that resolved upon discontinuation of drug therapy. If such reactions are observed, discontinue dorzolamide and evaluate the patient before considering restarting the drug.

Concomitant oral CA inhibitors: The concomitant administration of dorzolamide and oral CA inhibitors is not recommended.

230 OPHTHALMIC DRUG FACTS

Contact lenses: The preservative in dorzolamide solution, benzalkonium chloride, may be absorbed by soft contact lenses. Dorzolamide should not be administered while wearing soft contact lenses.

Corneal decompensation: Cases of corneal decompensation from dorzolamide have been reported in patients undergoing corneal transplants.

Drug Interactions:

Although acid-base and electrolyte disturbances were not reported in the clinical trials with dorzolamide, these disturbances have occurred with oral CA inhibitors and have, in some instances, resulted in drug interactions (eg, toxicity associated with high-dose salicylate therapy). Therefore, consider the potential for such drug interactions in patients receiving dorzolamide.

Adverse Reactions:

Ocular burning, stinging, or discomfort immediately following administration ($\approx$ 33%); bitter taste following administration ($\approx$ 25%); superficial punctate keratitis (10% to 15%); signs and symptoms of ocular allergic reaction ($\approx$ 10%); blurred vision, tearing, dryness, photophobia ($\approx$ 1% to 5%); headache, nausea, asthenia/fatigue (infrequent); skin rashes, urolithiasis, iridocyclitis (rare).

Overdosage:

Electrolyte imbalance, development of an acidotic state, and possible CNS effects may occur. Monitor serum electrolyte levels (particularly potassium) and blood pH levels. Significant lethality was observed in female rats and mice after single oral doses of 1927 and 1320 mg/kg, respectively.

Patient Information:

Dorzolamide is a sulfonamide and, although administered topically, it is absorbed systemically. Therefore, the same types of adverse reactions that are attributable to sulfonamides may occur with topical administration. Advise patients that if serious or unusual reactions or signs of hypersensitivity occur, they should discontinue use of the product.

Advise patients that if they develop any ocular reactions, particularly conjunctivitis and lid reactions, they should discontinue use and seek their physician's advice.

Instruct patients to avoid allowing the tip of the dispensing container to contact the eye or surrounding structures. Ocular solutions, if handled improperly or if the tip of the dispensing container contacts the eye or surrounding structures, can become contaminated by common bacteria known to cause ocular infections. Serious damage to the eye and subsequent loss of vision may result from using contaminated solutions.

Advise patients that if they develop an intercurrent ocular condition (eg, trauma, ocular surgery, infection), they should immediately seek their physician's advice concerning the continued use of the present multidose container.

If more than one topical ophthalmic drug is being used, administer the drugs 5 to 10 minutes apart with the drugs with sustained-release vehicles such as *Pilopine HS*, *Timoptic XE*, and *Betoptic S* administered last.

AGENTS FOR GLAUCOMA

Administration and Dosage:

Dosage: Instill 1 drop in the affected eye(s) 3 times daily; twice daily when used concomitantly with a beta blocker.

Concomitant therapy: Dorzolamide may be used concomitantly with other topical ophthalmic drug products to lower intraocular pressure. If more than 1 ophthalmic drug is being used, administer the drugs 5 minutes apart. Can be used twice daily with beta blocker or other aqueous-secretion inhibitor.

Rx	**Trusopt** (Merck)	**Solution:** 2%	In 5 and 10 mL.[1]

[1] 0.0075% benzalkonium Cl.

BRINZOLAMIDE

Actions:

Pharmacology: Brinzolamide is an inhibitor of carbonic anhydrase II (CA-II); an enzyme found in many tissues of the body including the eye. It catalyzes the reversible reaction involving the hydration of carbon dioxide and the dehydration of carbonic acid. Inhibition of carbonic anhydrase in the ciliary processes of the eye decreases aqueous humor secretion, presumably by slowing the formation of bicarbonate ions with subsequent reduction in sodium and fluid transport. The result is a reduction in IOP.

Pharmacokinetics: Elevated intraocular pressure is a major risk factor in the pathogenesis of optic nerve damage and glaucomatous visual field loss. Following topical ocular administration, brinzolamide is absorbed into the systemic circulation.

Clinical Trials: In 2, three-month studies, brinzolamide 1% dosed 3 times per day in patients with elevated intraocular pressure (IOP), produced significant reductions in IOPs (4 to 5 mm Hg). These IOP reductions are equivalent to the reductions observed with dorzolamide hydrochloride ophthalmic solution 2% dosed 3 times daily in the same studies.

In 2 clinical studies with elevated intraocular pressure, brinzolamide was associated with less stinging and burning upon instillation than dorzolamide hydrochloride.

Indications:

For the treatment of elevated IOP in patients with ocular hypertension or open-angle glaucoma.

Contraindications:

Hypersensitivity to any component of this product.

Warnings:

Systemic effects: Brinzolamide is a sulfonamide and, although administered topically, it is absorbed systemically. Therefore, the same types of adverse reactions that are attributed to sulfonamides may occur with the topical administration of brinzolamide. Fatalities have occurred, although rarely, due to severe reactions to sulfon-

232 OPHTHALMIC DRUG FACTS

amides including Stevens-Johnson syndrome, toxic epidermal necrolysis, fulminant hepatic necrosis, agranulocytosis, aplastic anemia, and other blood dyscrasias. Sensitization may occur when a sulfonamide is readministered irrespective of the route of administration. If signs of serious reactions or hypersensitivity occur, discontinue the use of this preparation.

Carcinogenesis: Carcinogenicity data on brinzolamide is not available.

Mutagenesis: The following tests for mutagenic potential were negative: (1) in vivo mouse micronucleus assay; (2) in vivo sister chromatid exchange assay; and (3) Ames *E. coli* test. The in vitro mouse lymphoma forward mutation assay was negative in the absence of activation, but positive in the presence of microsomal activation.

Fertility impairment: In reproductive studies of brinzolamide in rats, there were no adverse effects on the fertility or reproductive capacity of males or females at doses up to 18 mg/kg/day (375 times the recommended human ophthalmic dose).

Pregnancy: Category C. Developmental toxicity studies with brinzolamide in rabbits at oral doses of 1, 3, and 6 mg/kg/day (20, 62, and 125 times the recommended human ophthalmic dose) produced maternal toxicity at 6 mg/kg/day and a significant increase in the number of fetal variations, such as skull bones, which was only slightly higher than the historic value at 1 and 6 mg/kg. There are no adequate and well-controlled studies in pregnant women. Brinzolamide should be used during pregnancy only if the potential benefit to the mother justifies the potential risk to the fetus.

Lactation: It is not known whether this drug is excreted in breast milk. Because of the potential for serious adverse reactions to the nursing infant, a decision should be made whether to discontinue the nursing or discontinue the drug, taking into account the importance of the drug to the mother.

Children: Safety and efficacy have not been established.

Precautions:

Corneal endothelium effects: Carbonic anhydrase activity has been observed in the cytoplasm and around the plasma membranes of the corneal endothelium. The effects of continued administration of brinzolamide on the corneal endothelium has not been fully evaluated.

Acute angle-closure glaucoma: The management of acute angle-closure glaucoma requires therapeutic interventions in addition to ocular hypotensive agents. Brinzolamide has not been studied in patients with acute-closure glaucoma.

Severe renal impairment: Brinzolamide has not been studied in patients with severe renal impairment. Because brinzolamide and its metabolite are excreted predominantly by the kidney, it is not recommended in these patients.

Oral carbonic anhydrase inhibitors: There is potential for an additive effect on the known systemic effects of carbonic anhydrase inhibitors and brinzolamide. The concomitant administration of brinzolamide and oral carbonic anhydrase inhibitors is not recommended.

Drug Interactions:

Although brinzolamide 1% is a carbonic anhydrase inhibitor, acid-base and electrolyte alterations were not reported in the clinical trials. However, in patients treated with

AGENTS FOR GLAUCOMA

oral carbonic anhydrase inhibitors, rare instances of drug interactions have occurred with high-dose salicylate therapy. Therefore, consider the potential for such drug interactions.

Adverse Reactions:

The most frequently reported adverse events associated with brinzolamide were blurred vision and bitter, sour, or unusual taste. These events occurred in ≈ 5% to 10% of patients. Blepharitis, dermatitis, dry eye, foreign body sensation, headache, hyperemia, ocular discharge, keratitis, ocular pain, ocular pruritus, and rhinitis were reported at an incidence of 1% to 5%. The following adverse reactions were reported at an incidence of < 1%: allergic reactions; alopecia; chest pain; conjunctivitis; diarrhea; diplopia; dizziness; dry mouth; dyspepsia; eye fatigue; hypertonia; keratoconjunctivitis; keratopathy; kidney pain; lid margin crusting or sticky sensation; nausea; pharyngitis; tearing; and urticaria.

Overdosage:

Symptoms: Although there is no human data available, electrolyte imbalance, development of an acidotic state, and possible nervous system effects may occur following oral administration of an overdose. Serum electrolyte levels (particularly potassium) and blood pH levels should be monitored.

Patient Information:

Vision may be temporarily blurred following dosing with brinzolamide. Care should be exercised in operating machinery or driving a motor vehicle.

Instruct patients to avoid allowing the tip of the dispensing container to contact the eye or surrounding structures or surfaces, because the product can become contaminated by common bacteria known to cause ocular infections.

Patients should be advised that if they have ocular surgery or develop an intercurrent ocular condition (eg, trauma or infection), they should immediately seek their physician's advice concerning the continued use of the present multidose container.

Administration and Dosage:

Shake well before use. Instill 1 drop in the affected eye(s) 3 times daily.

Concurrent therapy: Brinzolamide may be used concurrently with other ophthalmic drug products to lower intraocular pressure. If more than one topical ophthalmic drug is being used, the drugs should be administered at ≥ 10 minutes apart.

Rx **Azopt** (Alcon)	**Suspension:** 1%	In 5, 10, and 15 mL plastic Drop-Tainer bottles with controlled dispensing tip.

234 OPHTHALMIC DRUG FACTS

PROSTAGLANDINS AND PROSTAMIDES

TRAVOPROST

Actions:

Pharmacology: Travoprost free acid is a selective FP prostanoid receptor agonist, which is believed to reduce intraocular pressure (IOP) by increasing uveoscleral outflow. The exact mechanism of action is unknown.

Pharmacokinetics: Travoprost is absorbed through the cornea as an isopropyl ester prodrug and is hydrolyzed by esterases in the cornea to its biologically active free acid. In humans, peak plasma concentrations of travoprost free acid (≤ 25 pg/ml) were reached within 30 minutes following topical ocular administration and were rapidly eliminated. Systemically, travoprost free acid is metabolized to inactive metabolites. Elimination as travoprost free acid from human plasma is rapid. Plasma levels are below the limit of quantitation (< 10 pg/mL) within 1 hour following ocular instillation.

Clinical Trials: Glaucoma or ocular hypertension patients with baseline pressure IOP of 25 to 27 mm Hg were dosed once daily in the evening and demonstrated 7 to 8 mm Hg reductions in IOP. In subgroup analyses, mean IOP reduction in black patients was up to 1.8 mm Hg greater than in non-black patients. It is not known at this time whether this difference is attributed to race or to heavily pigmented irides. In a multi-center, randomized, controlled trial, patients with mean baseline IOP of 24 to 26 mm Hg on timolol 0.5% twice daily were treated with travoprost 0.004% dosed every day adjunctively to timolol 0.5% twice daily demonstrated 6 to 7 mm Hg reductions in IOP.

Indications:

For the reduction of IOP in patients with open-angle glaucoma or ocular hypertension who are intolerant of other IOP-lowering medications or insufficiently responsive (failed to achieve target IOP determined after multiple measurements over time) to another IOP-lowering medication. Travoprost has not been evaluated for the treatment of angle closure, inflammatory, or neovascular glaucoma.

Contraindications:

Known hypersensitivity to travoprost, benzalkonium chloride, or any other ingredients of the product. Travoprost may interfere with the maintenance of pregnancy and should not be used by women during pregnancy or by women attempting to become pregnant.

Warnings:

Ocular changes: Travoprost has been reported to cause changes to pigmented tissues. The most frequently reported changes have been increased pigmentation of the iris and periorbital tissue (eyelid) and increased pigmentation and growth of eyelashes. These changes may be permanent.

AGENTS FOR GLAUCOMA

Mutagenesis: Travoprost was not mutagenic in the Ames test, mouse micronucleus test, and rat chromosome assay. A slight increase in the mutant frequency was observed in 1 of 2 mouse lymphoma assays in the presence of rat S-9 activation enzymes.

Fertility impairment: Travoprost did not affect mating or fertility indices in male or female rats at SC doses up to 10 mcg/kg/day (250 times the maximum recommended human ocular dose [MRHOD] of 0.04 mcg/kg/day on a mcg/kg basis). At 10 mcg/kg/day, the mean number of corpora lutea was reduced, and the post-implantation losses were increased. These effects were not observed at 3 mcg/kg/day (75 times the MRHOD).

Elderly: No overall differences in safety or effectiveness have been observed between elderly and other adult patients.

Pregnancy: Category C. Because prostaglandins are biologically active and may be absorbed through the skin, women who are pregnant or attempting to become pregnant should exercise appropriate precautions to avoid direct exposure to the contents of the bottle. In case of accidental contact with the contents of the bottle, thoroughly cleanse the exposed area with soap and water immediately.

Travoprost was teratogenic in rats, at an IV dose up to 10 mcg/kg/day (250 times the MRHOD), evidenced by an increase in the incidence of skeletal malformations as well as external and visceral malformations, such as fused sternebrae, domed head, andhydrocephaly. Travoprost was not teratogenic in rats at IV doses up to 3 mcg/kg/day (75 times the MRHOD), and in mice at SC doses up to 1 mcg/kg/day (25 times the MRHOD). Travoprost produced an increase in post-implantation losses and a decrease in fetal viability in rats at IV doses > 3 mcg/kg/day (75 times the MRHOD) and in mice at SC doses > 0.3 mcg/kg/day (7.5 times the MRHOD). In the offspring of female rats that received travoprost SC from day 7 of pregnancy to lactation day 21 at doses of ≥ 0.12 mcg/kg/day (3 times the MRHOD), the incidence of postnatal mortality was increased, and neonatal body weight gain was decreased. Neonatal development was also affected, evidenced by delayed eye opening, pinna detachment, and preputial separation, and by decreased motor activity.

No adequate and well-controlled studies have been performed in pregnant women. Travoprost may interfere with the maintenance of pregnancy and should not be used by women during pregnancy or by women attempting to become pregnant.

Lactation: A study in lactating rats demonstrated that radiolabeled travoprost or its metabolites were excreted in milk. It is not known whether this drug or its metabolites are excreted in human milk. Because many drugs are excreted in human milk, exercise caution when travoprost is administered to a nursing woman.

Children: Safety and efficacy not established.

Precautions:

Cornea: Reports of bacterial keratitis have been associated with the use of multiple-dose containers of topical ophthalmic products. These containers had been inadvertently contaminated by patients, who, in most cases, had a concurrent corneal disease or a disruption of the epithelial surface.

Iris pigmentation: Patients may slowly develop increased brown pigmentation of the iris. This change may not be noticeable for months to years (see Warnings). Iris pigmentation changes may be more noticeable in patients with mixed colored irdies (ie, blue-brown, grey-brown, yellow-brown, and green-brown); however, it has also been

236 OPHTHALMIC DRUG FACTS

observed in patients with brown eyes. The color change is believed to be due to increased melanin content in the stromal melanocytes of the iris. The exact mechanism of action is unknown at this time. Typically, the brown pigmentation around the pupil spreads concentrically towards the periphery in affected eyes, but the entire iris or parts of it may become more brownish. Until more information about increased brown pigmentation is available, examine patients regularly and, depending on the situation, treatment may be stopped if increased pigmentation ensues.

Iritis/Uveitis: Use with caution in patients with active intracocular inflammation.

Macular edema: Macular edema, including cystoid macular edema, has been reported during treatment with prostaglandin $F_{2\alpha}$ analogs. These reports have mainly occurred in aphakic patients, pseudophakic patients with a torn posterior lens capsule, or in patients with known risk factors for macular edema. Use travoprost with caution in these patients.

Contact lenses: Travoprost should not be administered while wearing contact lenses. Advise patients that travoprost contains benzalkonium chloride, which may be absorbed by the contact lenses. Remove contact lenses prior to the administration of the solution. Lenses may be reinserted 15 minutes following travoprost administration.

Adverse Reactions:

Ophthalmic: The most common ocular adverse event observed in controlled clinical studies with travoprost was ocular hyperemia, which was reported in 35% to 50% of patients. Approximately 3% of patients discontinued therapy because of conjunctival hyperemia.

Ocular adverse events reported at an incidence of 5% to 10% included decreased visual acuity, eye discomfort, foreign body sensation, pain, and pruritus.

Ocular adverse events reported at an incidence of 1% to 4% included abnormal vision, blepharitis, blurred vision, cataract, cells, conjunctivitis, dry eye, eye disorder, flare, iris discoloration, keratitis, lid margin crusting, photophobia, subconjunctival hemorrhage, and tearing.

Systemic: Nonocular adverse events reported at a rate of 1% to 5% were the following: Accidental injury, angina pectoris, anxiety, arthritis, back pain, bradycardia, bronchitis, chest pain, cold syndrome, depression, dyspepsia, GI disorder, headache, hypercholesterolemia, hypertension, hypotension, infection, pain, prostate disorder, sinusitis, urinary incontinence, and urinary tract infection.

Patient Information:

Patients should be advised concerning all the information contained in the Warnings and Precautions sections.

Instruct patients to avoid allowing the tip of the dispensing container to contact the eye or surrounding structures because this could cause the tip to become contaminated by common bacteria known to cause ocular infections. Serious damage to the eye and subsequent loss of vision may result from using contaminated solutions.

Advise patients that if they develop an intercurrent ocular condition (eg, trauma, infection) or have ocular surgery, they should immediately seek their physician's advice concerning the continued use of the multi-dose container.

AGENTS FOR GLAUCOMA

Advise patients that if they develop any ocular reactions, particularly conjunctivitis and lid reactions, they should immediately seek their physician's advice.

If more than 1 topical ophthalmic drug is being used, administer the drugs at least 5 minutes apart.

Administration and Dosage:

The recommended dosage is 1 drop in the affected eye(s) once daily in the evening. The travoprost dosage should not exceed once daily.

Reduction of IOP starts ≈ 2 hours after administration, and the maximum effect is reached after 12 hours.

Travoprost may be used concomitantly with other topical ophthalmic drugs to lower IOP. If more than 1 topical ophthalmic drugs is being used, the drugs should be administered at least 5 minutes apart.

Storage/Stability: Store between 2° to 25°C (36° to 77°F). Discard the container within 6 weeks of removing it from the sealed pouch.

Rx	**Travatan** (Alcon)	**Solution:** 0.004%	In 2.5 mL Drop-Tainers.[1]

[1] 0.015% benzalkonium chloride, EDTA.

BIMATOPROST

Actions:

Pharmacology: Bimatoprost is a synthetic prostamide structural analog with ocular hypotensive activity. It selectively mimics the effects of naturally occurring substances, prostamides. Bimatoprost is believed to lower IOP in humans by increasing outflow of aqueous humor through the trabecular meshwork and uveoscleral routes.

Pharmacokinetics: Bimatoprost was administered once daily to both eyes of healthy subjects for 2 weeks with peak blood concentrations within 10 minutes and below the lower limit of detection (0.025 ng/mL) within 1.5 hours. Steady-state levels were reached during the first week of ocular dosing. There was no significant systemic drug accumulation over time.

Bimatoprost is moderately distributed into body tissues with a steady-state volume of distribution of 0.67 L/kg. In human blood, bimatoprost resides mainly in the plasma. Approximately 12% of bimatoprost remains unbound in human plasma.

Clinical Trials: In clinical studies of patients with open angle glaucoma or ocular hypertension, bimatoprost once daily at bedtime reduced a mean baseline IOP of 26 mm Hg by 7 to 8 mm Hg. Bimatoprost once daily at bedtime was compared with timolol 0.5% twice daily in 2 randomized, double-masked trials. Bimatoprost reduced IOP 33% vs 23% for timolol and provided ≥ 2.5 mm Hg greater IOP reduction at all time points out to month 6. Of patients using bimatoprost, 64% reached a low IOP of ≤ 17 mm Hg vs 37% with timolol.

Indications:

For the reduction of elevated IOP in patients with open angle glaucoma or ocular hypertension who are intolerant of other IOP-lowering medications or insufficiently

238   OPHTHALMIC DRUG FACTS

responsive (failed to achieve target IOP determined after multiple measurements over time) to another IOP-lowering medication. Bimatoprost has not been evaluated for the treatment of angle closure, inflammatory, or neovascular glaucoma.

Contraindications:

Hypersensitivity to bimatoprost or any other ingredient of this product.

Warnings:

Ocular changes: Bimatoprost has been reported to cause changes to pigmented tissues. The most frequently reported changes have been increased pigmentation of the iris and periorbital tissue (eyelid) and increased pigmentation and growth of eyelashes. These changes may be permanent.

Eyelid skin darkening has been reported in association with the use of bimatoprost.

Bimatoprost may gradually change eyelashes in the treated eye; these changes include increased length, thickness, pigmentation, or number of lashes.

Inform patients who are expected to receive treatment in only 1 eye about the potential for increased brown pigmentation of the iris, periorbital, or eyelid tissue, and eyelashes in the treated eye and thus heterochromia between the eyes. Advise them of the potential for a disparity between the eyes in length, thickness, or number of eyelashes.

Pregnancy: Category C. There are no adequate and well controlled studies of bimatoprost administration in pregnant women. Bimatoprost was not mutagenic or clastogenic in the Ames test in the mouse lymphoma test or in the in vivo mouse micronucleus tests.

Lactation: It is not known whether bimatoprost is excreted in human milk, although in animal studies, bimatoprost has been shown to be excreted in breast milk. Because many drugs are excreted in human milk, exercise caution when bimatoprost is administered to a nursing woman.

Children: Safety and efficacy not established.

Precautions:

Bacterial keratitis: There have been reports of bacterial keratitis associated with the use of multiple-dose containers of topical ophthalmic products. These containers had been inadvertently contaminated by patients who, in most cases, had a concurrent corneal disease or a disruption of the ocular epithelial surface.

Active intraocular inflammation: Use bimatoprost with caution in patients with active intraocular inflammation (eg, uveitis).

Macular edema: Macular edema, including cystoid macular edema, has been reported during treatment with bimatoprost ophthalmic solution. Use bimatoprost with caution in aphakic patients, in pseudophakic patients with a torn posterior lens capsule, or in patients with known risk factors for macular edema.

Contact lenses: Do not administer bimatoprost while wearing contact lenses. Remove contact lenses prior to instillation of bimatoprost; lenses may be reinserted 15 min-

AGENTS FOR GLAUCOMA

239

utes after bimatoprost administration. Advise patients that bimatoprost contains benzalkonium chloride, which may be absorbed by soft contact lenses.

Adverse Reactions:

In clinical trials, the most frequent events associated with the use of bimatoprost occurring in ≈ 15% to 45% of patients included conjunctival hyperemia, growth of eyelashes, and ocular pruritus. Approximately 3% of patients discontinued therapy due to conjunctival hyperemia.

Ophthalmic: Adverse events that occurred in ≈ 3% to 10% of patients included the following: Ocular dryness, visual disturbances, ocular burning, foreign body sensation, eye pain, pigmentation of the periocular skin, blepharitis, cataract, superficial punctate keratitis, eyelid erythema, ocular irritation, and eyelash darkening. The following ocular adverse events were reported in ≈ 1% to 3% of patients: Eye discharge, tearing, photophobia, allergic conjunctivitis, asthenopia, increases in iris pigmentation, and conjunctival edema. In < 1% of patients, intraocular inflammation was reported as iritis.

Systemic: Systemic adverse events reported in ≈ 10% of patients were infectious (primarily colds and upper respiratory tract infections). The following systemic adverse events were reported in ≈ 1% to 5% of patients included headaches, abnormal liver function tests, asthenia, and hirsutism.

Patient Information:

Inform patients that bimatoprost may cause increased growth and darkening of eyelashes and darkening of the skin around the eye in some patients. Some patients may slowly develop darkening of the iris. These changes may be permanent.

Remove contact lenses prior to instillation of bimatoprost; lenses may be reinserted 15 minutes after bimatoprost administration. Advise patients that bimatoprost contains benzalkonium chloride, which may be absorbed by soft contact lenses.

Administration and Dosage:

The recommended dosage is 1 drop in the affected eye(s) once daily in the evening. The dosage should not exceed once daily because it has been shown that more frequent administration does not increase the IOP-lowering effect.

Reduction of IOP starts ≈ 4 hours after the first administration with maximum effect reached within ≈ 8 to 12 hours.

Bimatoprost may be used concomitantly with other topical ophthalmic drug products to lower IOP. If more than 1 topical drug is being used, administer the drugs at least 5 minutes apart.

Storage/Stability: Store in the original container at 15° to 25°C (59° to 77°F).

Rx **Lumigan** (Allergan)	**Solution:** 0.03%	In 2.5 and 5 mL.[1]	

[1] 0.05 mg benzalkonium chloride/mL.

OPHTHALMIC DRUG FACTS

UNOPROSTONE ISOPROPYL

Actions:

Pharmacology: Unoprostone is a prostaglandin $F_{2\alpha}$ analog that is believed to reduce elevated intraocular pressure (IOP) by increasing the outflow of aqueous humor, but the exact mechanism is unknown.

Pharmacokinetics:

>   *Absorption –* Unoprostone is absorbed through the cornea and conjunctival epithelium, where it is hydrolyzed by esterases to unoprostone-free acid. The systemic exposure of its metabolite unoprostone-free acid was minimal following the ocular administration.

>   *Excretion –* Elimination of unoprostone-free acid from human plasma is rapid, with a half-life of 14 minutes. Plasma levels of unoprostone-free acid dropped below the lower limit of quantitation (< 0.25 ng/mL) 1 hour following ocular instillation. The metabolites are excreted predominantly in the urine.

Clinical Trials: In patients with mean baseline IOP of 23 mm Hg, unoprostone lowers IOP by $\approx$ 3 to 4 mm Hg throughout the day. Unoprostone appears to lower IOP without affecting cardiovascular or pulmonary function.

Indications:

For the lowering of IOP in patients with open-angle glaucoma or ocular hypertension who are intolerant of other IOP-lowering medications or insufficiently responsive (failed to achieve target IOP determined after multiple measurements over time) to another IOP-lowering medication.

Contraindications:

Known hypersensitivity to unoprostone isopropyl, benzalkonium chloride, or any other ingredients of the product.

Warnings:

Ocular changes: Unoprostone has been reported to cause changes in pigmented tissue. These changes may be permanent.

It may gradually change eye color, increasing the amount of brown pigment in the iris. The long-term effects and consequences of potential injury to the eye are currently unknown. The change in iris color occurs slowly and may not be noticeable for months to several years. Inform patients of the possibility of iris color change.

Carcinogenesis: Unoprostone was not carcinogenic in rats administered oral doses up to 12 mg/kg/day for up to 2 years ($\approx$ 580- and 240-fold the recommended human dose).

Pregnancy: Category C. There are no adequate and well-controlled studies in pregnant women. Because animal studies are not always predictive of human response, use unoprostone during pregnancy only if the potential benefit to the mother justifies the potential risk to the fetus.

AGENTS FOR GLAUCOMA

Lactation: It is not known whether topical ocular administration could result in sufficient systemic absorption to produce detectable quantities in breast milk. Nevertheless, exercise caution when unoprostone is administered to a nursing mother.

Children: Safety and efficacy not established.

Precautions:

Bacterial keratitis: There have been reports of bacterial keratitis associated with the use of multiple-dose containers of topical ophthalmic products. These containers had been inadvertently contaminated by patients who, in most cases, had a concurrent corneal disease or a disruption of the ocular epithelial surface.

Active intraocular inflammation: Use unoprostone with caution in patients with active intraocular inflammation (eg, uveitis).

Contact lenses: Do not administer unoprostone to patients while they are wearing contact lenses. Advise patients that unoprostone contains benzalkonium chloride, which may be absorbed by contact lenses. Remove contact lenses prior to administration of the solution. Lenses may be reinserted 15 minutes following unoprostone administration.

Adverse Reactions:

Ophthalmic: The most common ocular adverse events were burning/stinging upon drug instillation, dry eyes, itching, increased length of eyelashes, and infection. These were reported in ≈ 10% to 25% of patients. Approximately 10% to 14% of patients were observed to have an increase in the length of eyelashes (≥ 1 mm) at 12 months, while 7% of patients were observed to have a decrease in the length of eyelashes.

Ocular adverse events occurring in ≈ 5% to 10% of patients were abnormal vision, eyelid disorder, foreign body sensation, and lacrimation disorder.

Ocular adverse events occurring in ≈ 1% to 5% of patients were blepharitis, cataract, conjunctivitis, corneal lesion, discharge from the eye, eye hemorrhage, eye pain, keratitis, irritation, photophobia, and vitreous disorder.

Other ocular adverse events reported in < 1% of patients were acute elevated IOP, color blindness, corneal deposits, corneal edema, corneal opacity, diplopia, hyperpigmentation of the eyelid, increased number of eyelashes, iris hyperpigmentation, iritis, optic atrophy, ptosis, retinal hemorrhage, and visual field effect.

Systemic: Flu syndrome (≈ 6%); accidental injury, allergic reaction, back pain, bronchitis, cough increased, diabetes mellitus, dizziness, headache, hypertension, insomnia, pharyngitis, pain, rhinitis, sinusitis (1% to 5%).

Overdosage:

If overdosage occurs, treatment should be symptomatic.

There is no published information available regarding overdosage with unoprostone. The risk of adverse effects caused by accidental oral ingestion is very low because the amount of active ingredient in each bottle is limited (7.5 mg in a 5 mL vial). Accidental ingestion of a vial by a child with 30 kg body weight will amount to a 0.25 mg/kg body weight.

OPHTHALMIC DRUG FACTS

Patient Information:

Instruct patients to avoid allowing the tip of the dispensing container to contact the eye or surrounding structures because this could cause the tip to become contaminated by common bacteria known to cause ocular infections. Serious damage to the eye and subsequent loss of vision may result from using contaminated solutions.

Advise patients that if they develop an intercurrent ocular condition (eg, trauma, infection) or have ocular surgery, they should immediately seek their physician's advice concerning the continued use of the multidose container.

Advise patients that if they develop any ocular reactions, particularly conjunctivitis and eyelid reaction, they should immediately seek their physician's advise.

If more than 1 topical ophthalmic drug is being used, administer the drugs at least 5 minutes apart.

Administration and Dosage:

The recommended dosage is 1 drop in the affected eye(s) twice daily. Unoprostone may be used concomitantly with other topical ophthalmic drug products to lower IOP. If 2 drugs are used, administer at least 5 minutes apart.

Storage/Stability: Store between 2° to 25°C (36° to 77°F).

Rx	**Rescula** (Novartis)	**Solution:** 0.15%	In 5 mL.[1]

[1] 0.015% benzalkonium chloride, EDTA, sodium hydroxide, hydrochloric acid.

LATANOPROST

Actions:

Pharmacology: Latanoprost is a prostanoid-selective FP receptor agonist for ophthalmic use. It is believed to reduce intraocular pressure by increasing the outflow of aqueous humor. Studies in animals and humans suggest that increased uveoscleral outflow is the main mechanism of action.

Pharmacokinetics: Latanoprost is absorbed through the cornea where the isopropyl ester prodrug is hydrolyzed to the acid form to become biologically active. Studies indicate that peak concentration in the aqueous humor is reached ≈ 2 hours after topical administration. The distribution volume in humans is 0.16 ± 0.02 L/kg. The acid of latanoprost could be measured in aqueous humor during the first 4 hours, and in plasma only during the first hour after local administration. Latanoprost is primarily metabolized by the liver with excretion by renal pathway. Approximately 88% and 98% of the dose is recovered in the urine after topical and intravenous dosing, respectively.

Animal studies – Latanoprost was shown to induce increased pigmentation of the iris in monkeys. The increased pigmentation is unlikely to be associated with proliferation of melanocytes and is believed to be caused by the stimulation of melanin production in melanocytes of the iris stroma. Doses of 4 times the daily human dose in cynomolgus monkeys demonstrated increased palpebral fissure. This effect has been reversible and occurred at doses above the standard clinical dose level.

AGENTS FOR GLAUCOMA

Clinical Trials: Patients with a mean baseline intraocular pressure of 24 to 25 treated with *Xalatan* 0.005% for 6 months demonstrated 6 to 8 mm Hg reductions in intraocular pressure. This was equivalent to the effect of timolol 0.5% twice daily.

Indications:

To lower intraocular pressure in patients with open-angle glaucoma and ocular hypertension who are intolerant of other intraocular pressure lowering medications or who insufficiently responded (failed to achieve target IOP determined after multiple measurements over time) to another intraocular pressure lowering medication.

Contraindications:

Hypersensitivity to latanoprost, benzalkonium chloride, or any other ingredient in the product.

Warnings:

Eye color change: Latanoprost may gradually change eye color by increasing the amount of brown pigmentation in the iris. This is caused by increasing the number of melanosomes (pigment granules) in melanocytes. The long term effects of this are currently unknown.

The color change occurs slowly and over a long period of time. Inform patients of the possibility of an increasing brown color in the eye. In patients receiving treatment in only one eye, heterochromia may occur between the eyes. The change in pigmentation may be permanent.

Renal/Hepatic function impairment: Use with caution in patients with renal or hepatic impairment as this drug has not been studied in these patients.

Carcinogenesis: Latanoprost was not carcinogenic in bacteria, mouse lymphoma, or mouse micronucleus tests or when mice and rats were given doses up to 2800 times the recommended human dose for 20 and 24 months, respectively.

Mutagenesis: Unscheduled DNA synthesis was negative in rats, both in vivo and in vitro.

Fertility impairment: Latanoprost was not found to have any effect on fertility in animal studies. Chromosome aberrations were observed in vitro with human lymphocytes.

Pregnancy: Category C. In rabbits receiving 80 times the maximum human dose, 4 of 16 females had no viable fetuses, with the highest nonembryocidal dose $\approx$ 15 times the maximum human dose. There are no adequate and well-controlled studies in pregnant women. Use during pregnancy only if the potential benefit to the mother justifies the potential risk to the fetus.

Lactation: It is not known whether latanoprost or its metabolites is excreted in breast milk. Because many drugs are excreted in human milk, exercise caution when administering to a nursing woman.

Children: Safety and efficacy have not been established.

OPHTHALMIC DRUG FACTS

Precautions:

Cornea: Latanoprost is hydrolyzed in the cornea. The effect of continued administration of latanoprost on the corneal endothelium has not been fully evaluated.

Bacterial keratitis: There have been reports of bacterial keratitis with the use of multidose containers or topical ophthalmic products due to the contamination of the containers by patients with concurrent corneal disease or a disruption of the ocular epithelial surface.

Brown pigmentation: Patients may develop increased brown pigmentation in the iris over several months to years. Usually, the brown pigmentation spreads toward the periphery of the affected eye, but the entire iris or parts of it may also become more brownish. Examine patients regularly. Treatment may be stopped if increased pigmentation occurs, depending upon the clinical situation. The increase in brown iris pigment did not progress further upon stopping treatment in clinical trials; however, the color change may be permament. Freckles and nevi of the iris did not appear to be affected by treatment.

Uveitis: Until further study, significant, previous bouts of uveitis are relative contraindications for the use of this drug.

Cystoid Macular Edema (CME): Previous bouts of CME are relative contraindications for the use of this drug.

Contact lenses: Do not administer latanoprost while wearing contact lenses.

Other conditions: There is no experience in the use of latanoprost for angle closure, inflammatory, or neovascular glaucoma, and only limited experience in pseudophakic patients.

Drug Interactions:

In vitro studies have shown that precipitation occurs when eyedrops containing thimerosal are mixed with latanoprost. If using these drugs concurrently, allow $\geq$ 5 minutes between applications.

Adverse Reactions:

Ophthalmic: Blurred vision, burning and stinging, conjunctival hyperemia, foreign body sensation, itching, increased pigmentation of iris, punctate epithelial keratopathy (5% to 15%); dry eye, excessive tearing, eye pain, lid crusting, lid edema, lid erythema, lid discomfort/pain, photophobia (1% to 4%); conjunctivitis, diplopia, discharge from eye (< 1%). Eye lash changes (increased length, thickness, pigmentation, and number of lashes). The following events occurred extremely rarely: Retinal artery embolus, retinal detachment, and vitreous hemorrhage from diabetic retinopathy.

Local conjunctival hyperemia occurred; however, less than 1% of patients discontinued therapy due to intolerance.

Systemic: Upper respiratory tract infection, cold, flu ($\approx$ 4%); muscle, joint, back, and chest pain, angina pectoris, rash, allergic skin reaction (1% to 2%).

AGENTS FOR GLAUCOMA

Overdosage:

Symptoms: Ocular irritation and conjunctival or episcleral hyperemia are the only ocular side effects of a latanoprost overdose. Transient bronchoconstriction has occurred in monkeys receiving large doses intravenously. However, no bronchoconstriction was induced in 11 patients with bronchial asthma receiving latanoprost. No adverse reactions were observed in healthy volunteers receiving 3 mcg/kg infused intravenously, but mean plasma concentrations were 200 times higher than during clinical ocular topical treatment. IV dosages of 5.5 to 10 mcg/kg caused abdominal pain, dizziness, fatigue, hot flushes, nausea, and sweating.

Treatment: Treat latanoprost overdosage symptomatically.

Patient Information:

The color of the iris can change due to an increase of the brown pigment. If only one eye is treated, a cosmetically different eye coloration may occur. Iris pigmentation changes may be more noticeable in patients with green-brown, blue/gray-brown, or yellow-brown irises.

Do not allow the dispensing container to touch the eye or surrounding structures to avoid contracting an eye infection from the resultant contamination of common bacteria. Serious damage to the eye and subsequent loss of vision can occur from using contaminated containers.

Patients should contact their physician concerning the continued use of the multidose container if they experience any eye trauma or infection or have ocular surgery.

Patients should contact their physician if they experience any ocular side effects, especially conjunctivitis and lid reactions.

Latanoprost contains benzalkonium chloride, which may be absorbed by contact lenses. Remove contact lenses prior to administering the latanoprost solution. Lenses can be reinserted 15 minutes after latanoprost administration.

If using > 1 topical ophthalmic drug, adminster drugs ≥ 5 minutes apart.

Administration and Dosage:

Administer 1 drop in the affected eye(s) once daily. Do not administer this medicine more frequently than once daily.

Reduction of intraocular pressure begins ≈ 3 to 4 hours after administration, with the maximum effect reached after 8 to 12 hours. Preliminary data suggest that maximal effect is not achieved in some patients for weeks or months.

Latanoprost may be used with other topical ophthalmic products to lower intraocular pressure. If using more than one topical ophthalmic drug, administer the drugs ≥ 5 minutes apart.

Storage/Stability: Protect from light. Store unopened bottle in refrigerator at 2° to 8°C (36° to 46°F). Opened container may be stored at room temperature up to 25°C (77°F) for 6 weeks.

| *Rx* | **Xalatan** (Pharmacia) | **Solution**: 0.005% | In 2.5 mL plastic ophthalmic dispenser bottle with dropper tip.[1] |

[1] With 0.02% benzalkonium chloride, sodium chloride, sodium dihydrogen phosphate monohydrate, disodium hydrogen phosphate anhydrous.

CARBONIC ANHYDRASE INHIBITOR/BETA-ADRENERGIC BLOCKING AGENT

DORZOLAMIDE HYDROCHLORIDE-TIMOLOL MALEATE

Actions:

Pharmacology: Comprised of two components, dorzolamide hydrochloride-timolol maleate decreases elevated intraocular pressure, whether associated with glaucoma, by reducing aqueous humor secretion. Elevated intraocular pressure is a major risk factor in the pathogenesis of optic nerve damage and glaucomatous visual field loss. The higher the level of intraocular pressure, the greater the likelihood glaucomatous field loss and optic nerve damage. Dorzolamide hydrochloride is an inhibitor of human carbonic anhydrase II. Timolol maleate is a $beta_1/beta_2$ (non-selective) adrenergic receptor blocking agent that does not have significant intrinsic sympathomimetic, direct myocardial depressant, or local anesthetic (membrane-stabilizing) activity. The combined effect of these two agents results in additional intraocular pressure reduction compared with either component administered alone, but the reduction is not as great when each are administered concomitantly.

Pharmacokinetics: Dorzolamide and timolol reach the systemic circulation when applied topically.

Dorzolamide accumulates in RBCs and is primarily excreted unchanged in the urine. Topical administration approximates an oral dose of 2 mg twice daily. Steady state is achieved in $\approx$ 8 weeks.

Timolol topical administration attains a mean peak plasma concentration following morning dosing of 0.46 ng/mL.

Indications:

For the reduction of elevated intraocular pressure in patients with open-angle glaucoma or ocular hypertension who are insufficiently responsive to beta-blockers (failed to achieve target IOP determined after multiple measurements over time).

Contraindications:

Hypersensitivity to any component of this product; bronchial asthma or history of bronchial asthma; severe chronic obstructive pulmonary disease; sinus bradycardia; second or third degree atrioventricular block; overt cardiac failure; cardiogenic shock.

Warnings:

Systemic exposure: Although administered topically, dorzolamide hydrochloride-timolol maleate is absorbed systemically. Therefore, severe reactions could occur due to the sulfonamide, dorzolamide (eg, allergic, hematologic, hepatic). In addition, severe respiratory reactions and cardiac reactions, including death due to broncho-

AGENTS FOR GLAUCOMA

spasm in patients with asthma, and rarely death in association with cardiac failure, have been reported following systemic or ophthalmic administration of timolol maleate. Refer to complete monographs on these agents for thorough descriptions.

Cardiac failure: Sympathetic stimulation may be essential for support of the circulation in individuals with diminished myocardial contractility and its inhibition by beta-adrenergic receptor blockade may precipitate more severe failure. Even in patients without a history of cardiac failure, continued myocardial depression with beta-blocking agents can, in some cases, lead to cardiac failure. At the first sign or symptom of cardiac failure, discontinue use.

Obstructive pulmonary disease: Patients with chronic obstructive pulmonary disease (eg, chronic bronchitis, emphysema) of mild to moderate severity, bronchospastic disease, or a history of bronchospastic disease should generally not receive beta-blocking agents.

Major surgery: Withdrawal of beta-adrenergic blocking agents prior to major surgery is controversial. Beta-adrenergic receptor blockade impairs the ability of the heart to respond to beta-adrenergically mediated reflex stimuli. This may augment the risk of general anesthesia in surgical procedures. Some patients receiving beta-adrenergic receptor blocking agents have experienced protracted severe hypotension during anesthesia. Difficulty in restarting and maintaining the heartbeat has also been reported. In patients undergoing elective surgery, some authorities recommend gradual withdrawal of beta-adrenergic receptor blocking agents. The anesthesiologist must be informed of this and any other drug therapy prior to surgery.

Diabetes mellitus: Administer beta-adrenergic blocking agents with caution in patients subject to spontaneous hypoglycemia or to diabetes (especially those with labile diabetes) who are receiving insulin or oral hypoglycemic agents. Beta-adrenergic receptor blocking agents may mask the signs and symptoms of acute hypoglycemia.

Thyrotoxicosis: Beta-adrenergic blocking agents may mask certain clinical signs (eg, tachycardia) of hyperthyroidism. Carefully manage patients suspected of developing thyrotoxicosis to avoid abrupt withdrawal of beta-adrenergic blocking agents that might precipitate a thyroid storm.

Pregnancy: Category C. This medication should only be used during pregnancy if the potential benefit to the mother justifies the potential risk to the fetus.

Lactation: It is not known if dorzolamide is excreted in human milk. Timolol maleate has been detected in human milk following oral and ophthalmic drug administration. Because of the potential for serious adverse reactions from this medicine in nursing infants, a decision should be made whether to discontinue nursing or to discontinue the drug, taking into account the importance of the drug to the mother.

Children: Safety and effectiveness have not been established.

Precautions:

Myasthenia gravis: Beta-adrenergic blockade has been reported to potentiate muscle weakness consistent with certain myasthenic symptoms (eg, diplopia, ptosis, generalized weakness). Timolol has been reported rarely to increase muscle weakness in some patients with myasthenia gravis or myasthenic symptoms.

Choroidal detachment: Choroidal detachment after filtration procedures has been reported with the administration of aqueous suppressant therapy (eg, timolol).

248   OPHTHALMIC DRUG FACTS

Bacterial keratitis: Bacterial keratitis is associated with the use of multidose containers of topical ophthalmic products. These containers have been inadvertently contaminated by patients who, in most cases, had a concurrent corneal disease or a disruption of the ocular epithelial surface.

Acid-based disturbances: Although acid-base and electrolyte disturbances were not reported in the clinical trials with dorzolamide hydrochloride ophthalmic solution, these disturbances have been reported with oral carbonic anhydrase inhibitors and have, in some instances, resulted in drug interactions (eg, toxicity associated with high-dose salicylate therapy). Consider the potential drug interactions in patients receiving this medicine.

Drug Interactions:

Ophthalmic Beta Blocker Drug Interactions			
Precipitant drug	Object drug*		Description
Dorzolamide/Timolol Maleate	Carbonic Anhydrase Inhibitors (oral)	↑	There is potential for an additive effect on the known systemic effects of carbonic anhydrase inhibition in patients receiving an oral carbonic anhydrase inhibitor and dorzolamide hydrochloride-timolol maleate. Concomitant administration is not recommended.
	Beta-adrenergic agents (oral)	↑	Observe patients who are receiving a beta-adrenergic blocking agent orally and dorzolamide hydrochloride-timolol maleate for potential additive effects of beta-blockade, both systemic and on intraocular pressure. Concomitant use is not recommended.
	Calcium antagonists	↔	Use caution in the coadministration of beta-adrenergic blocking agents and oral or intravenous calcium antagonists because of possible atrioventricular conduction disturbances, left ventricular failure, and hypotension. In patients with impaired cardiac function, avoid coadministration.
	Catecholamine-depleting drugs	↑	Close observation of the patient is recommended when a beta-blocker is administered to patients receiving catecholamine-depleting drugs, such as reserpine, because of possible additive effects, hypotension, or marked bradycardia, which may result in vertigo, syncope, or postural hypotension.
	Acid-base disturbances	↔	Although acid-base and electrolyte disturbances were not reported in the ophthalmic clinical trials, these disturbances have been reported with oral carbonic anhydrase inhibitors and have resulted in drug interactions (eg, toxicity associated with high-dose salicylate therapy). Consider potential drug interactions in patients receiving this medicine.

* ↑ = Object drug increased. ↔ = Undetermined effect.

Adverse Reactions:

Approximately 5% of 1035 patients discontinued therapy with this medicine because of adverse reactions. The most frequently reported adverse events were taste perversion (bitter, sour, unusual taste) or ocular burning or stinging in up to 30% of patients. Conjunctival hyperemia, blurred vision, superficial punctate keratitis, or eye itching were reported in 5% to 15% of patients.

The following adverse events were reported in 1% to 5% of patients:

    CNS – Dizziness; headache.

    GI – Abdominal pain; dyspepsia; nausea.

AGENTS FOR GLAUCOMA

GU – Urinary tract infection.

Ophthalmic – Blepharitis; cloudy vision; conjunctival discharge; conjunctival edema; conjunctival follicles; conjunctival injection; conjunctivitis; corneal erosion; corneal staining; cortical lens opacity; dryness of eyes; eye debris; eye discharge; eye pain; eye tearing; eyelid edema; eyelid erythema; eyelid exudate/scales; eyelid pain or discomfort; foreign body sensation; glaucomatous cupping; lens nucleus coloration; lens opacity; nuclear lens opacity; post-subcapsular cataract; visual field defect; vitreous detachment.

Miscellaneous – Back pain; hypertension; influenza.

Respiratory – Bronchitis; cough; pharyngitis; sinusitis; upper respiratory tract infection.

Dorzolamide:

Dermatologic – Contact dermatitis.

Hypersensitivity – Signs and symptoms of systemic allergic reactions including angioedema; bronchospasm; pruritus; urticaria.

Special Senses – Signs and symptoms of ocular allergic reaction; transient myopia.

Miscellaneous – Asthenia/fatigue.

Timolol (ocular and oral administration):

Cardiovascular – Arrhythmia; syncope; heart block; cerebral ischemia; worsening of angina pectoris; palpitation; cardiac arrest; pulmonary edema; claudication; Raynaud's phenomenon; cold hands and feet; worsening of arterial insufficiency; vasodilation.

CNS – Increase in signs and symptoms of myasthenia gravis, somnolence, insomnia, nightmares, behavioral changes and psychic disturbances including confusion, hallucinations, anxiety, disorientation, nervousness, memory loss; vertigo; local weakness; diminished concentration; reversible mental depression progressing to catatonia, an acute reversible syndrome characterized by disorientation for time and place; emotional liability; slightly clouded sensorium; decreased performance on neuropsychometrics.

Dermatologic – Alopecia; psoriasiform rash or exacerbation of psoriasis; pruritus; skin irritation; increased pigmentation; sweating.

Endocrine – Hyperglycemia; hypoglycemia (masked symptoms of hypoglycemia in diabetic patients).

GI – Anorexia; gastrointestinal pain; hepatomegaly; mesenteric arterial thrombosis; ischemic colitis.

GU – Retroperitoneal fibrosis; decreased libido; impotence; Peyronie's disease; urination difficulties.

Hematologic – Nonthrombocytopenic purpura; thrombocytopenic purpura; agranulocytosis.

Hypersensitivity – Erythematous rash; fever combined with aching and sore throat; laryngospasm with respiratory distress; signs and symptoms of systemic allergic reactions including angioedema, urticaria, localized and generalized rash.

250 OPHTHALMIC DRUG FACTS

Immunologic – Systemic lupus erythematosus.

Musculoskeletal – Arthralgia.

Respiratory – Bronchial bronchospasm (predominantly in patients with preexisting bronchospastic disease); bronchial obstruction; rales; respiratory failure.

Special Senses – Ptosis; decreased corneal sensitivity; cystoid macular edema; visual disturbances including refractive changes and diplopia; pseudopemphigoid; choroidal detachment following filtration surgery; tinnitus.

Miscellaneous – Asthenia/fatigue; extremity pain; decreased exercise tolerance; weight loss.

Patient Information:

Advise patients with bronchial asthma, a history of bronchial asthma, severe chronic obstructive pulmonary disease, sinus bradycardia, second or third degree atrioventricular block, or cardiac failure not to take this product.

If any ocular reactions develop, particularly conjunctivitis and lid reaction, patients should discontinue use and seek their physician's advice.

Patients should inform their physician and anesthesiologist when undergoing surgery about this and any other drug therapy.

Avoid allowing the tip of the dispensing container to contact the eye or surrounding structures. If handled improperly or if the tip of the dispensing container contacts the eye or surrounding structures, it can become contaminated by common bacteria known to cause ocular infections. Serious damage to the eye and subsequent loss of vision may result from using contaminated solutions.

If patients have ocular surgery or develop an intercurrent ocular condition (eg, trauma, infection), they should immediately seek their physician's advice concerning the continued use of the present multidose container.

If > 1 topical ophthalmic drug is being used, administer the drugs ≥ 10 minutes apart.

Dorzolamide hydrochloride-timolol maleate contains chloride, which may be absorbed by soft contact lenses. Contact lenses should be removed prior to administration of the solution. Lenses may be reinserted 15 minutes following administration.

Administration and Dosage:

Place 1 drop of dorzolamide hydrochloride-timolol maleate in the affected eye(s) 2 times daily.

If > 1 topical ophthalmic drug is being used, administer the drugs ≥ 10 minutes apart.

Storage/Stability: Store between 15° and 25°C (59° to 77°F). Protect from light.

Rx	**Cosopt** (Merck)	**Solution:** 20 mg dorzolamide, 5 mg timolol per mL	In 5 and 10 mL dispenser with controlled drop tip.[1]

[1] With sodium citrate, hydroxyethyl cellulose, sodium hydroxide, mannitol. Benzalkonium chloride 0.0075% is added as a preservative.

HYPEROSMOTIC AGENTS

Hyperosmotic agents (also referred to as osmotic agents) can be administered topically, orally, or intravenously to increase osmotic pressure of tears and plasma relative to that of the ocular structures. As a result of the osmotic gradient established, fluid moves from the eye to hyperosmotic tear fluid with topical instillation, or plasma of ocular blood vessels following oral or intravenous administration.

TOPICAL AGENTS

The clinical objective of topical osmotherapy is to enhance the rate of fluid movement from the edematous cornea. When these agents are applied to the eye, water is drawn from the cornea to the hyperosmolal tear film and eliminated through the usual tear flow mechanisms.

Sodium chloride, glycerol, and glucose have proven useful for reducing corneal edema of various etiologies, including bullous keratopathy and Fuchs' endothelial dystrophy.

Hypertonic solutions of sodium chloride or glucose can be useful for prolonged treatment of corneal edema. Sodium chloride appears less effective when the corneal epithelium is traumatized due to its increased ability to penetrate the epithelial barrier. Administer both sodium chloride and glucose at regular intervals for maximum clinical effect. Since vision is usually worse upon awakening, more frequent application during the first waking hours can be helpful.

Glycerol can reduce corneal edema within 1 to 2 minutes following topical instillation to the eye. Since application is painful, a topical anesthetic must be instilled prior to its use. The osmotic action of glycerol is transient since the molecules mix readily with water. Therefore, for diagnostic purposes, its primary clinical use is to facilitate ophthalmoscopy and gonioscopy with edematous corneas.

SYSTEMIC AGENTS

Hyperosmotic agents administered by oral and intravenous routes are useful for initial management of acute angle-closure glaucoma and prior to intraocular surgery to reduce intraocular pressure (IOP).

Following systemic administration, a relatively rapid increase in serum osmolarity can occur. Transfer of fluid from the eye to the circulation results in a decrease in IOP. Factors that determine the difference in osmotic pressure between the ocular fluids and plasma include the following:

OPHTHALMIC DRUG FACTS

- Molecular weight and concentration
- Dose administered
- Rate of absorption
- Distribution in body water
- Ocular penetration
- Rate of excretion
- Nature of diuresis

The integrity of the ocular tissues can also influence the osmotic effect. Inflammation may enhance ocular penetration and decrease the osmotic gradient, resulting in a reduction in the pressure-lowering effect of these agents.

Systemic administration can result in a significant drop in IOP within 15 to 60 minutes, depending on the dosage given. The effect of systemic osmotherapy can last up to 8 hours. The primary use of these agents is to treat or prevent acute rises in IOP such as acute angle-closure glaucoma and postoperative spiking of IOP. Chronic administration is contraindicated.

Osmotic Diuretic Pharmacokinetics								
Diuretic	Route	Onset (min)	Peak (hrs)	Duration (hrs)	Half-life	Metabolized (%)	Ocular penetration	Distribution
Glycerin	PO	10-30	1-1.5	4-5	30-45 minutes	80	poor	E[1]
Isosorbide	PO	10-30	1-1.5	5-6	5-9.5 hrs	0	good	TBW[2]
Mannitol	IV	30-60	1	6-8	15-100 minutes	7-10	very poor	E[1]
Urea	IV	30-45	1	5-6	N	N	good	TBW[2]

[1] E = extracellular water
[2] TBW = total body water

INTRAVENOUS ADMINISTRATION

Mannitol (*Osmitrol*) is currently the hyperosmotic of choice for intravenous use. It is not absorbed from the gastrointestinal tract and is ineffective by the oral route. Intravenous administration can reduce IOP within 20 to 30 minutes. The effect can last 4 to 8 hours. Mannitol exhibits minimal cellular penetration, is not metabolized, and is excreted in the urine. Therefore, it can be used in diabetic patients, but should be administered with caution in patients with renal disease. Since mannitol is confined to the extracellular fluid, dehydration and a profound diuresis can result following administration.

ORAL ADMINISTRATION

Glycerin (*Osmōglyn*) and isosorbide (*Ismotic*) are readily absorbed from the gastrointestinal tract and are effective when administered by the oral route.

Glycerin is metabolized in the body analogous to other carbohydrates and produces 4.32 kcal/g. Use caution when administering glycerin to diabetic patients because hyperglycemia and glycosuria can result. Although reduction in IOP is somewhat less than with mannitol, administration of the recommended dosage reduces pressure within 30 to 60 minutes. The osmotic effect can last for several hours.

Isosorbide is not metabolized, and $\approx$ 95% is excreted unchanged in the urine. Therefore, it provides no calories and, unlike glycerin, can be administered to diabetic patients. Isosorbide reduces IOP within 30 to 60 minutes. The effect can last as long as 5 to 6 hours.

HYPEROSMOTIC AGENTS

Although oral administration simplifies osmotherapy, both glycerin and isosorbide exhibit characteristics limiting their use. Neither agent can be administered to patients who are nauseated or vomiting. Since both agents have a sweet taste, they may induce nausea or vomiting. In addition, the increase in serum osmolarity can cause dehydration, headache, confusion, and disorientation.

Siret D. Jaanus, PhD
State University of New York

For More Information

Bartlett JD, Jaanus SD, eds. *Clinical Ocular Pharmacology*, ed. 4. Boston: Butterworth-Heinemann, 2001.

Becker B, et al. Hyperosmotic agents. In: Leopold IE, ed. *Symposium in Ocular Therapy*. St. Louis: C.V. Mosby Co., 1968.

Becker B, et al. Isosorbide: An oral hyperosmotic agent. *Arch Ophthalmol* 1967;78:147.

Galin MA, et al. Ophthalmological use of osmotic therapy. *Am J Ophthalmol* 1966;62:629.

Kolker AE. Hyperosmotic agents in glaucoma. *Invest Ophthalmol* 1970;9:418.

Lambert DW. Topical hyperosmotic agents and secretory stimulants. *Am J Ophthalmol* 1980;20:163.

Luxenberg MN, Green K. Reduction of corneal edema with topical hypertonic agents. *Am J Ophthalmol* 1970;9:418.

McCurdy DK, et al. Oral glycerol: The mechanism of intraocular hypotension. *Am J Ophthalmol* 1966;61:1244.

GLUCOSE, TOPICAL

Indications:

Corneal edema: Topical osmotherapy for reducing corneal edema.

Contraindications:

Hypersensitivity to any component of the product.

Precautions:

Irritation: If irritation develops, discontinue use.

Administration and Dosage:

May be used 2 to 6 times daily.

Depress lower lid with index finger while looking upward. Introduce a small amount of ointment behind depressed eyelid into conjunctival sac. Close and open eyes 2 times. Wipe off excess ointment. If eyelids are sticky, clean them before each application with a pledget of cotton and lukewarm boiled water.

Rx	Glucose-40 (Ciba Vision)	Ointment: 40%	White petrolatum, anhydrous lanolin, parabens. In 3.5 g.

GLYCERIN, TOPICAL

Actions:

Pharmacology: Glycerin ophthalmic solution is used only for topical application to the cornea. By virtue of its osmotic action (attraction of water through the semipermeable corneal epithelium), it promptly reduces edema and causes clearing of corneal haze. The action is transient and therefore is used primarily for diagnostic purposes.

Indications:

Edematous cornea: To clear an edematous cornea in order to facilitate ophthalmoscopic and gonioscopic examination in acute glaucoma, bullous keratitis, and Fuchs' endothelial dystrophy.

Contraindications:

Hypersensitivity to any component of the product.

Warnings:

Pregnancy: Category C. Safety for use during pregnancy has not been established. Use only when clearly needed.

HYPEROSMOTIC AGENTS

Lactation: It is not known whether glycerin is excreted in breast milk. Exercise caution when administering to a nursing mother.

Children: Safety and efficacy for use in children have not been established.

Precautions:

Irritation: Because glycerin is an irritant and may cause pain, instill a local anesthetic before use.

Adverse Reactions:

Some pain or irritation may occur upon instillation.

Administration and Dosage:

Instill 1 or 2 drops prior to examination. In gonioscopy of an edematous cornea, additional glycerin may be used as a lubricant.

Storage/Stability: Keep bottle tightly closed. Store at room temperature, 25°C (77°F). Discard product 6 months after dropper is first placed in the drug solution.

Rx	**Ophthalgan** (Wyeth)	**Solution:** Glycerin	0.55% chlorobutanol. In 7.5 mL.

SODIUM CHLORIDE, HYPERTONIC

Actions:

Pharmacology: A hypertonic (hyperosmolar) solution exerts an osmotic gradient greater than that present in body tissues and fluids, so that water is drawn from body tissues and fluids across semipermeable membranes. Applied topically to the eye, a hypertonicity agent creates an osmotic gradient that draws water out of the cornea.

Indications:

Corneal edema: Temporary relief.

Contraindications:

Hypersensitivity to any component of the product.

Adverse Reactions:

May cause temporary burning and irritation upon instillation.

Patient Information:

To avoid contamination, do not touch tip of container to any surface. Replace cap after using.

OPHTHALMIC DRUG FACTS

Do not use this product except under the advice and supervision of a physician. If you experience eye pain, changes in vision, continued redness or irritation of the eye, or if the condition worsens or persists, discontinue use and consult a physician.

Product may cause temporary burning and irritation when instilled into the eye.

Do not use if solution changes color or becomes cloudy.

Administration and Dosage:

Solution: Instill 1 or 2 drops in affected eye(s) every 3 or 4 hours, or as directed.

Ointment: Pull down lower eyelid of the affected eye(s) and apply a small amount ($\approx$ 0.25 inch) of ointment to the inside of the affected eye(s) every 3 or 4 hours, or as directed.

Storage/Stability: Store at 8° to 30°C (46° to 86°F). Keep tightly closed. Protect from light.

otc	**Adsorbonac** (Alcon)	**Solution:** 2%	In 15 mL.[1]
otc	**Muro 128** (Bausch & Lomb)		In 15 mL.[2]
otc	**Adsorbonac** (Alcon)	**Solution:** 5%	In 15 mL.[1]
otc	**AK-NaCl** (Akorn)		In 15 mL.[3]
otc	**Muro 128** (Bausch & Lomb)		In 15 and 30 mL.[4]
otc	**AK-NaCl** (Akorn)	**Ointment:** 5%	Preservative free. In 3.5 g.[5]
otc	**Muro 128** (Bausch & Lomb)		In 3.5 g single and twin packs.[6]

[1] With povidone, hydroxyethylcellulose 2910, PEG-90M, poloxamer 181, 0.004% thimerosal, EDTA.
[2] With hydroxypropyl methylcellulose 2910, 0.028% methylparaben, 0.012% propylparaben, propylene glycol, boric acid.
[3] With hydroxypropyl methylcellulose 2906, propylene glycol, 0.023% methylparaben, 0.01% propylparaben, boric acid.
[4] Boric acid, hydroxypropyl methylcellulose 2910, propylene glycol, 0.023% methylparaben, 0.01% propylparaben.
[5] With mineral oil, white petrolatum, lanolin oil.
[6] With mineral oil, white petrolatum, lanolin.

⚬ GLYCERIN (Glycerol)

Actions:

Pharmacology: An oral osmotic agent for reducing intraocular pressure. It adds to the tonicity of the blood until metabolized and eliminated by the kidneys.

Indications:

Glaucoma: Glycerin may be used to interrupt acute attacks.

Prior to and after ocular surgery: Where reduction of intraocular pressure is indicated, glycerin may be used prior to and after ocular surgery.

HYPEROSMOTIC AGENTS

Off-labeled: Glycerin has also been given by the IV route (with proper preparation) to lower intraocular and intracranial pressure.

Contraindications:

Well established anuria; severe dehydration; frank or impending acute pulmonary edema; severe cardiac decompensation; hypersensitivity to any of the ingredients.

Warnings:

Route of administration: For oral use only; not for injection.

Pregnancy: Category C. Safety for use during pregnancy has not been established. Use only when clearly needed and when the potential benefits to the mother outweigh the potential hazards to the fetus.

Precautions:

Special risk patients: Use cautiously in hypervolemia, confused mental states, congestive heart disease, diabetic patients, severely dehydrated individuals, and cardiac, renal, or hepatic disease.

Urinary retention: Avoid acute urinary retention in the preoperative period. Continued use may result in weight gain.

Adverse Reactions:

Nausea, vomiting, headache, confusion, and disorientation may occur. Severe dehydration, cardiac arrhythmias, or hyperosmolar nonketotic coma, which can result in death, have occurred.

Administration and Dosage:

1 to 2 g/kg 1 to 1.5 hours prior to surgery.

Rx **Osmōglyn** (Alcon)	**Solution:** 50% (0.6 g glycerin/mL)	Lime flavor. In 180 and 220 mL.	

ISOSORBIDE

Actions:

Pharmacology: Isosorbide is rapidly absorbed after oral administration. It is essentially nonmetabolized, and in the circulation, it contributes to the tonicity of the blood until it is eliminated by the kidneys unchanged. While in the blood, isosorbide acts as an osmotic agent to promote redistribution of water toward the circulation with ultimate elimination in the urine. The physical action is similar to that of other osmotic agents.

Indications:

For the short-term reduction of IOP prior to and after intraocular surgery.

OPHTHALMIC DRUG FACTS

May be used to interrupt an acute attack of glaucoma. Use where less risk of nausea and vomiting than that posed by other oral hyperosmotic agents is needed.

Contraindications:

Well-established anuria; severe dehydration; frank or impending acute pulmonary edema; severe cardiac decompensation; hypersensitivity to any component of this preparation.

Warnings:

Fluid/Electrolyte balance: With repeated doses, maintain adequate fluid and electro-lyte balance.

Urinary output: If urinary output continues to decrease, closely review the patient's clinical status. Accumulation may result in overexpansion of the extracellular fluid.

Pregnancy: Category B. There are no adequate data on whether this drug affects fer-tility in humans or has a teratogenic potential or other adverse fetal effects. Use dur-ing pregnancy only if clearly needed.

Precautions:

Repetitive doses: Use repetitive doses with caution, particularly in patients with dis-eases associated with salt retention. Ensure that the patient's bladder has been emp-tied prior to surgery.

Adverse Reactions:

Nausea; vomiting; headache; confusion; disorientation; gastric discomfort; thirst; hic-coughs; hypernatremia; hyperosmolarity; rash; irritability; syncope; lethargy; vertigo; dizziness; lightheadedness.

Administration and Dosage:

For oral use only.

Initial dose: 1.5 g/kg (equivalent to 1.5 mL/lb).

Dose range: 1 to 3 g/kg 2 to 4 times a day as indicated.

Palatability may be improved if the medication is poured over cracked ice and sipped.

Rx	**Ismotic** (Alcon)	**Solution:** 45% (100 g per 220 mL)	In 220 mL. With 4.6 mEq sodium and 0.9 mEq potassium per 220 mL. Alcohol, saccharin, sorbitol. Vanilla-mint flavor.

HYPEROSMOTIC AGENTS

MANNITOL

Actions:

Pharmacology: Mannitol is a nonelectrolyte osmotic diuretic that is pharmacologically inert.

IV mannitol is confined to the extracellular space. Only small amounts are metabolized. Mannitol is readily diffused through the glomeruli. Approximately 80% of a 100 g dose will appear in the urine in 3 hours, with lesser amounts thereafter. Even at peak concentrations, mannitol will exhibit < 10% of tubular reabsorption and is not secreted by tubular cells. Mannitol will hinder tubular reabsorption of water and enhance excretion of sodium and chloride by elevating the osmolarity of the glomerular filtrate.

This increase in extracellular osmolarity affected by the IV administration of mannitol will induce the movement of intracellular water to the extracellular and vascular spaces. This action underlies the role of mannitol in reducing intracranial pressure, intracranial edema, and elevated intraocular pressure (IOP).

Indications:

Reduction of elevated IOP when the pressure cannot be lowered by other means.

Contraindications:

Anuria due to severe renal disease; severe pulmonary congestion or frank pulmonary edema; active intracranial bleeding except during craniotomy; severe dehydration; progressive renal damage or dysfunction after instituting mannitol therapy, including increasing oliguria and azotemia; progressive heart failure or pulmonary congestion after mannitol therapy.

Warnings:

Fluid and electrolyte imbalance: By sustaining diuresis, mannitol may obscure and intensify inadequate hydration or hypovolemia. Excessive loss of water and electrolytes may lead to serious imbalances. Loss of water in excess of electrolytes can cause hypernatremia. Shift of sodium free intracellular fluid into the extracellular compartment following mannitol infusion may lower serum sodium concentration and aggravate preexisting hyponatremia. Also, movement of potassium ions from intracellular to extracellular space may cause hyperkalemia. Electrolyte measurements, including sodium and potassium, are therefore of vital importance in monitoring mannitol infusion.

Renal function impairment: Use a test dose (see Administration and Dosage); try a second test dose if there is an inadequate response, but do not attempt > 2 test doses.

If urine output continues to decline during infusion, closely review the patient's clinical status and suspend mannitol infusion, if necessary. Accumulation of mannitol may result in overexpansion of the extracellular fluid, which may intensify existing or latent CHF.

Osmotic nephrosis, a reversible vacuolization of the tubules of unknown clinical significance, may proceed to severe irreversible nephrosis; monitor renal function closely.

260 OPHTHALMIC DRUG FACTS

Pregnancy: Category C. It is not known whether mannitol can cause fetal harm when administered to a pregnant woman or can affect reproduction capacity. Give to a pregnant woman only if clearly needed.

Lactation: It is not known whether this drug is excreted in breast milk; exercise caution when administering to a nursing woman.

Children: Safety and efficacy for patients ≤ 12 years of age have not been established.

Precautions:

CHF: Carefully evaluate cardiovascular status before rapid administration of mannitol since sudden expansion of the extracellular fluid may lead to fulminating CHF.

Hypovolemia: By sustaining diuresis, mannitol may obscure and intensify inadequate hydration or hypovolemia.

Pseudoagglutination: Do not give electrolyte free mannitol solutions with blood. If blood is given simultaneously, add ≥ 20 mEq of sodium chloride to each liter of mannitol solution to avoid pseudoagglutination.

Hemoconcentration: The obligatory diuretic response following rapid infusion of 15%, 20%, or 25% mannitol may further aggravate preexisting hemoconcentration.

Adverse Reactions:

Cardiovascular: Edema; thrombophlebitis; hypotension; hypertension; tachycardia; angina-like chest pains; CHF.

CNS: Headache; blurred vision; convulsions; dizziness.

GI: Nausea; vomiting; diarrhea.

Metabolic: Fluid and electrolyte imbalance; acidosis; electrolyte loss; dehydration.

Renal: Urinary retention; osmotic nephrosis.

Miscellaneous: Pulmonary congestion; dry mouth; thirst; rhinitis; local pain; skin necrosis; chills; urticaria; fever.

Overdosage:

Symptoms: Larger than recommended doses may result in increased electrolyte excretion, particularly sodium, chloride, and potassium. Sodium depletion can result in orthostatic tachycardia or hypotension and decreased central venous pressure. Chloride metabolism closely follows that of sodium. Potassium deficit can impair neuromuscular function and cause intestinal dilation and ileus. If urine flow is inadequate, pulmonary edema or water intoxication may occur. Other symptoms include hypotension, polyuria that rapidly converts to oliguria, stupor, convulsions, hyperosmolality, and hyponatremia.

Treatment: Discontinue infusion immediately. Institute supportive measures to correct fluid and electrolyte imbalances. Hemodialysis is beneficial to clear mannitol and reduce serum osmolality.

HYPEROSMOTIC AGENTS

Administration and Dosage:

Reduction of intraocular pressure: 1.5 to 2 g/kg, as a 20% solution (7.5 to 10 mL/kg) or as a 15% solution (10 to 13 mL/kg) over a period as short as 30 minutes. When used preoperatively, administer 1 to 1.5 hours before surgery to achieve maximal effect.

Preparation of solution: When exposed to low temperatures, mannitol solution may crystallize. Concentrations > 15% have a greater tendency to crystallize. If crystals are observed, warm the bottle in a hot water bath, a dry heat oven, or autoclave, then cool to at or below body temperature before administering.

When infusing concentrated mannitol, the administration set should include a filter.

Rx	**Osmitrol** (Clintec)	**Injection:** 5%	In 1000 mL.
Rx	**Mannitol** (Various, eg, Astra)	**Injection:**10%	In 1000 mL.
Rx	**Osmitrol** (Clintec)		In 500 and 1000 mL.
Rx	**Osmitrol** (Clintec)	**Injection:** 15%	In 500 mL.
Rx	**Mannitol** (Various, eg, Astra)	**Injection:** 20%	In 250 and 500 mL.
Rx	**Osmitrol** (Clintec)		In 250 and 500 mL.
Rx	**Mannitol** (Various, eg, Astra)	**Injection:** 25%	In 50 mL.

SURGICAL ADJUNCTS

Irrigating solutions, viscoelastic agents, botulinum toxin type A, verteporfin (*Visudyne*), absorbable gelatin film, processed pericardium, and proteolytic enzymes are adjuncts to a variety of ophthalmologic procedures and surgeries.

INTRAOCULAR IRRIGATING SOLUTIONS

Irrigating solutions are aqueous solutions used to cleanse and to maintain moisture of ocular tissue. Ideally these solutions are isotonic. The optimum pH is 7.4. A pH < 7 or > 8 has caused cellular stress and cellular death when the tissues have been exposed for a prolonged period of time.

The commercially available intraocular irrigating solutions (eg, *BSS* and *BSS Plus*) are used during ocular surgery to protect the lens and corneal endothelium. Unlike physiological saline and Lactated Ringer's solution, these balanced salt solutions provide the ions magnesium and calcium as cellular nutrients. These nutrients are required for intercellular and intracellular function during prolonged ocular surgery. In addition to magnesium and calcium, bicarbonate, glucose, and glutathione are in these perfusion media (*BSS Plus*). These components help to maintain a deturgesced or thin cornea by avoiding corneal swelling.

For information on extraocular irrigating solutions, see the Nonsurgical Adjuncts chapter.

POVIDONE IODINE

An antimicrobial agent effective against a wide range of organisms, povidone iodine has become an important prophylactic adjunct to ophthalmic surgery. This agent is formulated for topical ophthalmic use on the skin of the eyelids and adnexal tissues. The ophthalmic preparation is commonly used to prep the periocular tissues (eyelids, brow, cheek) and to irrigate the ocular surface (cornea, conjuctiva, and fornices).

VISCOELASTIC AGENTS

Viscoelastic agents, sodium hyaluronate and hydroxypropyl methylcellulose, are used in many ophthalmic surgical procedures, including intraocular lens implantation and keratoplasty. In surgical procedures in the anterior segment of the eye, instillation maintains a deep anterior chamber, allowing for more efficient manipulation with less trauma to the corneal endothelium and surrounding tissues. The viscoelasticity of these agents helps push back the vitreous face and prevent formation of a postoperative flat chamber. The majority of the viscoelastic material is removed from the eye at the end of surgery to diminish the problems of glaucoma.

Viscoelastic agents are tissue-protective substances and do not interfere with normal wound healing. They are nonantigenic and do not contain proteins that may cause inflammation or foreign body reactions.

ABSORBABLE GELATIN FILM

In the dry state, absorbable gelatin film has the appearance and texture of cellophane. When moistened, it assumes a rubbery consistency and can be cut to desired size and shape and fitted to rounded or irregular surfaces.

It is used in many surgical procedures including glaucoma filtration operations (eg, iridencleisis and trephination), extraocular muscle surgery, and diathermy or scleral "buckling" operations for retinal detachment to aid in preventing formation of adhesions between contiguous ocular structures.

Absence of undue tissue reaction and absorption of gelatin film, with consequent decreased likelihood of developing adhesions, have been found to be of particular value in dural and ocular implants.

PROCESSED PERICARDIUM

Processed pericardium (*Tutoplast*) is a solvent dehydrated, gamma-irradiated preserved human pericardium. It is indicated for implantation with a specific spectrum of indications. Collagenous connective tissue with multidirectional fibers retains the mechanical strength and elasticity of native pericardium, while providing the basic formative structure to support replacement by new endogenous tissue. This tissue is indicated for use in a variety of surgical applications, including duraplasty (as a subsitute for human dura mater), and in abdominal, urological, ophthamological, and vascular surgery.

INTRAOCULAR ACETYLCHOLINE AND CARBACHOL

Both acetylcholine and carbachol are available for intracameral use to produce complete and rapid miosis following intraocular surgery. Because carbachol is a potent miotic, the intracameral formulation is considerably less concentrated than the solutions prepared for topical use. Intracameral carbachol is available as a 0.01% sterile balanced salt solution with no preservatives and is supplied in a 1.5 mL sterile glass disposable vial. The dose is 0.5 mL applied by gentle irrigation. Acetylcholine is available as a 1:100 solution when reconstituted in a dual chamber vial. The dose is generally 0.5 to 2 mL. Patients treated with intracameral carbachol after phacoemulsification and posterior chamber lens implantation often demonstrate lower IOP during the first postoperative day.

POLYDIMETHYLSILOXANE

Polydimethylsiloxane (silicone oil) is used by retinal surgeons to produce retinal tamponade in selected cases of retinal detachment. This agent is injected directly into the vitreous space in cases of complicated retinal detachment, such as may occur in patients with proliferative vitreoretinopathy, proliferative diabetic retinopathy, cytomegalovirus (CMV) retinitis, giant retinal tears, and following perforating injuries. Silicone oil can also be used as primary therapy in detachments associated with AIDS-relatied CMV retinitis.

SURGICAL ADJUNCTS

BOTULINUM TOXIN TYPE A

Botulinum toxin is a form of purified botulinum toxin type A produced from a culture of the Hall strain of *Clostridium botulinum*. Botulinum toxin type A blocks neuromuscular conduction by binding to receptor sites on motor nerve terminals, entering the nerve terminals, and inhibiting the release of acetylcholine. When injected IM at therapeutic doses, the drug produces localized chemical denervation muscle paralysis. When the muscle is chemically denervated, it atrophies and may develop extrajunctional acetylcholine receptors. There is evidence that the nerve can sprout and reinnervate the muscle, with reversible weakness. The paralytic effect on muscles injected with botulinum toxin type A is useful in reducing the excessive, abnormal contractions associated with blepharospasm.

SURGICAL ENZYMES

Alpha-chymotrypsin is a proteolytic surgical enzyme used to dissolve zonules of the lens during intracapsular cataract surgery. Destruction of the equatorial pericapsular membrane of the lens occurs in 5 minutes. Zonular fibers are lysed within 10 to 15 minutes of application; complete lysis of the entire zonular membrane may take ≤ 30 minutes.

Many chemicals and natural body fluids are capable of inactivating alpha-chymotrypsin. Examples of products that may cause zonulysis to fail include the following: Serum, blood, detergents, alkali, acids, antiseptics, and epinephrine 1:100. These products may be used to inactivate alpha-chymotrypsin after zonulysis is complete. Pilocarpine (eg, *Isopto Carpine*), tetracaine (eg, *Pontocaine HCl*), acetylcholine (*Miochol*), and epinephrine 1:1000 will not inactivate this surgical enzyme.

Two other enzymes have been used during ocular surgery: Hyaluronidase and urokinase. Hyaluronidase is added to local anesthetic solutions to increase drug absorption and dispersion. This enzyme hydrolyzes hyaluronic acid in the connective tissue, which increases tissue permeability.

Urokinase has been used to irrigate hyphemas and to treat acute retinal artery and vein occlusions. The conversion of plasminogen to the proteolytic enzyme plasmin by urokinase causes degradation of plasma proteins, fibrinogen, and fibrin clots.

Tissue plasminogen activator (tPA) is an enzyme that has the property of fibrin-enhanced conversion of plasminogen to plasmin. It produces limited conversion of plasminogen in the absence of fibrin. When introduced into the systemic circulation of pharmacologic concentration, it binds to fibrin in a thrombus and converts the entrapped plasminogen to plasmin. This initiates local fibrinolysis with limited systemic proteolysis.

VERTEPORFIN

Choroidal neovascularization associated with age-related macular degeneration is a major cause of visual impairment. This disease is difficult to treat with conventional laser procedures because normal retinal tissues can be destroyed, resulting in central vision loss. Photodynamic therapy offers the opportunity to selectively eradicate neovascular membranes while producing minimal damage to normal retinal and choroidal tissues.

The procedure involves intravenous administration of verteporfin (*Visudyne*) for 10 minutes. Verteporfin is a potent photosensitizing dye. Five minutes after the conclusion of dye administration, during which the drug selectively accumulates in the abnormal, neovascular tissue, nonthermal light at 689 nm is applied to the abnormal tissues for 83 seconds. When activated by light, verteporfin causes the production of singlet oxygen and free radicals that produce cell death and occlusion of abnormal vessels. The use of verteporfin in the photodynamic therapy of neovascular age-related macular degeneration has been shown to be effective in stabilizing the disease in animal models and in human clinical trials.

J. James Rowsey, MD
Saint Luke's Cataract and Laser Institute
Tarpon Springs, FL

For More Information

Duane TD, ed. *Clinical Ophthalmology*. Philadelphia: Lippincott-Raven, 1987.

Ellis PP. *Ocular Therapeutics and Pharmacology*, ed. 7. St. Louis: C.V. Mosby, 1985.

Goodman & Gilman's. *The Pharmacological Basis of Therapeutics*, ed. 9. New York: McGraw-Hill, 1996.

Havener WH. *Ocular Pharmacology*, ed. 5. St Louis: C.V. Mosby, 1983.

Whikehart Dr. Irrigating Solutions. In: Bartlett JD, Jaanus SD, eds. *Clinical Ocular Pharmacology*, ed. 3. Boston: Butterworth-Heinemann, 1995.

SURGICAL ADJUNCTS

INTRAOCULAR IRRIGATING SOLUTIONS

Actions:

Pharmacology: Sterile irrigating solution is a sterile physiological balanced salt solution, each mL containing sodium chloride 0.64%, potassium chloride 0.075%, calcium chloride dihydrate 0.048%, magnesium chloride hexahydrate 0.03%, sodium acetate trihydrate 0.39%, sodium citrate dihydrate 0.17%, sodium hydroxide or hydrochloric acid (to adjust pH), and water. This solution is isotonic to ocular tissue and contains electrolytes required for normal cellular metabolic functions.

Indications:

Irrigation: For irrigation during various ocular surgical procedures. Some products may also be used for ears, nose, and throat (consult specific product labeling).

Warnings:

Route of administration: Not for injection or IV infusion. Use aseptic technique only.

Precautions:

Preservative free solutions: Do not use for > 1 patient.

Corneal clouding and edema: Corneal clouding and edema have occurred following ocular surgery in which balanced salt solution was used as an irrigating solution. Take appropriate measures to minimize trauma to the cornea and other ocular tissues.

Concomitant medication: Addition of any medication to balanced salt solution may result in damage to intraocular tissue.

Diabetics: Studies suggest that intraocular irrigating solutions which are iso-osmotic with normal aqueous fluids should be used with caution in diabetic patients undergoing vitrectomy as intraoperative lens changes have been observed.

Adverse Reactions:

When corneal endothelium is abnormal, irrigation or any other trauma may result in bullous keratopathy. Postoperative inflammatory reactions and corneal edema and decompensation have occurred. Relationship to balanced salt solution is not established.

Administration and Dosage:

Use balanced salt solution according to the established practices for each surgical procedure. Follow the manufacturer directions for the particular administration set to be used. For products with separate solutions for reconstitution, never use Part I or Part II alone; this could result in damage to the eye.

Storage/Stability: Store at 8° to 30°C (46° to 86°F). Avoid excessive heat. Do not freeze. Discard prepared solution after 6 hours. Do not use if cloudy or if seal or packaging is damaged. Do not use reconstituted solution if it is discolored or contains a precipitate.

268 OPHTHALMIC DRUG FACTS

Rx	Balanced Salt Solution (B. Braun)	Solution: 0.64% NaCl, 0.075% KCl, 0.03% magnesium chloride, 0.048% calcium chloride, 0.39% sodium acetate, 0.17% sodium citrate, sodium hydroxide or hydrochloric acid	In 500 mL.
Rx	BSS (Alcon)		Preservative free. In 15, 30, 250, and 500 mL.
Rx	Iocare Balanced Salt (Ciba Vision)		Preservative free. In 15 mL.
Rx	BSS Plus (Alcon)	Solution: Mix aseptically just prior to use. Part I: 7.44 mg NaCl, 0.395 mg KCl, 0.433 mg dibasic sodium phosphate, 2.19 mg sodium bicarbonate, hydrochloric acid or sodium hydroxide/mL	Preservative free. In 240 mL.
		Part II: 3.85 mg calcium chloride dihydrate, 5 mg magnesium chloride hexahydrate, 23 mg dextrose, 4.6 mg glutathione disulfide/mL	Preservative free. In 10 mL.
Rx	B-Salt Forte (Akorn)	Solution: Mix aseptically just prior to use. Part I: 7.14 mg NaCl, 0.38 mg KCl, 0.154 mg calcium chloride dihydrate, 0.2 mg magnesium chloride hexahydrate, 0.92 mg dextrose, hydrochloric acid or sodium hydroxide/mL	Preservative free. In 515 mL.
		Part II: 1081 mg sodium bicarbonate, 216 mg dibasic sodium phosphate (anhydrous), 95 mg glutathione disulfide (oxidized glutathione)/vial	Preservative free. In 60 mL.

POVIDONE IODINE

Actions:

Pharmacology: Povidone iodine has broad-spectrum antimicrobial action.

Indications:

Ophthalmic preoperative prep: Used prior to eye surgery to prep the periocular region (lids, brow, and cheek) and irrigate the ocular surface (cornea, conjunctiva, and palpebral fornices).

Contraindications:

Hypersensitivity to iodine.

Warnings:

For external use only: Not for intraocular injection or irrigation.

Pregnancy: Category C. Safety for use during pregnancy has not been established. Use only when clearly needed.

Lactation: Because of the potential for adverse reactions in nursing infants, decide whether to discontinue nursing or discontinue the drug, taking into account the importance of the drug to the mother.

SURGICAL ADJUNCTS

269

Children: Safety and efficacy have not been established.

Precautions:

Thyroid disorders: Use with caution in patients with thyroid disorders because of the possibility of iodine absorption.

Adverse Reactions:

Local sensitivity has been exhibited by some individuals.

Administration and Dosage:

Do not use in an open globe, as endothelial toxicity may ensue.

Transfer solution to a sterile prep cup. Apply to lashes and lid margins with sterile applicator; repeat once. Apply to lids, brow, and cheek in an ever-expanding circular fashion with sterile applicator; repeat 3 times. While separating the lids, irrigate cornea, conjunctiva, and palpebral fornices with solution and leave in for 2 minutes; flush with sterile saline solution.

Rx	**Betadine 5% Sterile Ophthalmic Prep Solution** (Alcon)	**Solution:** 5% povidone iodine	In 50 mL.[1]

[1] Glycerin, sodium chloride, sodium hydroxide, and sodium phosphate.

SODIUM HYALURONATE

Actions:

Pharmacology: Sodium hyaluronate and sodium chondroitin sulfate are widely distributed in extracellular matrix of connective tissues. They are found in the synovial fluid, skin, umbilical cord, and vitreous and aqueous humor. The cornea is the ocular tissue with the greatest concentration of sodium chondroitin sulfate; the vitreous and aqueous humor contain the greatest concentration of sodium hyaluronate.

This preparation is a specific fraction of sodium hyaluronate developed for use in anterior segment and vitreous procedures as a viscoelastic agent. It has high molecular weight, is nonantigenic, does not cause inflammatory or foreign body reactions, and has a high viscosity. The 1% solution is transparent and remains in the anterior chamber for < 6 days. It protects corneal endothelial cells and other ocular structures. It does not interfere with epithelialization and normal wound healing.

Indications:

Surgical aid: As a surgical aid in cataract extraction (intra- and extracapsular), intraocular lens implantation (IOL), corneal transplant, glaucoma filtration, retinal attachment surgery, and posterior segment surgery to gently separate, maneuver, and hold tissues.

To maintain a deep anterior chamber in surgical procedures in the anterior segment of the eye, allowing for efficient manipulation with less trauma to the corneal endothelium and other surrounding tissues.

To push back the vitreous face and prevent formation of a postoperative flat chamber.

To create a clear field of vision, facilitating intra- and postoperative inspection of the retina and photocoagulation.

Off-labeled: Sodium hyaluronate has been used in the treatment of refractory dry eye syndrome.

Warnings:

Hypersensitivity: Because this preparation is extracted from avian tissues and contains minute amounts of protein, risks of hypersensitivity exist.

Precautions:

For intraocular use: Use only if solution is clear. Do not reuse cannulas.

Postoperative intraocular pressure (IOP): Postoperative IOP may be elevated as a result of pre-existing glaucoma, compromised outflow, and by operative procedures and sequelae, including enzymatic zonulysis, absence of an iridectomy, trauma to filtration structures, and by blood and lenticular remnants in the anterior chamber. Because the exact role of these factors is difficult to predict in any individual case, the following precautions are recommended:

> *Do not overfill the anterior chamber* – Do not overfill the anterior chamber (except in glaucoma surgery). (See Administration and Dosage.)

> *Monitoring* – Carefully monitor IOP, especially during the immediate postoperative period. Treat significant increases appropriately.

> *Posterior segment surgery* – In posterior segment surgery, in aphakic diabetics, exercise special care to avoid using large amounts of the drug. Remove some of the preparation by irrigation or aspiration at the close of surgery (except in glaucoma surgery). (See Administration and Dosage.)

> Avoid trapping air bubbles behind the drug.

Cloudiness/Precipitate: Reports indicate that the drug may become cloudy or form a slight precipitate after instillation. The clinical significance is not known because the majority of reports do not indicate any harmful effects on ocular tissues. Be aware of this phenomenon and remove cloudy or precipitated material by irrigation or aspiration. In vitro studies suggest that this phenomenon may be related to interactions with certain concomitantly administered ophthalmic medications.

ProVisc: The device used to obtain *ProVisc* material may cause an allergic reaction in susceptible patients.

Adverse Reactions:

Although well tolerated, a transient postoperative increase of IOP has been reported (see Precautions).

Other reactions that have occurred include postoperative inflammatory reactions (iritis, hypopyon), corneal edema, and corneal decompensation.

SURGICAL ADJUNCTS

271

Administration and Dosage:

Cataract surgery - IOL implantation: Slowly introduce a sufficient amount (using cannula or needle) into anterior chamber. Inject before or after delivery of lens. Injection before lens delivery protects corneal endothelium from possible damage from removal of the cataractous lens. May use to coat surgical instruments and the IOL prior to insertion. May inject additional amounts during surgery to replace any of the drug lost.

Glaucoma filtration surgery: In conjunction with the performance of the trabeculectomy, inject slowly and carefully through a corneal paracentesis to reconstitute the anterior chamber. Further injection can be continued to allow it to extrude into the subconjunctival filtration site through and around the sutured outer scleral flap.

Corneal transplant surgery: After removal of the corneal button, fill the anterior chamber with the drug. Then, suture the donor graft in place. An additional amount may be injected to replace the lost amount as a result of surgical manipulation.

Sodium hyaluronate has also been used in the anterior chamber of the donor eye prior to trepanation to protect the corneal endothelial cells of the graft.

Retinal attachment surgery: Slowly introduce into the vitreous cavity. The injection may be directed to separate membranes from retina for safe excision and release of traction. Also serves to maneuver tissues into desired position (eg, to gently push back a detached retina or unroll a retinal flap); aids in holding retina against the sclera for reattachment.

Storage/Stability:

Amvisc/Amvisc Plus, Healon/Healon GV – Store at 2° to 8°C (36° to 46°F).

AMO Vitrax – Store at room temperature (15° to 30°C; 59° to 86°F). Do not freeze. Protect from light.

ProVisc – Drug should reach room temperature before use ($\approx$ 20 to 40 minutes, depending on quantity). Store in refrigerator at 2° to 8°C (36° to 46°F).

Rx	**Biolon** (Akorn)	**Injection:** 10 mg/mL[1]	In 0.5 or 1 mL disposable syringes.
Rx	**Healon** (Pharmacia)		In 0.4, 0.55, and 0.85 mL disp. syringes.
Rx	**ProVisc** (Alcon)		In 0.4, 0.55, and 0.85 mL disp. glass syringes.
Rx	**Amvisc** (Chiron)	**Injection:** 12 mg/mL[2]	In 0.5 or 0.8 mL disp. syringes.
Rx	**Healon GV** (Pharmacia)	**Injection:** 14 mg/mL[1]	In 0.85 mL disp. syringes.
Rx	**Amvisc Plus** (Chiron)	**Injection:** 16 mg/mL[2]	In 0.5 or 8 mL disp. syringes.
Rx	**AMO Vitrax** (Allergan)	**Injection:** 30 mg/mL[3]	In 0.65 mL disp. syringe.

[1] With 8.5 mg NaCl per mL.
[2] With 9 mg NaCl per mL.
[3] With 3.2 mg NaCl, 0.75 mg KCl, 0.48 mg calcium chloride, 0.3 mg magnesium chloride, 3.9 mg sodium acetate, and 1.7 mg sodium citrate per mL.

SODIUM HYALURONATE AND CHONDROITIN SULFATE

Refer to the Sodium Hyaluronate monograph for more complete information.

Indications:

Surgical aid: A surgical aid in anterior segment procedures, including cataract extraction and intraocular lens implantation.

Off-labeled: Topical treatment of severe dry eye disorders.

Administration and Dosage:

The higher viscosity materials remain longer in the anterior chamber and will be more difficult to remove from the eye. However, they provide better endothelial protection during phacoemulsification in the presence of Fuch dystrophy.

Carefully introduce (using a 27-gauge cannula) into the anterior chamber. May inject prior to or following delivery of the crystalline lens. Instillation prior to lens delivery provides additional protection to corneal endothelium, protecting it from possible damage arising from surgical instrumentation. May also be used to coat intraocular lens and tips of surgical instruments prior to implantation surgery. Intravitreal injection through the pars plana is helpful in torn capsules to avoid lens sublaxation. May inject additional solution during anterior segment surgery to fully maintain the chamber or to replace solution lost during surgery. At the end of surgery, remove solution by thoroughly irrigating the eye with a balanced salt solution. Alternatively, the solution may be left in the eye when used as directed.

Storage/Stability: Store at 2° to 8°C (36° to 46°F). Do not freeze.

Rx	**Viscoat** (Alcon)	**Solution:** ≤ 40 mg sodium chondroitin sulfate, 30 mg sodium hyaluronate per mL	In 0.5 mL disposable syringes.[1]

[1] 0.45 mg sodium dihydrogen phosphate hydrate, 2 mg disodium hydrogen phosphate, 4.3 mg sodium chloride per mL.

HYDROXYPROPYL METHYLCELLULOSE

Actions:

Pharmacology: Hydroxypropyl methylcellulose is an isotonic, nonpyrogenic viscoelastic solution with a high molecular weight (> 80,000 daltons). It maintains a deep chamber during anterior segment surgery and allows for more efficient manipulation with less trauma to the corneal endothelium and other ocular tissues. The viscoelasticity helps the vitreous face to be pushed back, preventing formation of a postoperative flat chamber. It is also used as a demulcent agent.

Indications:

For professional use in gonioscopic examinations.

Precautions:

Intraocular pressure (IOP): Transient increased IOP may occur following surgery because of pre-existing glaucoma or because of the surgery itself. If the postoperative IOP increases above expected values, administer appropriate therapy.

SURGICAL ADJUNCTS

Adverse Reactions:

Although well tolerated, a transient, postoperative increase in IOP has been reported (see Precautions). Other reactions that have occurred include postoperative inflammatory reactions (iritis, hypopyon), corneal edema, and corneal decompensation.

Administration and Dosage:

Gonioscopic examinations: Fill gonioscopic prism with 2.5% solution, as necessary.

Storage/Stability: If this solution dries on optical surfaces, let them stand in cool water before cleansing. If solution changes color or becomes cloudy, do not use. Not for use with hot laser treatment as solution clouding will occur.

To avoid contamination, do not touch tip of container to any surface. Replace cap after using. Keep container tightly closed. Store at room temperature 15° to 30°C (59° to 86°F). Avoid excessive heat over 60°C (140°F). Protect from light.

otc	**Gonak** (Akorn)	**Solution:** 2.5%	In 15 mL.[1]
otc	**Goniosol** (Novartis)		In 15 mL.[2]

[1] With 0.01% benzalkonium chloride, boric acid, KCl, sodium borate, hydrochloric acid or sodium hydroxide, and EDTA.
[2] With 0.01% benzalkonium chloride, boric acid, KCl, EDTA.

HYDROXYETHYLCELLULOSE

Indications:

Gonioscopic bonding: For use in bonding gonioscopic prisms to the eye.

Administration and Dosage:

Storage/Stability: Store at room temperature 15° to 30°C (59° to 86°F).

Rx	**Gonioscopic** (Alcon)	**Solution:** Hydroxyethylcel-lulose	In 15 mL Drop-Tainers.[1]

[1] With 0.004% thimerosal, 0.1% EDTA.

ABSORBABLE GELATIN FILM, STERILE

Actions:

Pharmacology: A sterile, absorbable gelatin film for use in ocular surgery.

In the dry state it has the appearance and texture of cellophane of equivalent thickness; when moistened, it assumes a rubbery consistency and can be cut to desired size and fitted to rounded or irregular surfaces. The rate of absorption after implantation ranges from 1 to 6 months, depending upon the size of the implant and the site of implantation. Pleural and muscle implants are completely absorbed in 8 to 14 days; dural and ocular implants usually require ≤ 2 to 5 months for complete absorp-

OPHTHALMIC DRUG FACTS

tion. The absence of undue tissue reactions, with the consequent decreased likelihood of developing adhesions, has been of particular value in the case of dural and ocular implants.

Indications:

Ocular surgery: In glaucoma filtration operations (ie, iridencleisis and trephination), extraocular muscle surgery, and diathermy or scleral "buckling" operations for retinal detachment. There is a remarkable lack of cellular reaction to the film implanted subconjunctivally or used as a seton into the anterior chamber. Evidence shows that implants help prevent formation of adhesions between contiguous ocular structures.

Contraindications:

Because the rate of absorption is likely to be increased in the presence of purulent exudation, do not implant in grossly contaminated or infected surgical wounds.

Administration and Dosage:

Preparation: Immerse in sterile saline solution; soak until quite pliable; cut to the desired size and shape; apply as follows:

As a seton in iridencleisis: Place a small piece ($\approx$ 4 mm $\times$ 10 mm) over the prolapsed iris pillar parallel to the limbus; Tenon's capsule and the conjunctiva are then closed with continuous absorbable sutures closely spaced to ensure tight wound closure.

Diathermy or scleral "buckling" operations: Place film over the sclera, then suture the muscle and the conjunctiva over the underlying film.

Extraocular muscle surgery: Place film over and beneath the muscle before Tenon's capsule and the conjunctiva are closed in layers.

Storage/Stability: Store at room temperature 15° to 30°C (59° to 86°F). To ensure sterility, use immediately after withdrawal from the envelope.

Rx	**Gelfilm** (Pharmacia)	100 mm × 125 mm	In 1s.
Rx	**Gelfilm Ophthalmic** (Pharmacia)	25 mm × 50 mm	In 6s.

MIOTICS, DIRECT-ACTING

For complete prescribing information, see the Miotics, Direct-Acting monograph in the Agents for Glaucoma chapter.

Actions:

Pharmacology: The direct-acting miotics are parasympathomimetic (cholinergic) drugs that duplicate the muscarinic effects of acetylcholine. When applied topically, these drugs produce pupillary constriction, stimulate the ciliary muscles, and increase aqueous humor outflow facility.

SURGICAL ADJUNCTS

ACETYLCHOLINE CHLORIDE, INTRAOCULAR

Indications:

To produce complete miosis within seconds after delivery of the lens in cataract surgery. In penetrating keratoplasty, iridectomy, and other anterior segment surgery where rapid, complete miosis may be required.

Administration and Dosage:

Solution: Instill the solution into the anterior chamber before or after securing at least 1 suture. The pupil is rapidly constricted and the peripheral iris drawn away from the angle of the anterior chamber if there are no mechanical hindrances. Any anatomical hindrance to miosis may require surgery to permit desired drug effect.

Dose of 0.5 to 2 mL produces satisfactory miosis. Solution need not be flushed from the chamber after miosis occurs. Because acetylcholine has a short duration of action, pilocarpine may be applied topically before dressing to maintain miosis.

Preparation of solution: The aqueous solution of acetylcholine chloride is unstable. Prepare solution immediately before use. Do not use solution that is not clear and colorless. Discard any solution that has not been used. Do not gas sterilize.

Storage/Stability: Store at room temperature 15° to 30°C (59° to 86°F). Do not freeze.

Rx **Miochol-E** (Novartis)	**Solution:** 1:100 acetylcholine chloride when reconstituted	In 2 mL dual chamber univial (lower chamber 20 mg lyophilized acetylcholine chloride and 56 mg mannitol; upper chamber 2 mL electrolyte diluent[1] and sterile water for injection).

[1] Sodium chloride, potassium chloride, magnesium chloride hexahydrate, calcium chloride dihydrate.

CARBACHOL, INTRAOCULAR

For complete prescribing information, refer to the Miotics, Direct-Acting group monograph in the Agents for Glaucoma chapter. The following section is included here for completeness to show all of the clinical uses of this drug class.

Indications:

Miosis: Intraocular use for miosis during surgery.

Administration and Dosage:

For single-dose intraocular use only. Discard unused portion.

Open under aseptic conditions only.

Gently instill no more than 0.5 mL into the anterior chamber before or after securing sutures. Miosis is usually maximal 2 to 5 minutes after application.

Storage/Stability: Store at room temperature 15° to 30°C (59° to 86°F).

Rx	**Carbastat** (Novartis)	**Solution:** 0.01%	In 1.5 mL vials.[1]
Rx	**Miostat** (Alcon)		In 1.5 mL vials.[1]

[1] With 0.64% sodium chloride, 0.075% potassium chloride, 0.048% calcium chloride dihydrate, 0.03% magnesium chloride hexahydrate, 0.39% sodium acetate trihydrate, 0.17% sodium citrate dihydrate, sodium hydroxide, hydrochloric acid.

POLYDIMETHYLSILOXANE (Silicone Oil)

Actions:

Pharmacology: Polydimethylsiloxane, an oil that is injected into the vitreous space of the eye, is used as a prolonged retinal tamponade in select cases of retinal detachment.

Clinical Trials:

>*Anatomic reattachment rates* – Successful reattachment of the retina occurred in 64% to 75% of the patients who were treated with polydimethylsiloxane. This rate varied depending on the specific etiology of the disease and the severity of the condition. In AIDS CMV retinitis patients receiving silicone oil as a primary means for reattaching the retina, attachment rates were as high as 90% within an average 6-month follow-up period.

>*Visual acuity outcomes* – At 6 months, 45% to 70% of patients showed improvements in visual acuity. In ≈ 15% to 26% of patients, visual acuity did not change and in ≈ 15% to 30%, worsening of visual acuity occurred. Deterioration of visual acuity in treated patients appeared to be related to redetachment of the retina, further progression of retinal disease, or to keratopathy and cataract complications. In AIDS CMV retinitis patients, improvement or maintenance of visual acuity was documented in 57% of the patients within an average 6-month follow-up period. In AIDS patients, further decline in visual acuity was seen due to continuing progression of retinal and optic nerve disease and development of oil related cataracts in 33% of patients within 4 to 5 months of oil instillation.

Indications:

Retinal detachments: Prolonged retinal tamponade in selected cases of complicated retinal detachments or early phthisis where other interventions are not appropriate for patient management. Complicated retinal detachments or recurrent retinal detachments occur most commonly in eyes with proliferative vitreoretinopathy (PVR), proliferative diabetic retinopathy (PDR), cytomegalovirus (CMV) retinitis, giant tears, and following perforating injuries.

For primary use in detachments due to AIDS-related CMV retinitis and other viral infections.

Contraindications:

Pseudophakic patients with silicone intraocular lens (silicone oil can chemically interact and opacify silicone elastomers).

SURGICAL ADJUNCTS

Warnings:

Cataract: Approximately 50% to 70% of phakic patients developed a cataract within 12 months of oil instillation. Approximately 33% of phakic AIDS CMV retinitis patients developed some degree of cataract within an average 4 to 5 month time frame from oil instillation.

Anterior chamber oil migration: In 17% to 20% of patients, oil emulsification or migration into the anterior chamber was observed. Migration into the anterior chamber occurred in both phakic and aphakic patients.

Keratopathy: From 8% to 20% of patients developed keratopathy (0.6%, AIDS patients). This complication occurred most frequently in aphakic patients (18% to 21%) and in the patients in whom oil had migrated into the anterior chamber (30%); the keratopathy in these cases was attributed to prolonged physical contact between the corneal endothelium and the silicone oil.

Glaucoma: Approximately 19% to 20% (0.06%, AIDS patients) of patients developed a persistent elevation in intraocular pressure (> 23 to 25 mm Hg). The neovascular glaucoma rate was $\approx$ 8%. Moderate temporary postoperative increases occurred within the first 3 weeks of treatment. Thereafter, secondary ocular hypertension occurred by several mechanisms. Glaucoma complications occurred in $\approx$ 30% of patients in which anterior chamber oil is noted. Patients with proliferative diabetic retinopathy were at highest risk for development of glaucoma following silicone oil instillation into the vitreous space.

Precautions:

Long-term use: The safety and efficacy of long-term use have not been established.

Adverse Reactions:

Miscellaneous: The most common adverse reactions include the following: Cataract (50% to 70%); anterior chamber oil migration (17% to 20%); keratopathy (8% to 20%); glaucoma (19% to 20%). See Warnings.

Other adverse reactions ranked by frequency of occurrence include the following: Redetachment, optic nerve atrophy, rubeosis iritis, temporary IOP increase, macular pucker, vitreous hemorrhage, phthisis, traction detachment, angle block (> 2%); subretinal strands, retinal rupture, endophthalmitis, subretinal silicone oil, choroidal detachment, aniridia, PVR reproliferation, cystoid macular edema, enucleation (< 2%).

Administration and Dosage:

Polydimethylsiloxane can be used in conjunction with or following standard retinal surgical procedures including scleral buckle surgery, vitrectomy, membrane peeling, and retinotomy or relaxing retinectomy.

Avoid introduction of air bubbles into the oil by careful withdrawal or decanting of the oil into the syringe. The oil can be injected into the vitreous from the syringe via a single-use cannulated infusion line or syringe needle. Subretinal fluid can be drained with a flute needle concurrent with polydimethylsiloxane infusion. The vitreous space can be filled with the oil to between 80% and 100% while exchanging for fluid or air, taking necessary precautions to avoid high intraocular pressure from developing during the exchange. Because the polydimethylsiloxane is less dense than the eye aqueous fluid, a basal iridectomy at the 6 o'clock meridian (Ando iridec-

278 OPHTHALMIC DRUG FACTS

tomy) is recommended to minimize oil-induced pupillary block and early angle-closure glaucoma. Upon choice of the physician, it may be desirable to have the patient assume a face-down posture during the first 24 hours following surgery.

Monitor the patient closely for development of glaucoma, cataract, and keratopathy complications and schedule for follow-up re-examination at regular intervals.

It is recommended that polydimethylsiloxane be removed at an appropriate interval within 1 year following instillation if the retina is stable, attached, and without significant remnants of proliferation. Although there is insufficient clinical evidence to support justification for longer term tamponade, whether or not the oil should be removed in patients at high risk for redetachment or the development of phthisis and shrinkage due to hypotony must be determined individually by the physician. In order to minimize the number of invasive traumatic experiences for patients with AIDS and CMV retinitis at high risk for redetachment and who have a shortened expected lifespan, avoid silicone oil removal procedures if the patient concurs.

Polydimethylsiloxane can be removed from the posterior chamber by withdrawal with a normal 10 mL syringe and a wide bore 1 mm cannula. By repeated oil-fluid exchange, most of the remaining small silicone oil droplets can subsequently be mobilized and removed from the eye. Alternatively, oil may be passively removed by infusion of an appropriate aqueous solution under the oil bubble, while allowing the oil to effuse out of a sclerotomy incision, or limbal incision in aphakic patients.

As there is a possible correlation between the migration of polydimethylsiloxane into the anterior chamber and the appearance of corneal changes such as edema, hazing or opacification, Descemet folds, or decompensation, perform regular monitoring of the patient's corneal status and take early corrective action if necessary, including extraction of the oil from the anterior chamber. Large bubbles or droplets of oil in the anterior chamber can be removed manually by syringe. Further standard practice for medical treatment of the keratopathy is recommended.

Temporary pressure increases > 3 weeks after surgery that can normalize spontaneously or be corrected by surgical treatment are those in which the polydimethylsiloxane causes a mechanical blockage of the pupil or inferior iridectomy or causes chamber angle closure by forcing its way anteriorly. In these situations, some of the oil may be withdrawn to relieve the mechanical force of the oil interface. Presence of polydimethylsiloxane droplets in the anterior chamber may also cause a chronic outflow obstruction of the trabecular meshwork. In such situations, elevated intraocular pressure can be managed with antiglaucoma medication in the majority of outflow obstruction patients.

Admixture incompatibility: Do not admix with any other substances prior to injection.

Storage/Stability: Store at room or cool temperature 8° to 24°C (46° to 75°F). Polydimethylsiloxane is supplied in a sterile vial intended for single use only and contains no preservative. Do not resterilize. Discard unused portions. Discard product after expiration date.

| *Rx* | **AdatoSil 5000**
(Escalon Ophthalmics) | **Injection:** Polydimethylsiloxane oil | In single-use 10 and 15 mL vials. |

SURGICAL ADJUNCTS

BOTULINUM TOXIN TYPE A

Actions:

Pharmacology: Botulinum toxin is a sterile, lyophilized form of purified botulinum toxin type A, produced from a culture of the Hall strain of *Clostridium botulinum* grown in a medium containing N-Z amine and yeast extract. Botulinum toxin type A blocks neuromuscular conduction by binding to receptor sites on motor nerve terminals, entering the nerve terminals, and inhibiting the release of acetylcholine. When injected IM at therapeutic doses, botulinum toxin type A produces a localized chemical denervation muscle paralysis. When the muscle is chemically denervated, it atrophies and may develop extrajunctional acetylcholine receptors. There is evidence that the nerve can sprout and reinnervate the muscle, reversing the weakness.

The paralytic effect on muscles injected with botulinum toxin type A is useful in reducing the excessive, abnormal contractions associated with blepharospasm.

When used for the treatment of strabismus, the administration of botulinum toxin type A may affect muscle pairs by inducing an atrophic lengthening of the injected muscle and a corresponding shortening of the muscle's antagonist. Following periocular injection of botulinum toxin type A, distant muscles show electrophysiologic changes, but no clinical weakness or other clinical change for a period of several weeks or months, parallel to the duration of local clinical paralysis.

Clinical Trials: In 1 study, botulinum toxin was evaluated in 27 patients with essential blepharospasm; 26 had previously undergone drug treatment utilizing benztropine mesylate, clonazepam, or baclofen without adequate clinical results. Three of these patients then underwent muscle stripping surgery still without an adequate outcome. Upon using botulinum toxin, 25 of the 27 patients reported improvement within 48 hours. One of the other patients was later controlled with a higher dosage. The remaining patient reported only mild improvement but remained functionally impaired.

In another study, 12 patients with blepharospasm were evaluated in a double-blind, placebo-controlled study. All patients receiving botulinum toxin (n = 8) improved compared with no improvements in the placebo group (n = 4). The mean dystonia score improved 72%, the self-assessment score rating improved 61%, and a videotape evaluation rating improved 39%. The effects of the treatment lasted a mean of 12.5 weeks.

Patients with blepharospasm (n = 1684) evaluated in an open trial showed clinical improvement lasting an average of 12.5 weeks prior to need for retreatment.

Patients with strabismus (n = 677) treated with ≥ 1 injection of botulinum toxin type A were evaluated in an open trial; 55% were improved to an alignment of 10 prism diopters when evaluated ≥ 6 months following injection. These results are consistent with results from additional open label trials.

Indications:

Treatment of strabismus and blepharospasm associated with dystonia, including benign essential blepharospasm or VII nerve disorders in patients ≥ 12 years of age.

Contraindications:

Hypersensitivity to any ingredient in the formulation.

Warnings:

Strabismus: The efficacy of botulinum toxin type A in deviations > 50 prism diopters, in restrictive strabismus, in Duane syndrome with lateral rectus weakness, and in secondary strabismus caused by prior surgical over-recession of the antagonist is doubtful, or multiple injections over time may be required. Botulinum toxin type A is ineffective in chronic paralytic strabismus except to reduce antagonist contracture in conjunction with surgical repair.

Dosage: Do not exceed the recommended dosages and frequencies of administration. There have been no reported instances of systemic toxicity resulting from accidental injection or oral ingestion of botulinum toxin type A. Should accidental injection or oral ingestion occur, medically supervise the patient for several days on an outpatient basis for signs or symptoms of systemic weakness or muscle paralysis. The entire contents of a vial is below the estimated dose for systemic toxicity in humans weighing $\geq$ 6 kg.

Hypersensitivity: As with all biologic products, epinephrine and other precautions should be available should an anaphylactic reaction occur.

Pregnancy: Category C. It is not known whether botulinum toxin type A can cause fetal harm when administered to a pregnant woman or can affect reproduction capacity. Administer to pregnant women only if clearly needed.

Lactation: It is not known whether this drug is excreted in breast milk. Exercise caution when botulinum toxin type A is administered to a nursing woman.

Children: Safety and efficacy in children < 12 years of age have not been established.

Precautions:

Safe and effective use: Safe and effective use of botulinum toxin type A depends upon proper storage of the product, selection of the correct dose, and proper reconstitution and administration techniques. Physicians administering botulinum toxin type A must understand the relevant neuromuscular and orbital anatomy and any alterations to the anatomy caused by prior surgical procedures, and standard electromyographic techniques.

Retrobulbar hemorrhages: During the administration of botulinum toxin type A for the treatment of strabismus, retrobulbar hemorrhages sufficient to compromise retinal circulation have occurred from needle penetrations into the orbit. Have appropriate instruments to decompress the orbit accessible. Ocular (globe) penetrations by needles have also occurred. An ophthalmoscope to diagnose this condition should be available.

Reduced blinking: Reduced blinking from botulinum toxin type A injection of the orbicularis muscle can lead to corneal exposure, persistent epithelial defect, and corneal ulceration, especially in patients with VII nerve disorders. One case of corneal perforation in an aphakic eye requiring corneal grafting has occurred because of this effect. Carefully test corneal sensation in eyes previously operated upon, avoid injection into the lower lid area to avoid ectropion, and vigorously treat any epithelial defect. This may require protective drops, ointment, therapeutic soft contact lenses, or closure of the eye by patching or other means.

Antibodies: Presence of antibodies to botulinum toxin type A may reduce the effectiveness of therapy. In clinical studies, reduction in effectiveness due to antibody production has occurred in 1 patient with blepharospasm receiving 3 doses over a

SURGICAL ADJUNCTS

6-week period totaling 92 U and in several patients with torticollis who received multiple doses experimentally, totaling over 300 U in 1 month. For this reason, keep the dose of botulinum toxin type A for strabismus and blepharospasm as low as possible, in any case < 200 U in a 1-month period.

Drug Interactions:

Aminoglycosides: The effect of botulinum toxin may be potentiated by aminoglycoside antibiotics or any other drug that interferes with neuromuscular transmission. Exercise caution when botulinum toxin type A is used in patients taking these drugs.

Adverse Reactions:

Ophthalmic:

> *Strabismus* – Inducing paralysis in ≥ 1 extraocular muscle may produce spatial disorientation, double vision, or past-pointing. Covering the affected eye may alleviate these symptoms. Extraocular muscles adjacent to the injection site are often affected, causing ptosis or vertical deviation, especially with higher doses. Side effects in 2058 adults who received 3650 injections for horizontal strabismus included ptosis (15.7%) and vertical deviation (16.9%). The incidence of ptosis was much less after inferior rectus injection (0.9%) and much greater after superior rectus injection (37.7%).

Side effects persisting for > 6 months in an enlarged series of 5587 injections of horizontal muscles in 3104 patients included ptosis lasting over 180 days (0.3%) and vertical deviation > 2 prism diopters lasting over 180 days (2.1%).

In these patients, the injection procedure caused 9 scleral perforations. A vitreous hemorrhage occurred and later cleared in 1 case. No retinal detachment or visual loss occurred in any case; 16 retrobulbar hemorrhages occurred. Decompression of the orbit after 5 minutes was done to restore retinal circulation in 1 case. No eye lost vision from retrobulbar hemorrhage. Five eyes had pupillary change consistent with ciliary ganglion damage (Adies pupil).

> *Blepharospasm* – In 1684 patients who received 4258 treatments (involving multiple injections) for blepharospasm, incidence of adverse reactions per treated eye was: Ptosis (11%); irritation/tearing, includes dry eye, lagophthalmos, and photophobia (10%); ectropion, keratitis, diplopia, and entropion occurred rarely (< 1%).

Ecchymosis occurs easily in the soft eyelid tissues. This can be prevented by applying pressure at the injection site immediately after the injection. In 2 cases of VII nerve disorder (1 case of an aphakic eye), reduced blinking from botulinum toxin type A injection of the orbicularis muscle led to serious corneal exposure, persistent epithelial defect, and corneal ulceration. Perforation requiring corneal grafting occurred in 1 case, an aphakic eye (see Precautions).

Two patients previously incapacitated by blepharospasm experienced cardiac collapse attributed to over-exertion within 3 weeks following botulinum toxin type A therapy. Caution sedentary patients to resume activity slowly and carefully following the administration of botulinum toxin type A.

Local: Diffuse skin rash (n = 7) and local swelling of the eyelid skin (n = 2) lasting for several days following eyelid injection have occurred.

Overdosage:

In the event of overdosage or injection into the wrong muscle, additional information may be obtained by contacting Allergan Pharmaceuticals at (800) 347-5063 from 8 am to 4 pm Pacific Time, or at (714) 724-5954 for a recorded message at other times.

Patient Information:

Patients with blepharospasm may have been extremely sedentary for a long time. Caution these patients to resume activity slowly and carefully follow administration.

Administration and Dosage:

Strabismus: Botulinum toxin type A is intended for injection into extraocular muscles utilizing the electrical activity recorded from the tip of the injection needle as a guide to placement within the target muscle. Do not attempt Injection without surgical exposure or electromyographic guidance. Physicians should be familiar with electromyographic technique.

> *Preparation* – An injection of botulinum toxin type A is prepared by drawing into a sterile 1 mL tuberculin syringe an amount of the properly diluted toxin (see Dilution Table) slightly greater than the intended dose. Air bubbles in the syringe barrel are expelled and the syringe is attached to the electromyographic injection needle, preferably a 1½-inch, 27-gauge needle. Injection volume in excess of the intended dose is expelled through the needle into an appropriate waste container to ensure patency of the needle and to confirm that there is no syringe-needle leakage. Use a new, sterile needle and syringe to enter the vial on each occasion for dilution or removal of botulinum toxin type A.

To prepare the eye for botulinum toxin type A injection, give several drops of a local anesthetic and an ocular decongestant several minutes prior to injection.

> *Note* – The volume of botulinum toxin type A injected for treatment of strabismus should be between 0.05 to 0.15 mL per muscle.

The initial listed doses of the diluted botulinum toxin type A (see Dilution table) typically create paralysis of injected muscles beginning 1 to 2 days after injection and increasing in intensity during the first week. The paralysis lasts for 2 to 6 weeks and gradually resolves over a similar time period. Overcorrections lasting > 6 months have been rare. Aprroximately 50% of patients will require subsequent doses because of inadequate paralytic response of the muscle to the initial dose, or because of mechanical factors such as large deviations or restrictions, or because of the lack of binocular motor fusion to stabilize the alignment.

> 1. Initial doses in units (U). Use the lower listed doses for treatment of small deviations. Use the larger doses only for large deviations.
>   a. For vertical muscles, and for horizontal strabismus of < 20 prism diopters: 1.25 to 2.5 U in any one muscle.
>   b. For horizontal strabismus of 20 to 50 prism diopters: 2.5 to 5 U in any one muscle.
>   c. For persistent VI nerve palsy of ≥ 1 month duration: 1.25 to 2.5 U in the medial rectus muscle.
>
> 2. Subsequent doses for residual or recurrent strabismus.
>   a. Re-examine patients 7 to 14 days after each injection to assess the effect of that dose.

SURGICAL ADJUNCTS

b. Patients experiencing adequate paralysis of the target muscle who require subsequent injections should receive a dose comparable to the initial dose.

c. Subsequent doses for patients experiencing incomplete paralysis of the target muscle may be increased up to 2-fold the previously administered dose.

d. Subsequent injections should not be administered until the effects of the previous dose have dissipated as evidenced by substantial function in the injected and adjacent muscles.

e. Maximum recommended dose as a single injection for any one muscle is 25 U.

Blepharospasm: Diluted botulinum toxin type A (see Dilution table) is injected using a sterile, 27- to 30-gauge needle without electromyographic guidance. Initially, 1.25 to 2.5 U (0.05 to 0.1 mL volume at each site) injected into the medial and lateral pre-tarsal orbicularis oculi of the upper lid and into the lateral pre-tarsal orbicularis oculi of the lower lid is the initial recommended dose.

In general, the initial effect of the injections is seen within 3 days and reaches a peak at 1 to 2 weeks post-treatment. Each treatment lasts ≈ 3 months, following which the procedure can be repeated indefinitely. At repeat treatment sessions, the dose may be increased up to 2-fold if the response from the initial treatment is considered insufficient (usually defined as an effect that does not last > 2 months). However, there appears to be little benefit obtainable from injecting > 5 U per site. Some tolerance may be found when botulinum toxin type A is used in treating blepharospasm if treatments are given any more frequently than every 3 months; it is rare to have the effect become permanent.

The cumulative dose of botulinum toxin type A in a 30-day period should not exceed 200 U.

Dilution technique: To reconstitute lyophilized botulinum toxin type A, use sterile normal saline without a preservative; 0.9% Sodium Chloride Injection is the recommended diluent. Draw up the proper amount of diluent in the appropriate size syringe. Because botulinum toxin type A is denatured by bubbling or similar violent agitation, inject the diluent into the vial gently. Discard the vial if a vacuum does not pull the diluent into the vial. Record the date and time of reconstitution on the space on the label. Administer within 4 hours after reconstitution.

During this time period, store reconstituted botulinum toxin type A in a refrigerator at 2° to 8°C (36° to 46°F). Reconstituted botulinum toxin type A should be clear, colorless, and free of particulate matter. The use of 1 vial for > 1 patient is not recommended because the product and diluent do not contain a preservative.

Dilution of Botulinum Toxin Type A	
Diluent added (0.9% Sodium Chloride Injection)	Resulting dose
1 mL	10 units
2 mL	5 units
4 mL	2.5 units
8 mL	1.25 units

These dilutions are calculated for an injection volume of 0.1 mL. A decrease or increase in the botulinum toxin type A dose is also possible by administering a smaller or larger injection volume – from 0.05 mL (50% decrease in dose) to 0.15 mL (50% increase in dose).

Storage/Stability: Store the lyophilized product in a freezer at or below -5°C (23°F). Administer within 4 hours after the vial is removed from the freezer and reconsti-

284 OPHTHALMIC DRUG FACTS

tuted. During these 4 hours, store reconstituted botulinum toxin type A in a refrigerator at 2° to 8°C (36° to 46°F). Reconstituted botulinum toxin type A should be clear, colorless, and free of particulate matter.

Rx	Botox (Allergan)	Powder for Injection (lyophilized): 100 units of lyophilized *Clostridium botulinum* toxin type A[1])	Preservative free. 0.05 mg albumin (human), 0.9 mg sodium chloride. In vials.

[1] One unit corresponds to the calculated median lethal intraperitoneal dose (LD_{50}) in mice of the reconstituted drug injected.

VERTEPORFIN

Actions:

Pharmacology: Verteporfin is a light-activated drug used in photodynamic therapy. It consists of a 2-stage process requiring administration of verteporfin for injection and nonthermal red light.

Verteporfin is transported in the plasma primarily by lipoproteins. Once it is activated by light in the presence of oxygen, highly reactive, short-lived singlet oxygen and reactive oxygen radicals are generated.

Light activation of verteporfin results in local damage to neovascular endothelium, resulting in vessel occlusion. Damaged endothelium is known to release procoagulant and and vasoactive factors through the lipo-oxygenase (leukotriene) and cyclo-oxygenase (eicosanoids such as thromboxane) pathways, resulting in platelet aggregation, fibrin clot formation, and vasoconstriction. Verteporfin appears to preferentially accumulate in neovasculature, including choroidal neovasculature. However, animal models indicate that the drug is also present in the retina. Therefore, there may be collateral damage to retinal structures following photoactivation including retinal pigmented epithelium and outer nuclear layer of the retina. The temporary occlusion of choroidal neovascularization (CNV) following verteporfin therapy has been confirmed in humans by fluorescein angiography.

Indications:

Age-related macular degeneration: Treatment of age-related macular degeneration in patients with predominantly classic subfoveal choroidal neovascularization (CNV).

During clinical studies, older patients ($\approx$ 75 years of age), patients with dark irides, patients with occult lesions, or patients with < 50% classic CNV were less likely to benefit from verteporfin therapy.

Contraindications:

Patients with porphyria or a known hypersensitiviy to any component of this preparation.

Warnings:

Photosensitivity: Following verteporfin injection, avoid exposure of skin or eyes to direct sunlight or bright indoor light for 5 days. If emergency surgery is necessary within 48 hours after treatment, protect as much of the internal tissue as possible from intense light.

SURGICAL ADJUNCTS

Ocular changes: Do not retreat patients who experience severe decrease of vision of ≥ 4 lines within 1 week after treatment, at least until their vision completely recovers to pretreatment levels and the potential benefits and risks of subsequent treatment are carefully considered by the treating physician.

Lasers: Use of incompatible lasers that do not provide the required characteristics of light for the photactivation of verteporfin could result in incomplete treatment because of partial photoactivation of verteporfin, overtreatment due to overactivation of verteporfin, or damage to surrounding normal tissue.

Elderly: A reduced treatment effect was seen with increasing age.

Pregnancy: Category C. There are no adequate and well-controlled studies in pregnant women. Use during pregnancy only if the benefit to the mother justifies the potential risk to the fetus.

Lactation: It is not known if verteporfin is excreted in breast milk. Use caution when verteporfin is administered to a woman who is nursing.

Precautions:

Extravasation: Standard precautions to avoid extravasation include the following:

- ◆ Establish a free-flowing IV line before starting infusion and carefully monitor the line.
- ◆ Because of the possible fragility of vein walls in some elderly patients, use the largest arm vein possible, preferably antecubital.
- ◆ Avoid small veins in the back of the hand.

If extravasation does occur, stop the infusion immediately and apply cold compresses. In the event of extravasation during infusion, the extravasation area must be thoroughly protected from direct light until the swelling and discoloration have faded in order to prevent the occurrence of a local burn, which could be severe.

Hepatic Function Impairment: Carefully consider verteporfin therapy in patients with moderate to severe hepatic impairment; there is no clinical experience with verteporfin in these patients.

Adverse Reactions:

The most frequently reported adverse events are headaches; injection site reactions (eg, extravasation and rashes); and visual disturbances (eg, blurred vision, decreased visual acuity, and visual field defects).

Severe vision decrease, equivalent of ≥ 4 lines, within 7 days after treatment has been reported. Partial recovery of vision was observed in many patients.

Photosensitivity reactions occurred in the form of skin sunburn following exposure to sunlight.

The higher incidence of back pain in the verteporfin group occurred primarily during infusion.

Overdosage:

Symptoms: Overdose of drug or light in the treated eye may result in nonperfusion of normal retinal vessels with the possibility of severe decrease in vision that could be

286 OPHTHALMIC DRUG FACTS

permanent. An overdose will also result in the prolongation of the period during which the patient remains photosensitive to bright light.

Treatment: Extend photosensitivity precautions for a time proportional to the overdose.

Patient Information:

Advise patients who receive verteporfin that they will become temporarily photosensitive after the infusion. Advise the patient to avoid exposure of unprotected skin, eyes, or other body organs to direct sunlight or bright indoor light for 5 days after treatment. Sources of bright light include, but are not limited to, tanning salons, bright halogen lighting, and high power lighting used in surgical operating rooms and dental offices.

Instruct patients to protect all parts of their skin and their eyes by wearing protective clothing and dark sunglasses if they must go outdoors in daylight during the first 5 days after treatment. UV sunscreens are not effective in protecting against photosensitivity reactions because photoactivation of the residual drug in the skin can be caused by visible light.

Encourage patients not to stay in the dark and to expose their skin to ambient indoor light, as it will help inactivate the drug in the skin through a process called photobleaching.

Administration and Dosage:

A course of verteporfin therapy is a 2-step process: IV infusion of verteporfin and activation of verteporfin with light from a nonthermal diode laser.

Reevaluate patients every 3 months; if choroidal neovascular leakage is detected on fluorescein angiography, repeat therapy.

Verteporfin administration: Reconstitute each vial of verteporfin with 7 mL Sterile Water for Injection to produce 7.5 mL containing 2 mg/mL. Inspect visually for particulate matter and discoloration prior to adminstration; reconstituted verteporfin is an opaque, dark green solution.

Withdraw the volume of reconstituted verteporfin required to achieve the desired dose of 6 mg/m^2 and dilute with 5% Dextrose for Injection to a total infusion volume of 30 mL. The full infusion volume is administered IV over 10 minutes at a rate of 3 mL/minute, using an appropriate syringe pump and in-line filter.

Take precautions to prevent extravasation at the injection site. If extravasation occurs, protect the site from light.

Light administration: Initiate 689 nm wavelength laser light delivery to the patient 15 minutes after the start of the 10-minute verteporfin infusion.

Photoactivation of verteporfin is controlled by total light dose delivered. In the treatment of choroidal neovascularization, the recommended light dose is 50 J/cm^2 of neovasular lesion administered at an intensity of 600 mW/cm^2. This dose is administered over 83 seconds.

Light dose, light intensity, ophthalmic lens magnification factor, and zoom-lens setting are important parameters for the appropriate delivery of light to the predetermined treatment spot. Follow the laser system manuals for procedure set up and operation.

SURGICAL ADJUNCTS

287

The laser system must deliver a stable power output at a wavelength of 689 ± 3 nm. Light is delivered to the retina as a single circular spot via a fiber optic and and a slit lamp, using a suitable ophthalmic magnification lens.

Concurrent bilateral treatment: The controlled trials allowed only the treatment of 1 eye per patient. In patients who present with eligible lesions in both eyes, evaluate the potential benefits and risks of treating both eyes, concurrently. If the patient has already received previous verteporfin therapy in 1 eye with an acceptable safety profile, both eyes can be treated concurrently after a single administration of verteporfin. Treat the more aggressive lesion first at 15 minutes after the start of infusion. Immediately at the end of light application to the first eye, adjust the laser settings to introduce the treatment parameters for the second eye, with the same light dose and intensity as for the first eye, starting ≤ 20 minutes from the start of infusion.

In patients who present for the first time with eligible lesions in both eyes without prior verteporfin therapy, it is prudent to treat only 1 eye (the most aggressive lesion) at the first course. One week after the first course, if no significant safety issues are identified, the second eye can be treated using the same treatment regimen after a second verteporfin infusion. Approximately 3 months later, both eyes can be evaluated and concurrent treatment following a new verteporfin infusion can be started if both lesions still show evidence of leakage.

Storage/Stability: Use within 4 hours of reconstitution. Store between 20° and 25°C (68° and 77°F). Protect from light.

| Rx | **Visudyne** (Novartis) | **Lyophilized cake:** 15 mg (reconstituted to 2 mg/mL) | Egg phosphatidylglycerol. In single-use vials. |

Nonsurgical Adjuncts

Dapiprazole HCl, extraocular irrigating solutions, lid scrubs, and vitamins and minerals are adjuncts to a variety of ophthalmic procedures and conditions.

DAPIPRAZOLE HYDROCHLORIDE

Dapiprazole is classified pharmacologically as an alpha-adrenergic antagonist. This drug demonstrates rapid reversal of mydriasis produced by phenylephrine and, to a lesser extent, tropicamide. The miosis produced by dapiprazole 0.5% begins 10 minutes following instillation and results in a significant reduction in pupil size. Approximately 50% of the pupils of treated eyes will achieve their premydriatic diameter within 2 hours of dilation with phenylephrine 2.5% and tropicamide 1%. The rate of pupillary constriction may be slightly slower in individuals with blue or green irides than in patients with brown irides. The most significant side effect is conjunctival hyperemia associated with the alpha-receptor blockade of the conjunctival vasculature. The conjunctival injection lasts ≈ 20 minutes in > 80% of patients, and burning or stinging on instillation of the drug is reported in ≈ 50% of the patients.

EXTRAOCULAR IRRIGATING SOLUTIONS

Extraocular irrigating solutions are sterile isotonic solutions for general ophthalmic use. Office uses include irrigating procedures following tonometry, gonioscopy, foreign body removal, or use of fluorescein. They are also used to soothe and cleanse the eye, and in conjunction with hard contact lenses. Because these solutions have a short contact time with the eye, they do not need to provide nutrients to cells. Unlike intraocular irrigants, irrigants for extraocular use contain preservatives that prevent bacterial contamination. However, the preservatives are exceedingly toxic to the corneal endothelium, and intraocular use of extraocular irrigating fluids is contraindicated.

LID SCRUBS

The mainstay of therapy for blepharitis is generally considered to be careful eyelid hygiene. This is easily accomplished at home by the patient. Although baby shampoo is frequently used for this purpose, commercially available eyelid cleansers are now available and are known to be effective with potentially less ocular stinging, burning, and toxicity. Commercial lid scrub products are designed to aid in the removal of oils, debris, or desquamated skin associated with the inflamed eyelid. The lid scrubs can also be used for hygienic eyelid cleansing in contact lens wearers. These products are designed to be used full strength on eyelid tissues but must not be instilled

OPHTHALMIC DRUG FACTS

directly into the eyes. Some of the commercial products are packaged with gauze or cotton pads, which provide an abrasive action to augment the cleansing properties of the detergent solution.

VITAMINS AND MINERALS

Deficiencies of vitamin A and zinc have sometimes been associated with certain adverse ocular effects. Beyond replacement of documented deficiencies, however, treatment or prevention of ophthalmic diseases using vitamins and minerals is not clearly established. Recently, various investigators have explored the use of vitamins A, C, and E, as well as zinc, as preventative measures for degenerative ophthalmic conditions often associated with the aging process. The primary mechanisms of action offered to explain the effectiveness of such therapy include antioxidation and free radical scavenging. Several products are now commercially available for the prevention and treatment of macular degeneration, but considerably more data will be required before the efficacy of these products becomes well established.

Jimmy D. Bartlett, OD, DOS
University of Alabama at Birmingham

For More Information

Blaho K. Adjunctive agents. In: Bartlett JD, Jaanus SD, eds. *Clinical Ocular Pharmacology*, ed. 4. Boston: Butterworth-Heinemann, 2001.

Doughty MJ, Lyle WM. A review of the clinical pharmacokinetics of pilocarpine, moxisylyte (thymoxamine), dapiprazole in the reversal of diagnostic pupillary dilation. *Optom Vis Sci* 1992;69:358-68.

Allison RW, et al. Reversal of mydriasis by dapiprazole. *Ann Ophthalmol* 1990;92:131-38.

Bartlett JD, Classe JG. Dapiprazole: Will it affect the standard of care for pupillary dilation? *Optom Clin* 1992;2(3):65-75.

Whikehart DR. Irrigating solutions. In: Bartlett JD, Jaanus SD, eds. *Clinical Ocular Pharmacology*, ed. 4. Boston: Butterworth-Heinemann, 2001.

Polack FM, Goodman DF. Experience with a new detergent lid scrub in the management of chronic blepharitis. *Arch Ophthalmol* 1988;106:719-20.

Sperduto RD. Do we have a nutritional treatment for age-related cataract or macular degeneration? *Arch Ophthalmol* 1990;108:1403-05.

NONSURGICAL ADJUNCTS

DAPIPRAZOLE HYDROCHLORIDE

Actions:

Pharmacology: Dapiprazole acts by blocking the alpha-adrenergic receptors in smooth muscle and produces miosis through an effect on the dilator muscle of the iris.

The drug does not have any significant activity on ciliary muscle contraction and, therefore, does not induce a significant change in the anterior chamber depth or the thickness of the lens.

Dapiprazole has demonstrated safe and rapid reversal of mydriasis produced by phenylephrine and, to a lesser degree, tropicamide. In patients with decreased accommodative amplitude caused by treatment with tropicamide, the miotic effect of dapiprazole may partially increase the accommodative amplitude.

Eye color affects the rate of pupillary constriction. In individuals with brown irides, the rate of pupillary constriction may be slightly slower than in individuals with blue or green irides. Eye color does not appear to affect the final pupil size.

Dapiprazole does not significantly alter intraocular pressure (IOP) in normotensive eyes or in eyes with elevated IOP.

Indications:

Mydriasis: Treatment of iatrogenically-induced mydriasis produced by adrenergic (phenylephrine) or parasympatholytic (tropicamide) agents.

Contraindications:

Hypersensitivity to any component of this preparation.

When constriction is undesirable, such as in acute iritis.

Warnings:

For topical ophthalmic use only: Not for injection.

Frequency of use: Do not use more frequently than once a week.

IOP reduction: Not indicated for the reduction of IOP or in the treatment of open-angle glaucoma.

Vision reduction: May cause difficulty in dark adaptation and may reduce field of vision. Patients should exercise caution in night driving or when performing other activities in poor illumination.

Pregnancy: Category B. There are no adequate and well controlled studies in pregnant women. Use during pregnancy only when clearly needed and when potential benefits to the mother outweigh the potential hazards to the fetus.

Lactation: It is not known whether this drug is excreted in breast milk. Exercise caution when dapiprazole is administered to a nursing woman.

Children: Safety and efficacy for use in children have not been established.

Adverse Reactions:

Conjunctival injection lasting 20 minutes (> 80%); burning on instillation ($\approx$ 50%); ptosis, lid erythema, lid edema, chemosis, itching, punctate keratitis, corneal edema, browache, photophobia, headaches (10% to 40%); dryness of the eye, tearing, blurring of vision (less frequent).

Patient Information:

May cause difficulty in dark adaptation and may reduce field of vision. Exercise caution when driving at night or performing other activities in poor illumination.

To avoid contamination, do not touch tip of container to any surface.

Do not use more frequently than once a week.

Discard any solution that is not clear and colorless.

Administration and Dosage:

Shake container for several minutes to ensure mixing.

Instill 2 drops into the conjunctiva of each eye followed 5 minutes later by 2 additional drops. Administer after the ophthalmic examination to reverse the diagnostic mydriasis.

Storage/Stability: Store at room temperature 15° to 30°C (59° to 86°F) for 21 days after reconstitution.

Rx **Rēv-Eyes** (Lederle)	**Powder, lyophilized**: 25 mg (0.5% solution when reconstituted)	In vial with 5 ml diluent and dropper.[1]

[1] With 2% mannitol, 0.4% hydroxypropyl methylcellulose, 0.01% EDTA, 0.01% benzalkonium chloride, sodium chloride.

EXTRAOCULAR IRRIGATING SOLUTIONS

Actions:

Pharmacology: These sterile isotonic solutions are for general ophthalmic use. Office uses include irrigating procedures following tonometry, gonioscopy, foreign body removal, or use of fluorescein; they are also used to soothe and cleanse the eye. Because these solutions have a short contact time with the eye, they do not need to provide nutrients to cells. Unlike intraocular irrigants, irrigants for extraocular use contain preservatives which prevent bacteriostatic contamination. However, the preservatives are exceedingly toxic to the corneal endothelium and intraocular use of extraocular irrigating fluids is contraindicated.

Indications:

Irrigation: For irrigating the eye to help relieve irritation by removing loose foreign material, air pollutants (smog or pollen), or chlorinated water.

NONSURGICAL ADJUNCTS

Contraindications:

Hypersensitivity to any component of the formulation; as a saline solution for rinsing and soaking contact lenses; injection or intraocular surgery.

Patient Information:

If you experience eye pain, changes in vision, continued redness or irritation of the eye, or if the condition worsens or persists, consult a doctor.

Obtain immediate medical treatment for all open wounds in or near the eyes.

If solution changes color or becomes cloudy, do not use.

Do not use these products with contact lenses.

To avoid contamination, do not touch tip of the container to any surface. Replace cap after using.

Administration and Dosage:

Solution: Flush the affected eye(s) as needed, controlling the rate of flow of solution by pressure on the bottle.

Eyecup: Fill the sterile eyecup halfway with eye wash. Apply the cup tightly to the affected eye and tilt the head backward. Open eyes wide, rotate eye, and blink several times to ensure that the solution completely floods the eye. Discard the wash. Rinse the cup with clean water and if necessary, repeat the procedure with the other eye.

Rinse the eyecup before and after every use. Avoid contamination of the rim or inside surfaces of the cup.

Storage/Stability: If solution changes color or becomes cloudy, do not use.

otc	**AK-Rinse** (Akorn)	**Solution:** Sodium carbonate, KCl, boric acid, EDTA, 0.01% benzalkonium Cl	In 30 and 118 mL.
otc	**Collyrium for Fresh Eyes Wash** (Wyeth-Ayerst)	**Solution:** Boric acid, sodium borate, benzalkonium Cl	In 120 mL.
otc	**Dacriose** (Novartis)	**Solution:** NaCl, KCl, sodium phosphate, sodium hydroxide, 0.01% benzalkonium Cl, EDTA	In 15 and 120 mL.
otc	**Eye Stream** (Alcon)	**Solution:** 0.64% NaCl, 0.075% KCl, 0.03% magnesium Cl hexahydrate, 0.048% calcium Cl dihydrate, 0.39% sodium acetate trihydrate, 0.17% sodium citrate dihydrate, 0.013% benzalkonium Cl	In 30 and 118 mL.
otc	**Eye Wash** (Bausch & Lomb)	**Solution:** Boric acid, KCl, EDTA, sodium carbonate, 0.01% benzalkonium Cl	In 118 mL.
otc	**Eye Wash** (Zenith-Goldline)	**Solution:** Boric acid, KCl, EDTA, anhydrous sodium carbonate, 0.01% benzalkonium Cl	In 118 mL.
otc	**Eye Wash** (Lavoptik)	**Solution:** 0.49% NaCl, 0.4% sodium biphosphate, 0.45% sodium phosphate, 0.005% benzalkonium Cl	In 180 mL with eyecup.

otc	**Eye Irrigating Solution** (Rugby)	**Solution**: Sodium borate, NaCl, boric acid, sorbic acid, EDTA	In 118 mL.
otc	**Optigene** (Pfeiffer)	**Solution**: NaCl, mono- and dibasic sodium phosphate, EDTA, benzalkonium Cl	In 118 mL.

LID SCRUBS

Indications:

Eyelid cleansing: To aid in the removal of oils, debris, or desquamated skin.

Precautions:

For external use only: Do not instill directly into eye.

Administration and Dosage:

Close eye(s) and gently scrub on eyelid(s) and lashes using lateral side-to-side strokes; rinse thoroughly.

otc	**Eye•Scrub** (Ciba Vision)	**Solution**: PEG-200 glyceryl tallowate, disodium laureth sulfosuccinate, cocoamidopropylamine oxide, PEG-78 glyceryl cocoate, benzyl alcohol, EDTA	In UD 30s (pads) and kit (120 mL and 60 pads).
otc)	**Lid Wipes-SPF** (Akorn)	**Solution**: PEG-200 glyceryl tallowate, PEG-80 glyceryl cocoate, laureth-23, coco-amidopropylamine oxide, NaCl, glycerin, sodium phosphate, sodium hydroxide	Preservative free. In UD 30s (pads).
otc)	**OCuSOFT** (OCuSOFT)	**Solution**: PEG-80, sorbitan laurate, sodium trideceth sulfate, PEG-150 distearate, coco-amidopropyl hydroxysultaine, lauroampho-carboxyglycinate, sodium laureth-13 carboxylate, PEG-15 tallow polyamine, quaternium-15	Alcohol and dye free. In UD 30s (pads), 30, 120 and 240 mL and compliance kit (120 mL and 100 pads).

TEAR TEST STRIPS

Indications:

Schirmer Tear Test:

> *Test I* – To diagnose dry eye syndrome, to evaluate lacrimal gland function in contact lens wearers, to check tear production prior to eyelid surgery and prior to corneal transplantation and cataract surgery.

> *Test II* – To assess the adequacy of reflex lacrimation.

Sno-Strips: Perform test on eye before any topical medication (especially anesthetic) is administered or other procedures are carried out (eg, manipulation of eyelids).

Zone-Quick: To indicate tear volume. No anesthesia required. If eyedrops have been used, perform test ≥ 5 minutes later. Test may be performed during contact lens wear.

NONSURGICAL ADJUNCTS

Precautions:

Zone-Quick: Tear volume may vary. Repeat testing on different days will give a more accurate volume representation.

Zone-Quick may induce a slight mechanical irritation leading to lacrimination in some patients (rarely). In those patients it may be necessary to use another tear test in addition to *Zone-Quick*.

Administration and Dosage:

Schirmer Tear Test: Strips are placed at the junction of the middle and temporal one-third of the eyelid margin. To avoid increased reflex lacrimation and pain, do not touch the cornea.

Sno-Strips: Apply to lower temporal lid margin of eye. The distance between notch and shoulder of strip is 10 mm, which should be wetted in $\approx$ 3 minutes. Repeat if > 5 minutes; > 10 minutes indicates reduced tear secretion.

Zone-Quick: Test eyes one at a time. Thread is placed on the palpebral conjunctiva. Patient should look straight ahead and blink normally for 15 seconds. After 15 seconds, gently pull the lower eyelid down and remove thread with upward motion. Measure entire length of red portion of thread in millimeters.

Storage/Stability: Store in dark place at room temperature.

otc	**Sno-Strips** (Akorn)	**Strips:** Sterile tear flow test strips	In 100s.
otc	**Schirmer Tear Test** (Alcon)	**Strips:** Sterile test strips	In 250s.
otc	**Zone-Quick** (Menicon USA)	**Threads:** Phenol red threads (PRT)	In 50 aluminum pkg sets (100 threads).

ZINC SULFATE SOLUTION

Indications:

Astringent: A mild astringent for temporary relief of minor eye irritation.

Warnings:

Irritation/Eye pain: If irritation persists or increases, or if eye pain or a change in vision occurs, discontinue use and consult physician.

Administration and Dosage:

Instill 1 to 2 drops into eye(s) up to 4 times daily. If solution discolors or becomes cloudy, do not use.

otc	**20/20 Eye Drops** (S. S. S.)	**Solution:** 0.25%	In 15 mL.[1]
otc	**Clear Eyes ACR Eye Drops** (Ross)		In 15 and 30 mL.[2]
otc	**Vasoclear A Eye Drops** (Novartis)		In 15 mL.[3]
otc	**Visine AC** (Pfizer)		In 15 mL.[4]
otc	**Zincfrin** (Alcon)		In 15 mL.[5]

[1] With 0.4% glycerin, 0.012% naphazoline HCl, EDTA, KCl, and camphor.
[2] With 0.2% glycerin, 0.012% naphazoline HCl, benzalkonium chloride, boric acid, EDTA, NaCl, and sodium citrate.
[3] With 0.02% naphazoline HCl, 1% polyethylene glycol 40, 0.0025% PVA, NaCl, and EDTA.
[4] With 0.05% tetrahydrozoline HCl, boric acid, NaCl, and EDTA.
[5] With 0.12% phenylephrine HCl, 0.01% benzalkonium chloride, polysorbate 80, sodium citrate, citric acid, and sodium hydroxide.

VITAMINS AND MINERALS

Actions:

Pharmacology: Certain vitamin and mineral deficiencies have been associated with adverse ocular effects, most notably vitamin A and zinc. Beyond replacement of documented deficiency, treatment or prevention of ophthalmic diseases with vitamins and minerals is not well established.

However, investigators are beginning to explore this area. Some claims are being made for vitamins A, C, and E, and zinc as preventatives for degenerative ophthalmic changes often associated with aging. The principal mechanisms of action are offered as antioxidation and free radical scavenging.

Much more data are required before actual recommendations can be made. However, products labeled with such claims are available.

Administration and Dosage:

Take with meals.

Adults: 1 to 2 tablets 1 or 2 times daily or as directed by a physician.

Storage/Stability: Store at room temperature 15° to 30°C (59° to 86°F) .

otc	**Vitamin A Palmitate** (Freeda)	**Tablets:** 10,000 IU	In 100s and 250s.
		15,000 IU	In 100s and 250s.
		25,000 IU	In 100s.
otc	**Beta Carotene** (Freeda)	**Tablets:** 10,000 IU	In 100s, 250s, and 500s.
otc	**Palmitate-A** (Akorn)	**Tablets:** 15,000 IU vitamin A palmitate	In 100s.
otc	**Palmitate-A 5000** (Akorn)	**Tablets:** 5000 IU vitamin A palmitate	In 100s.

NONSURGICAL ADJUNCTS

otc	**Icaps Plus** (Alcon)	**Tablets:** 6000 IU vitamin A^1, 200 mg C, 20 mg B_2, 60 IU E, 40 mg Zn^2, 2 mg Cu, 5 mg Mn, 20 mcg Se	In 120s.
otc	**Icaps Time Release** (Alcon)	**Tablets:** 7000 IU vitamin A^1, 200 mg C, 20 mg B_2, 100 IU E, 40 mg Zn^2, 2 mg Cu, 20 mcg Se	In 60s.
otc	**AntiOxidants** (Akorn)	**Caplets:** 5000 IU vitamin A^1, 400 mg C^3, 200 IU E^4, 40 mg Zn^5, 5 mg L-glutathione, 3 mg sodium pyruvate, 2 mg Cu^6, 40 mcg Se^7	In 60s.
otc	**Oxi-Freeda** (Freeda)	**Tablets:** 5000 IU beta carotene, 150 IU E, 20 mg B_1, 20 mg B_2, 20 mg B_6, 10 mcg B_{12}, 15 mg elemental Zn, 50 mcg Se, 20 mg calcium pantothenate, 40 mg glutathione, 40 mg B_3, 100 mg C, 75 mg L-cysteine	In 100s and 250s.
otc	**One-A-Day Extras Antioxidant** (Bayer)	**Capsules, softgel:** 5000 IU vitamin A^1, 200 IU E, 250 mg C, 7.5 mg Zn, 1 mg Cu, 15 mcg Se, 1.5 mg Mn	(One-A-Day). Tartrazine. In 50s.
otc	**OCuSoft VMS** (OCu-SOFT)	**Tablets:** 5000 IU vitamin A, 30 IU E, 60 mg C, 40 mg Zn, 2 mg Cu, 40 mcg Se	Film coated. In 60s.
otc	**Ocuvite** (Bausch & Lomb)	**Tablets:** 40 mg elemental Zn^8, 2 mg elemental Cu^9, 40 mcg elemental Se^{10}, 5000 IU vitamin A^1, 30 IU E^4, 60 mg C^3	In 75s.
otc	**Ocuvite Extra** (Bausch & Lomb)	**Tablets:** 40 mg elemental Zn^8, 2 mg elemental Cu^9, 200 mg C, 50 IU E, 6000 IU vitamin A^1, 40 mcg elemental Se, 3 mg B_2, 40 mg B_3, 5 mg elemental Mn, 5 mg L-glutathione	In 50s.

[1] As beta carotene.
[2] As zinc acetate.
[3] As ascorbic acid.
[4] As dl-alpha tocopheryl acetate.
[5] As zinc ascorbate.
[6] As copper ascorbate.
[7] As L-selenomethionine.
[8] As zinc oxide.
[9] As cupric oxide.
[10] As sodium selenate.

Contact Lens Care

More than 25 million Americans wear contact lenses. Contact lenses can offer patients a natural appearance, increased visual performance, and convenience. They can correct most refractive errors such as myopia, hyperopia, and astigmatism. Bifocal contact lenses are available for the presbyopic patient. Tinted contact lenses enhance or completely change the color of a patient's eyes. Research and development by major ophthalmic corporations have produced a variety of new lens materials and designs. With new contact lens products and patient education, contact lens use should continue to grow.

The number of contact lens care products has also increased dramatically. Patients may become confused because there are more than 100 different products sold for contact lens care.

CONTACT LENS MATERIALS AND COMPOSITION

Three types of contact lenses are manufactured: Hard (PMMA), rigid gas permeable (RGP), and soft.

HARD CONTACT LENSES

Hard contact lenses are made from polymethylmethacrylate (PMMA). PMMA does not transmit the oxygen needed for normal corneal integrity. Hard contact lenses have caused chronic corneal edema, corneal distortion, edematous corneal formations, spectacle blur, polymegethism, and corneal abrasions. Because of these ocular complications, hard lenses should not be the lenses of choice for a new contact lens patient. Less than 1% of the contact lens population wear hard contact lenses.

RIGID GAS PERMEABLE LENSES (RGP)

Approximately 20% of contact lens patients wear rigid gas permeable (RGP) lenses. These lenses are oxygen permeable; therefore, the RGP patient does not have the severe physiological complications of the hard lens patient. Several lens polymers with a high degree of oxygen permeability have been FDA-approved for extended wear. RGP lenses provide the patient with good vision, durability, and easy care.

The first successful RGP lens materials were introduced in 1979 and were of silicone/acrylate (S/A) composition. Also referred to as silicone-based, these copolymers have excellent oxygen permeability characteristics, and actually contain the element silicon as siloxane bonds in side branches of the main carbon-carbon polymer chain. Unlike

OPHTHALMIC DRUG FACTS

homogenous PMMA lens materials, S/A materials are polymers with silicone, methacrylate, wetting agents, and cross-linking agents; the latter 2 ingredients are important because of the dryness (hydrophobicity) and flexibility of silicone. Wetting agents, including HEMA and methacrylic acid (the most common), achieve their effect through their strong affinity with water molecules. Cross-linking agents have the ability to strengthen the material; therefore, the flexibility is decreased, machining characteristics are improved, and the material is less sensitive to the effect of solvents.

As it became apparent that higher oxygen permeable (ie, Dk) lens materials would be necessary to meet the cornea's daily wear oxygen requirements and allow for flexible/extended wear schedules, higher Dk lens materials were introduced. However, increasing the siloxane bonding to increase oxygen permeability increased the hydrophobic properties and the flexibility of the lens, resulting in such problems as corneal desiccation, surface deposits, warpage, and flexure with subjective symptoms such as dryness and reduced vision. Increasing the amount of wetting agent to offset these problems typically results in excessive material hydration, causing poor contact lens stability; an excess of cross-linking agents to enhance stability could result in a brittle material. Most of the lenses in use today are fluoro-silicone/acrylate (F-S/A) lens materials. They are similar to silicone/acrylates with the notable exception of the addition of fluorine. Fluorine, known for its nonstick properties in Teflon-coated cooking materials, increases the deposit resistance of the lens material by promoting tear film interaction with the lens surface. In addition, low surface tension (energy) is present; in other words, there is a reduced affinity of polarized tear components to become adherent to the contact lens surface. Therefore, the primary problem experienced with S/A lens material—dryness—is often reduced with F-S/A materials. F-S/A lens materials can essentially be divided into three categories based upon their oxygen permeability. Low Dk (ie, 25 to 50) materials typically provide the greatest stability and surface wettability. They are recommended for myopic daily wear and borderline dry eye patients. High Dk (ie, 51 to 100) materials recommended for hyperopic daily wear and myopic flexible wear and extended wear patients. Hyper Dk (ie, > 100) materials are recommended for RGP extended wear patients.

HYDROGEL (SOFT) CONTACT LENSES

A hydrogel contact lens, sometimes referred to as a soft contact lens, is a flexible lens made of plastic that is able to absorb or bind water. When placed on the eye, it will conform to the shape of the cornea. The water content allows oxygen permeability; the higher the water content, the greater the oxygen permeability. This benefit is often somewhat negated by the greater center thickness often necessary in high water content lens materials reducing the overall oxygen transmission. Introduced in the US in 1971, today soft lenses are manufactured from polymers that contain 38% to 79% water.

Hydrogel lenses are categorized into 4 groups based upon their water content and surface reactivity. Lenses with < 50% water content are labeled "low water;" lenses with > 50% water content are labeled "high water." Less reactive surfaces are termed "nonionic" and more reactive materials are labeled "ionic."

HYDROGEL LENS CLASSIFICATION
Group 1: Low Water (< 50% H_2O) Nonionic Polymers
Group 2: High Water (> 50% H_2O) Nonionic Polymers
Group 3: Low Water (< 50% H_2O) Ionic Polymers
Group 4: High Water (> 50% H_2O) Ionic Polymers

Daily wear soft contact lenses are designed to be worn all day (12 to 14 hours), but must be removed nightly to be cleaned and disinfected. Extended wear soft lenses can be worn for > 24 hours. The FDA and most eye care practitioners recommend a maxi-

CONTACT LENS CARE

301

mum wearing period of 7 days. The lenses must then be removed overnight for cleaning and disinfection. The primary advantage of extended wear lenses is convenience. The popularity of extended wear soft lenses has decreased in recent years, because of the reported risk of infection resulting primarily from corneal hypoxia, surface contamination, and limbal compression. The former problem should be minimized by the recent introduction of hyper Dk silicone-hydrogel lens materials.

Disposable soft contact lenses are designed to eliminate the complications of lens deposits by replacing lenses at frequent intervals. Lens deposits can interfere with vision, cause corneal irritation, and contribute to ocular infection. In addition, disposable lenses offer the patient the convenience of reduced lens care. Soft toric and bifocal lens designs have recently been introduced.

Some disposable lenses are approved for daily wear and others for extended wear. It is recommended that conventional soft lenses be discarded after 12 weeks of wear. Disposable lenses should be replaced every 1 to 2 weeks. Planned replacement lenses are replaced every 1, 3, or 6 months. The doctor will prescribe the replacement schedule for each patient. If a disposable lens is not discarded immediately after lens removal, it should be cleaned with a surfactant cleaner and stored in a disinfection solution. The new silicone-hydrogel lenses (ie, Purevision, Bausch & Lomb) offer promise as a hyper Dk extended wear lens material that can be replaced on a monthly basis.

Recently, 3 companies have introduced a 1-day single-use soft lens. This lens is designed to be worn 1 time and then thrown away. The patient will apply a fresh, clean, sterile lens each day of lens wear. Contact lens care products (ie, lens case, cleaning solution, disinfection solution) are not needed with these new soft lenses.

COMPLIANCE

Contact lens success is dependent upon patient compliance in caring for their contact lenses. Surveys indicate that 31% to 80% of patients do not care for their lenses in the manner prescribed. Often this pertains to failure to clean or disinfect the lenses as recommended by their practitioner. In some cases this may be the result of failure to use the quantity of solution as recommended by the manufacturer. It has been found that patients actually spend < 25% on contact lens solutions as they should be spending if they were following manufacturers' recommendations.

The key factor to optimizing patient compliance is thorough education. Patients should understand every component of lens care (ie, wetting, cleaning, disinfection) and why it is important. In addition, they should be able to restate the exact care procedures prior to leaving the office with their contact lenses. When they return for follow-up visits, they should be questioned as to their compliance with lens care (ie, solutions they are using, cleaning upon removal, using fresh solution, cleaning case). In one study it was found that with patients who did not have their care instructions repeated at follow-up visits, 50% of their solutions, lenses, and cases were contaminated. For those individuals who had these instructions repeated at follow-up visits, only 6% contamination was found. Another method to ensure they will comply with using the recommended solutions is to provide a large quantity (ie, a 2 to 3 month supply) initially of solutions and to sell solutions in the office.

The temptation to use a cheaper saline, or even use homemade saline with salt tablets, must be addressed. Homemade saline should never be used. Patients must recognize that contamination of these solutions can result in a serious eye infection. Likewise, the use of tap water for any purpose—but especially for wetting, rewetting, or storage—should be avoided because the risk of *Acanthamoeba* keratitis. For the same reason, contact lenses should not be used while swimming or when using a hot tub or sauna.

With soft lenses in particular, it is important that the disinfection system is compatible with the type of lens material. Disinfection of low water content FDA Group 1 and Group 3 lenses can usually be performed safely and effectively by thermal, chemical, or hydrogen peroxide systems. High water content Group 2 and Group 4 lenses should not be thermally disinfected, but chemical or hydrogen peroxide systems are usually safe and effective. However, some Group 4 ionic polymers may react negatively with sorbic acid-preserved solutions.

It is becoming more evident that lens case contamination can result in ocular irritation and infection. Contact lens wearers with eye infections are often found to have lens cases that are contaminated with the same organism as is involved in the eye infection. The most frequently cited source of contamination of the lens case is the patient's own fingers. Therefore, washing hands prior to contact lens application is quite important. Case contamination increases with the number of weeks the patient uses the same case. It is, therefore, important to recommend regular case replacement and to even provide patients with several cases to encourage disposal. Lens cases should be cleaned regularly to prevent a build-up of muco-protein material, which serves as a good culture medium for microbial growth. Once cleaned, sterile saline should be used to rinse the case.

Doctors, pharmacists, and opticians must have a comprehensive understanding of all contact lens materials and systems. With this knowledge, they can educate the patient, increase compliance and, therefore, decrease lens and solution-related complications. Compliance has been defined by the FDA as the use of an approved contact lens care regimen in agreement with the manufacturer's instructions and consistent with good general hygiene. Compliance must meet 4 criteria:

1. The patient should always wash his or her hands before lens manipulation;

2. The patient should use an FDA-approved care system in an appropriate manner;

3. The patient should wear lenses only on a daily wear schedule unless the lenses are approved by the FDA for extended wear;

4. All solutions should be free of bacterial contamination.

CONTACT LENS GUIDELINES

- Proper contact lens care will increase success and decrease complications.
- Cleaning does not disinfect lenses.
- Disinfecting does not clean lenses.
- Enzyme solutions are not a substitute for disinfection.
- Wash and rinse hands thoroughly before handling contact lenses.
- Do not insert contact lenses if eyes are red or irritated. If eyes become painful or vision worsens while wearing lenses, remove lenses and consult eye care practitioner immediately.
- Do not wear contact lenses while sleeping unless they have been prescribed for extended wear.
- For soft lens care, use only products designed for soft lenses.
- For rigid lens care, use only products designed for rigid lenses.
- Do not change or substitute products from a different manufacturer without consulting a doctor.
- Always follow label directions or doctor's recommendations.
- Do not store lenses in tap water.
- Never use saliva to wet contact lenses.
- Keep lens care products out of the reach of children.
- Do not instill topical medications while contact lenses are being worn unless directed by a doctor.

CONTACT LENS CARE

303

CONTACT LENS GUIDELINES
◆ Do not get cosmetic lotions, creams, or sprays in eyes or on lenses. It is best to put on lenses before putting on makeup and remove them before removing makeup. Water-based cosmetics are less likely to damage lenses than oil-based products. ◆ Schedule and keep follow-up appointments with an eye-care practitioner (approximately every 6 to 12 months or as recommended). ◆ Contact lenses wear out with time and should be replaced regularly. Throw away disposable lenses after the recommended wearing period.

CONTACT LENS NON-COMPLIANCE AND MANAGEMENT		
Compliance Problem	Cause(s)	Management
Discoloration	Inadequate cleaning	Emphasize cleaning upon removal
	Improper solution use	Have patient repeat care instructions
	If oily film, may be lanolin-based	Avoid hand creams/ lanolin-based soaps
Lens Parameter Change	Group 4 lenses with long H_2O_2 soak cycles	Use non-H_2O_2 or short cycle H_2O_2
	Use of improper H_2O_2 (ie, *AOSept* patient uses another brand)	Patient education on solution compliance
	Soaking lenses in alcohol-based cleaner	Advise patient of consequences
	Patient uses vigorous digital cleaning of RGPs causing warpage or increase in minus power	Advise patient to clean carefully in palm of hand
Corneal Staining	Improper preservative use (ie, *BAK* with soft lenses; purchases improper solutions)	Patient education on proper solution use; provide patient with large initial supply of appropriate solutions; sell solutions in-office
	Patient sensitivity to a specific preservative	Change patient to another preserved system
	Inadequate buffering/ neutralization of H_2O_2	Reeducate patient on proper use and disposal of H_2O_2 solutions
	Uses topical medications that are absorbed by the contact lenses	Discontinue contact lens wear
	Does not rinse off cleaner adequately or inserts lens with a cleaning/soaking solution (ie, *Claris*)	Comply with instructions on use of cleaner
Bacterial Infection	Case contamination	Clean, rinse with saline every night; dispose of frequently
	Inadequate cleaning	Patient education on proper cleaning upon removal
	Lenses not discarded as often as scheduled	Emphasize proper wear and discard schedule
	Patient "tops off" solution every night	Educate patient to discard old solution and use fresh
	Poor hygiene	Emphasize importance of clean lenses/wash hands prior to lens application
	RGP lenses stored dry	Remind patient of need to disinfect RGP lenses
	Inadequate disinfection (ie, does not disinfect after cleaning)	Ensure at follow-up visits that patient understands all steps in lens care
	Expired solutions or leaves cap off	Advise patient about the consequences of contamination

CONTACT LENS NON-COMPLIANCE AND MANAGEMENT		
Compliance Problem	Cause(s)	Management
Acanthamoeba Keratitis	Tap water used for wetting/rewetting/soaking	Tap water use is prohibited
	Patient wears lenses in hot tub or while swimming	Lens wear is not advised for these activities
	Patient makes own saline with salt tablets	Salt tablet use is not recom- mended
Unilateral redness/re- duced wearing time	Left Lens Syndrome	Patient educated to clean left lens as long as right

PRECAUTIONS FOR CONTACT LENS USE

ACANTHAMOEBA KERATITIS

Acanthamoeba penetration into the cornea can cause a necrotizing stromal melt and corneal performations. If not diagnosed in an early state—and it is a difficult condition to detect early—it can result in the need for a corneal transplant. Numerous species of *Acanthamoeba* have been identified; the 2 most common forms associated with contact lens adherence are *castellani* and *polyphaga*. *Acanthamoeba* can be present in 2 forms: the trophozoite (characteristic ameba presentation) and the rounded cyst form. The latter form is more resistant to disinfection than the trophozoite.

The overall incidence of *Acanthamoeba* infection with contact lens wear is extremely low when compared with the 28 million people in the US who wear contact lenses. It appears that Group 4 (high water ionic) soft lenses are most often associated with *Acanthamoeba* adherence. The least adherent materials are Group 1 (low water non-ionic) soft lenses and RGP lens materials.

It is most associated with the use of tap water for storing or wetting/rewetting the lenses. Likewise, it often occurs with people who use salt tablets to develop their own saline. There is also a relationship with hot tub water and this infection as well as wearing soft lenses while swimming.

The most effective disinfection method for killing *Acanthamoeba* is heat; however, many lens materials are not compatible with heat disinfection. The use of hydrogen peroxide has a variable effect against *Acanthamoeba*. More than 10 minutes of storage in hydrogen peroxide is necessary for effective killing of the trophozoite form. Hydrogen peroxide does not appear to be effective against the cystic form. Chemical disinfection via non-hydrogen peroxide solutions such as *Opti-Free* and *ReNu* appear to exhibit poor antiacanthamoebal activity. However, when combined with digital cleaning and rinsing, the effect is much greater. The use of *MiraFlow*, with 20% isopropyl alcohol, as a cleaner is highly effective. Guidelines for minimizing the risk of *Acanthamoeba* infection are listed below.

STEPS TO MINIMIZE RISK OF *ACANTHAMOEBA* KERATITIS ASSOCIATED WITH CONTACT LENS WEAR
Do not wear contact lenses while swimming
Do not wear contact lenses while in hot tub or spa
Never use tap water, distilled water, mineral water, or saliva with contact lenses
Use only sterile contact lens solutions
Clean lenses upon removal
Disinfect lenses after cleaning
Do not use homemade saline (ie, salt tablets)
Wash hands prior to handling lenses
Clean contact lens case daily by rinsing with sterile saline
Replace lens case frequently

HUMAN IMMUNODEFICIENCY VIRUS (HIV)

With as many as 1 in 300 individuals HIV-affected, and the potential impact of the AIDS virus, it is understandable that concern is expressed about contact lens implications. HIV has been isolated in bodily fluids, including tears, and has been located in the conjunctiva, cornea, and on contact lenses. For patients who have the HIV virus, contact lens wear may not be appropriate as the lenses themselves can act as a highly desirable medium for bacteria.

Disinfection of trial lenses and cases used during these fittings is important if, in fact, the lenses are not disposable. Hydrogen peroxide systems approved for contact lenses can be used to disinfect RGP and hydrogel lenses. Heat disinfection is recommended for those lenses compatible with this form of disinfection. Chemical disinfection alone appears to have a minimal effect on the AIDS virus.

IN-OFFICE DISINFECTION

Most trial lenses in use today are used once and then discarded. This is the most acceptable method of diagnostic lens use because there would be no danger of ocular infection spread from one patient to the next because the lenses are packaged in sterile containers. However, there are still some diagnostic lenses that are reused after being disinfected, which does not produce a sterile lens. Large thermal disinfection units are available to disinfect lenses in glass vials, which is an acceptable method of disinfection; however, some lens materials contraindicate thermal disinfection use, primarily those with > 55% water content. Oxidative disinfection, although an excellent method of disinfection, is difficult to use for diagnostic lenses because of the necessity of disinfecting the lens in a special case and transferring the disinfected lens to a glass vial. The lens may become contaminated in the transfer process or the vial may become contaminated. It is acceptable to store lenses in a glass vial in a chemical disinfecting solution; however, their effects on *Acanthamoeba* and the AIDS virus are questionable. Diagnostic lenses redisinfected with *AOSept* or *ReNu MultiPurpose* solutions (versus thermal disinfection) should be redisinfected at least once a month to prevent contamination.

Arguably the most effective system is a combination. *Opti-Free Express*, as a result of both the preservative action and the omission of a surfactant, may be used and is approved for use in heat disinfection. The other chemical disinfection systems, conversely, contain a surfactant that, after repeated thermal disinfection cycles, may result in a cloudy lens. As with any lens worn by the patient, the lens should be thoroughly cleaned and rinsed prior to disinfection. Lenses of > 55% water content may be stored in *Opti-Free Express* or other chemical disinfecting solution without thermal disinfection. The practitioner must keep in mind the limitations of the systems. Any lens used on a known AIDS patient or a patient exposed to *Acanthamoeba* should be disposed of and not reused, even though at the present time it is thought that the risk of transmission via the tears is low. In addition to disinfection of diagnostic lenses after use, diagnostic lenses that are stored in-office and have been opened should be disinfected, at minimum, every month to prevent contamination of the lenses and the vials.

Edward Bennett, OD, MS, ED
Co-Chief, Contact Lens Service
School of Optometry
University of Missouri-St. Louis
St. Louis, MO

For More Information

Bartlett JD, Jaanus SD. Clinical Ocular Pharmacology, ed 4. Boston: Butterworth-Heinemann, 2001.

Bennett ES, Henry VA. Clinical Manual of Contact Lenses (2nd edition). Philadelphia, J.B. Lippincott.

Bennett ES, Weissman BA. Clinical Contact Lens Practice (1993 & 1996 Updates). Philadelphia, J.B. Lippincott.

Chun MW, Weissman BA. Compliance in contact lens care. *Am J Optom Physiol Opt* 1987; 64:274-6.

Collins MJ, Carney LG, Patient compliance and its influence on contact lens wearing problems. *Am J Optom Physiol Opt*1986;63:952-6.

Hom MM. Manual of Contact Lens Prescribing and Fitting with CD-ROM. Boston; Butterworth-Heinemann. 2000.

Lowther GE, Shannon BJ, Weisbarth R. The Pharmacist's Guide to Contact Lenses and Lens Care. Atlanta, CIBAVision Corporation, 1988.

RGP Lens Institute. RGP Lens Product Guide. Contact Lens Manufacturers Association, 2000.

Thompson TT. Tyler's quarterly soft contact lens parameter guide. 2001:18(1).

White P, Scott C. Contact Lenses and Solutions Summary. Contact Lens Spectrum (supplement); 1998;13(7).

CONTACT LENS CARE

307

COMPONENTS IN CONTACT LENS SOLUTIONS

PRESERVATIVES:

Chlorhexidine: Chlorhexidine is bactericidal in action and has been used traditionally in a concentration of 0.005% in hydrogel lens chemical disinfection solutions. However, as gradual binding to hydrogel lenses has been problematic, chlorhexidine is used primarily with RGP lenses today. The binding capacity of chlorhexidine to RGP lenses appears to be limited because of the wettability of RGP lenses and to chlorhexidine's large molecular structure with a weak cationic action. Although chlorhexidine has been reported to have an excellent spectrum of antimicrobial activity, it has limited effectiveness against yeast and fungi; therefore, it often has been combined with EDTA or thimerosal for greater effectiveness. In addition, chlorhexidine has been found to be relatively ineffective against *Serratia marcescens*.

Benzalkonium Chloride: Benzalkonium chloride is a quaternary ammonium compound that is effective against a wide spectrum of bacteria and fungi and normally is used at a concentration of 0.004% in some RGP lens solutions. The effectiveness of BAK is enhanced when used in combination with EDTA, allowing a lower concentration than otherwise necessary. It is not used as a preservative with hydrogel lens solutions because the hydrogel plastic will bind the preservative and actually concentrate it, thereby allowing it to potentially reach toxic levels and cause ocular injury.

Thimerosal: Thimerosal is an organic mercurial compound that at one time was a commonly used hydrogel lens solution preservative. However, some patients are sensitive to organic mercurial compounds and experience a burning sensation and associated clinical signs of redness and superficial punctuate keratitis. In addition, it is slow-acting in nature and, in low concentrations, may be ineffective against *Pseudomonas*. Although thimerosal has been found to be compatible with RGP lenses, exhibiting only rare sensitivity reactions, for optimal antimicrobial effectiveness it should be used in combination with another preservative such as chlorhexidine.

Ethylenediamine Tetra Acetate (EDTA): Ethylenediamine tetra acetate is a chelating agent and not a true preservative. However, it is commonly used in combination with BAK and other preservatives in the rigid contact lens solutions because of its synergistic ability to enhance the bacterial action of pure preservatives against *Pseudomonas*.

Benzyl Alcohol: Benzyl Alcohol was originally considered for use as a solvent for contact lens materials; however, it also was found to have good disinfection capabilities. Pure benzyl alcohol possesses certain physicochemical characteristics that are regarded as ideal for an ophthalmic preservative, including low molecular weight, bipolarity, and water solubility. It is used in some RGP lens combination cleaning/disinfecting solutions. Caution must be used to not wet and insert a lens with a benzyl alcohol-preserved solution because a hypersensitivity reaction may occur.

Polyaminopropyl Biguanide: Polyaminopropyl biguanide (PAPB) is a high molecular weight preservative that alters the phospholipid groups found in bacterial cell walls. It has been used as a preservative in hydrogel lens disinfection regimens (as DYMED) because of its low sensitivity rate. It has replaced chlorhexidine as a preservative in one of the RGP care systems because it exhibits greater antimicrobial effectiveness, notably against *Serratia marcescens*. Some toxic reactions were experienced by patients when it was initially introduced in an RGP wetting/soaking solution. However, when reduced in concentration by two-thirds, it has demonstrated both excellent antimicrobial activity and minimal toxicity when compared with other systems.

308 OPHTHALMIC DRUG FACTS

Polyquad: Used in both soft and RGP lens formulations, polyquad is similar to BAK in composition and action, but appears to minimize the incidence of any adverse reactions. Like PAPB, it's high molecular weight prevents it from being absorbed into the contact lens matrix.

Sorbic acid: Typically used in 0.1% concentrations, sorbic acid is a bacteriostatic agent that produces a low incidence of hypersensitive reactions. It is a relatively unstable compound that breaks down into an aldehyde; therefore, through this process it can cause soft lens discoloration when used with hydrogen peroxide.

Actions:

> *Pharmacology* – There are numerous preservatives currently in common use, all differing in their mode of action and effectiveness. They are capable of either killing (bactericidal agents) or inhibiting the growth (bacteriostatic agents) of microorganisms. Preservatives are the active ingredients and should perform the following functions:
>
> 1. Effectively provide the necessary degree of disinfection in the environment in which it is to be used.
>
> 2. Not cause toxic reactions.
>
> 3. Be compatible with the lens materials, avoiding adverse effects on surface wettability and lens parameters.
>
> 4. Be compatible with the tear film.

Indications: To be used in contact lens salines, chemical disinfection solutions, and cleaners for the purpose of inhibiting microbial growth in these solutions.

Contraindications: Hypersensitivity to any specific preservative used in the formulation.

BUFFERS

Actions:

Pharmacology: A weak acid or base and its corresponding salt typically compose the buffer in a contact lens solution. Buffers can be identified by the suffix "-ate" on the label. The borate buffer commonly used in contact lens solutions—which also has some antimicrobial activity—consists of boric acid and sodium borate. Bicarbonate and citrate are other buffers used in these solutions.

Indications:

Buffers are indicated in contact lens solutions to maintain a fairly neutral pH level (ie, 6 to 8). Because of their phosphate concentration, the tear layer naturally assists in maintaining a neutral pH.

Contraindications:

None.

CONTACT LENS CARE

309

WETTING AGENTS

Polyvinyl Alcohol (PVA):

Polyvinyl alcohol has several properties that make it a beneficial additive to RGP lens solutions. It is water soluble and is relatively nonviscous and nontoxic to ocular tissues. It has good viscosity-building properties and exhibits good tear spreading on the eye and lens surfaces. It also does not retard regeneration of corneal epithelium.

Methylcellulose:

Methylcellulose derivatives have been used successfully as wetting agents in more viscous RGP solutions. They add greater viscosity—and therefore, longer term wettability—than PVA; however, methylcellulose retards epithelial regeneration.

Poloxamer 407:

Poloxamer 407 is used as a viscosity builder and wetting agent in some rewetting drop formulations. It has mucomimetic properties.

Actions:

Pharmacology: RGP wetting/rewetting and soft lens rewetting solutions often have wetting agents in the solution itself. These substances typically have good viscosity-building properties and exhibit good spreading and wettability on the eye and lens surfaces.

Indications:

To enhance surface wettability of contact lens materials.

Contraindications:

None.

Wetting/soaking solutions typically contain either polyvinyl alcohol or a methylcellulose derivative as a wetting agent.

CONTACT LENS CARE PRODUCTS

Products for use with contact lenses possess the same general characteristics of all ophthalmic products; they are sterile, isotonic, and free of particulate matter. Additionally, product formulations contain various components to achieve specific goals of contact lens care. Although all contact lenses serve similar functions in correcting visual defects, each type of lens material requires a unique lens care program. In selecting appropriate lens care solutions, correctly identifying the type of lens material a patient is wearing is essential.

Individual drug monographs are on the following pages.

OPHTHALMIC DRUG FACTS

RIGID GAS PERMEABLE (RGP) LENSES

Products for use with RGP lenses include: disinfecting/wetting/soaking, disinfecting/cleaning, surfactant cleaners, enzymatic cleaners, and rewetting drops. All have important functions in maintaining/enhancing the wettability, sterility, and cleanliness of RGP lens materials.

DISINFECTING/WETTING/SOAKING SOLUTIONS, RGP LENSES

Actions:

Pharmacology: These solutions are formulated for comfort and compatibility with ocular tissues. Therefore, the pH of the solution should be near physiologic pH, or only slightly buffered to allow the pH to rapidly adjust to that of tear film. A wetting agent such as PVA and possibly a viscosity-building agent such as methylcellulose will be used to enhance the tear spreading properties over the surface of the lens. Preservative use is such to disinfect the lens while not being toxic to the eye.

Indications:

These solutions are used for both insertion and soaking/disinfection of RGP lenses. They enhance lens surface wettability, maintain lens hydration similar to that achieved during contact lens wear, disinfect the lens, and act as a mechanical buffer between the lens and the cornea.

Warnings:

Almost all of these solutions are not compatible with soft lens material.

otc	**Boston Advance Comfort Formula Conditioning Solution** (Polymer Tech)	**Solution:** Buffered, slightly hypertonic. 0.05% EDTA, 0.003% chlorhexidine gluconate, 0.0005% polyaminopropyl biguanide. Cationic cellulose derivative polymer, PEG, cellulosic viscosifier, polyvinyl alcohol.	In 30 and 120 mL.
otc	**Boston Original Formula Conditioning Solution** (Polymer Tech)	**Solution:** Buffered, slightly hypertonic, low viscosity. 0.05% EDTA, 0.006% chlorhexidine gluconate. Cationic cellulose derivative polymer, polyvinyl alcohol, hydroxyethyl cellulose.	In 30 and 120 mL.
otc	**Boston Simplicity Multi-Action Solution** (Polymer Tech)	**Solution:** Buffered, slightly hypertonic. 0.05% EDTA, 0.003% chlorhexidine gluconate, 0.0005% polyaminopropyl biguanide. PEO sorbitan monolaurate, betaine surfactant, silicone glycol copolymer, PEG, cellulosic viscosifier.	In 60 and 120 mL.
otc	**ComfortCare GP Wetting & Soaking Solution** (Allergan)	**Solution:** Buffered, isotonic. 0.02% EDTA, 0.005% chlorhexidine gluconate. Oxyethylene, povidone, polyvinyl alcohol, propylene glycol, NaCl, hydroxyethylcellulose, phosphates.	In 120 and 240 mL.
otc	**Flex-Care Rinsing, Disinfecting and Storage Solution Especially for Sensitive Eyes** (Alcon)	**Solution:** Buffered, isotonic. 0.1% EDTA, 0.005% chlorhexidine gluconate. NaCl, sodium borate, boric acid.	Thimerosal free. In 118, 237, and 355 mL.

CONTACT LENS CARE

311

otc	**Opti-Soak Daily Cleaner Especially for Sensitive Eyes** (Alcon)	**Solution:** Buffered, isotonic. 0.1% EDTA, 0.001% polyquad. Polysorbate 21, polymeric cleaning agents.	Thimerosal free. In 15 mL.
otc	**Optimum C/D/S Solution** (Lobob)	**Solution:** 0.1% EDTA, 0.1% benzyl alcohol, 0.05% sorbic acid, 0.02% sodium bisulfite. NaCl, potassium chloride, PVA, PVP, hydroxyethylcellulose.	In 120 mL.
otc	**Wet-N-Soak Plus Wetting and Soaking Solution** (Allergan)	**Solution:** Buffered, isotonic. 0.003% benzalkonium chloride, polyvinyl alcohol, EDTA.	In 120 and 180 mL.
otc	**Wetting and Soaking Solution** (Bausch & Lomb)	**Solution:** Buffered, slightly hypertonic, low viscosity. 0.05% EDTA, 0.006% chlorhexidine gluconate. Cationic cellulose derivative polymer.	In 120 mL.

DISINFECTING/CLEANING SOLUTIONS, RGP LENSES

Actions:

Pharmacology: These solutions incorporate a mild surfactant cleaner into a preserved-disinfecting solution. With the exception of 1 product (ie, *Boston Simplicity*, an all-in-one product with wetting, cleaning, and disinfecting functions), these solutions are not intended for wetting/rewetting use. Because of the nature and composition of the surfactant cleaning agent(s), these solutions can induce a punctate keratitis if directly instilled into the eye.

Indications:

These solutions are used for disinfecting and cleaning of RGP lenses. It may be necessary to add an enzymatic cleaner to the care regimen in some patients.

Warnings:

With the exception of *Boston Simplicity* (Polymer Tech), which is also a wetting solution, these solutions should not be directly instilled into the eye or a toxic reaction to the surfactant cleaner may result.

otc	**Boston Simplicity Multi-Action** (Polymer Tech)	**Solution:** Buffered, slightly hypertonic. 0.05% EDTA, 0.003% chlorhexidine gluconate, 0.0005% polyaminopropyl biguanide. PEO sorbitan monolaurate, betaine surfactant, silicone glycol copolymer, PEG, cellulosic viscosifier.	In 60 and 120 mL.
otc	**Claris Cleaning and Soaking Solution** (Allergan)	**Solution:** 0.5% trisodium edetate, 0.3% benzyl alcohol. Lauryl sulfate salt of imidazoline, octylphenoxypolyethoxyethanol.	In 120 mL.
otc	**ContaClair** (Accugel)	**Solution:** Buffered , isotonic. 0.0031% biguanide copolymer. EDTA.	In 355 mL.
otc	**Optimum Extra Strength Cleaner** (Lobob)	**Solution:** 0.5% EDTA, 0.1% benzyl alcohol. Lauryl sulfate salt.	In 120 mL.

SURFACTANT CLEANING SOLUTIONS, RGP LENSES

Actions:

Pharmacology: These solutions use cleaners that typically consist of nonionic surfactant (detergents). Mild abrasive particles are added in some formulations for greater effect against bound muco-protein deposit complexes.

Indications:

All RGP wearing patients should use some type of cleaning solution upon lens removal because lipids, mucus, proteins, and other substances such as cosmetics and hand creams can adhere to the lens surface resulting in blurred vision and possibly reduced wearing time. These solutions help maintain a clean, wettable surface and good optics. If an abrasive cleaner is used do not clean the lens forcefully between the fingers, because increases in minus power and warpage have been reported over time.

Warnings:

Solutions used strictly for cleaning should never be used for wetting/rewetting RGP lenses or chemical keratitis may result.

otc	**Boston Advance Cleaner** (Polymer Tech)	**Solution:** Concentrated homogenous surfactant. Alkyl ether sulfate, ethoxylated alkyl phenol, tri-quaternary cocoa-based phospholipid, titanium dioxide, silica gel.	In 10 and 30 mL.
otc	**Boston Original Formula Cleaner** (Polymer Tech)	**Solution:** Concentrated homogenous surfactant. Alkyl ether sulfate, silica gel, titanium dioxide.	In 10 and 30 mL.
otc	**Claris Cleaning and Soaking Solution** (Allergan)	**Solution:** 0.5% trisodium EDTA, 0.3% benzyl alcohol. Lauryl sulfate salt of imidazoline, octylphenoxypolyethoxyethanol.	In 120 mL.
otc	**Concentrated Cleaner** (Bausch & Lomb)	**Solution:** Concentrated homogenous surfactant. Alkyl ether sulfate, ethoxylated alkyl phenol, tri-quaternary cocoa-based phospholipid, silica gel.	In 10 and 30 mL.
otc	**LC-65 Daily Contact Lens Cleaner** (Allergan)	**Solution:** Buffered, surface-active. Cocoamphocarboxyglycinate, sodium lauryl sulfate, hexylene glycol, NaCl, sodium phosphate, EDTA.	In 15 and 60 mL.
otc	**Opti-Clean II Daily Cleaner Especially for Sensitive Eyes** (Alcon)	**Solution:** Buffered, isotonic. 0.1% EDTA, 0.001% polyquad. Polysorbate 21, polymeric cleaning agents.	Thimerosal free. In 15 and 30 mL.
otc	**Opti-Soak Daily Cleaner Especially for Sensitive Eyes** (Alcon)	**Solution:** Buffered, isotonic. 0.1% EDTA, 0.001% polyquad. Polysorbate, polymeric cleaning agents.	Thimerosal free. In 15 mL.
otc	**Resolve/GP Daily Cleaner** (Allergan)	**Solution:** Buffered. Cocoamphocarboxyglycinate, sodium lauryl sulfate, hexylene glycol, alkyl ether sulfate, fatty acid amide surfactants.	Preservative free. In 30 mL.

CONTACT LENS CARE

313

ENZYMATIC CLEANERS, RGP LENSES

Actions:

Pharmacology: An enzymatic cleaner acts chemically to dissolve adherent mucoprotein complexes on the surface of the lens. Specific enzymes currently in use include papain (from papaya fruit), pancreatin (from hog pancreas), and Subtilisin A and B (produced by microorganisms).

Indications:

Enzyme cleaners are used as an adjunct to surfactant cleaning for the removal of adherent deposits. They are especially beneficial in dry eye patients who are more prone to deposit formation and for individuals who are not compliant with regular surfactant cleaning. Commonly available in tablet form, which dissolves in saline, they are currently available in a liquid form as marketed by 2 companies (*Boston One-Step Liquid Enzyme Cleaner* for weekly use from Polymer Technology; *Opti-Free Supra-Clens Daily Protein Removal* for daily use from Alcon). The liquid enzyme has the benefit of promoting patient compliance the simplicity of adding a drop of the enzyme solution to the disinfecting solution in each case well for overnight use.

Warnings:

Enzyme solutions are not to be used for wetting or rewetting of RGP lenses or chemical keratitis may result.

otc	**Boston One-Step Liquid Enzymatic Cleaner** (Polymer Tech)	**Solution:** Subtilisin A. Glycerol.	Preservative free. In 1 and 2.4 mL.
otc	**Opti-Free Supra Clens Daily Protein Remover** (Alcon)	**Solution:** Propylene glycol, sodium borate, highly purified porcine pancreatin enzymes.	Preservative free. In 1.5 and 5 mL.
otc	**Opti-Zyme Enzymatic Cleaner Especially for Sensitive Eyes** (Alcon)	**Tablets:** Highly purified pork pancreatin. *To make solution for soaking, dilute in preserved saline or sterile unpreserved saline solution.*	Preservative free. In 8s, 24s, 36s, and 56s.
otc	**ProFree/GP Weekly Enzymatic Cleaner** (Allergan)	**Tablets:** Papain, NaCl, sodium carbonate, sodium borate, EDTA.	In 16s and 24s with vials.

REWETTING SOLUTIONS, RGP LENSES

Actions:

Pharmacology: Rewetting drops are usually isotonic or slightly hypertonic. They typically contain a viscosity agent or wetting agent to enhance surface wettability.

Indications:

Rewetting solutions are needed when an RGP wearing patient experiences dryness or redness. These solutions rewet the lens surface, rinse away trapped debris, and break up loosely-adherent deposits.

OPHTHALMIC DRUG FACTS

Warnings:

One formulation, *Boston Rewetting Drops*, is not compatible for use with soft lenses.

otc	**Boston Rewetting Drops** (Polymer Tech)	**Solution:** Buffered, slightly hypertonic. 0.05% EDTA, 0.006% chlorhexidine gluconate. Cationic cellulose derivative polymer, polyvinyl alcohol, hydroxyethyl cellulose.	In 10 mL.
otc	**Claris Rewetting Drops** (Allergan)	**Solution:** Buffered, isotonic. 0.006% polixetonium chloride, hydroxyethyl cellulose, borate buffer.	In 15 mL.
otc	**Lens Drops** (Ciba Vision)	**Solution:** Buffered, isotonic. 0.2% EDTA, 0.15% sorbic acid. NaCl, borate buffer, carbamide, poloxamer 407.	Thimerosal free. In 15 mL.
otc	**Opti-Tears Soothing Drops** (Alcon)	**Solution:** Isotonic. 0.1% EDTA, 0.001% polyquad. Dextran, NaCl, potassium chloride, hydroxypropyl methylcellulose.	Thimerosal free. In 15 mL.
otc	**Optimum C/D/S Solution** (Lobob)	**Solution:** 0.1% EDTA, 0.1% benzyl alchol, 0.05% sorbic acid, 0.02% sodium bisulfite. NaCl, potassium chloride, PVA, PVP, hydroxyethycellulose.	In 120 mL.
otc	**Sterile Sereine Wetting Solution** (Optikem)	**Solution:** Buffered. 0.1% EDTA, 0.01% benzalkonium chloride.	In 120 mL.

HYDROGEL (SOFT) LENSES

Hydrogel contact lens care systems are designed to clean, disinfect, and rewet the lenses. Lenses are cleaned gently in the palm of the hand prior to disinfection. Disinfection of hydrogel lenses is the most important step in the care process. Disinfection is achieved by using a thermal (heat), chemical (non-hydrogen peroxide), or hydrogen peroxide (oxidative) system.

DISINFECTION, CHEMICAL NON-HYDROGEN PEROXIDE, SOFT LENSES

Actions:

Pharmacology: These solutions disinfect via the use of preservatives compatible with hydrogel lens materials. Because many of these solutions combine wetting and, in a few cases, cleaning, they incorporate buffers and a mild surfactant. Typically, a minimum of 4 hours is recommended for disinfection. One faster system, *Quick Care* (Ciba Vision), allows for disinfection and cleaning in a 5-minute period. The starting solution is hypertonic with a surfactant and isopropyl alcohol. Then it is stored for 1 minute in a saline solution with a trace amount of hydrogen peroxide.

Indications:

For disinfection of hydrogel lenses. Other functions—including wetting, rinsing, and cleaning—may be present as well.

Warnings:

Some patients may exhibit a sensitivity to the preservatives in a given system.

CONTACT LENS CARE

otc	**Clear Conscience Multi-purpose Solution** (Clear Conscience)	**Solution:** Buffered, isotonic. 0.0001% poly-hexamethylene biguanide, EDTA. Polyoxy-ethylene polyoxypropylene block copolymer, phosphate salt, NaCl.	Thimerosal free. In 355 mL.
otc	**ContaClair** (Accugel)	**Solution:** Buffered, isotonic. 0.0031% bigua-nide copolymer. EDTA.	In 355 mL.
otc	**Flex-Care Rinsing, Disin-fecting and Storage Solution Especially for Sensitive Eyes** (Alcon)	**Solution:** Buffered, isotonic. 0.1% EDTA, 0.005% chlorhexidine gluconate. NaCl, sodium borate, boric acid.	Thimerosal free. In 355 mL.
otc	**Opti-Free Express Multi-Purpose Disinfecting Solution** (Alcon)	**Solution:** Buffered, isotonic. 0.05% EDTA, 0.001% polyquad, 0.0005% myristamido-propyl dimethylamine. Sodium citrate, NaCl, boric acid, sorbitol, AMP-95, tetronic 1304.	In 118, 355, and 473 mL.
otc	**Opti-Free Rinsing, Disin-fecting and Storage Solution** (Alcon)	**Solution:** Buffered, isotonic. 0.05% EDTA, 0.001% polyquad. Citrates, NaCl.	In 118, 237, 355, and 473 mL.
otc	**Opti-One Multi-Purpose Solution** (Alcon)	**Solution:** Buffered, isotonic. 0.05% EDTA, 0.0011% polyquad. Borates, citrates, manni-tol, NaCl, surfactants.	In 355 mL.
otc	**Purilens UV Disinfec-tion System** (Purilens)	**Solution:** Uses cleaning unit with UV-C radiation to disinfect lenses.	
otc	**Quick CARE** (Ciba Vision)	**Disinfecting Solution:** NaCl, disodium lauro-amphodiacetate.	Thimerosal free. In 15 mL.
		Rinse and Neutralizer: Isotonic. Sodium borate, boric acid, sodium perborate (gener-ating up to 0.006% hydrogen peroxide), phosphonic acid.)	In 360 mL.
otc	**ReNu Multi-Purpose Solution** (Bausch & Lomb)	**Solution:** Isotonic. 0.00005% polyaminopro-pyl biguanide. Boric acid, EDTA, polox-amine, sodium borate, NaCl.	In 118, 237, and 355 mL.
otc	**SOLO-care Multi-Pur-pose Solution** (Ciba Vision)	**Solution:** Isotonic. 0.025% EDTA, 0.0001% polyhexanide. NaCl, polyoxyethylene poly-oxypropylene block copolymer, sodium phosphate dibasic, sodium phosphate monobasic.	Thimerosal free. In 118 and 355 mL.

DISINFECTION, HYDROGEN PEROXIDE (OXIDATIVE), SOFT LENSES

Actions:

Pharmacology: Oxidative disinfection consists of a 3% hydrogen peroxide solution; neutralizing solution, tablet, or disc; saline; and cleaner. Hydrogen peroxide does not result in clinically significant sensitivity problems when used properly because it breaks down into water and oxygen. It is important that some method of neutraliza-tion is present to prevent this acidic solution from direct contact with the eye. Pre-sent formulations are stable and newer systems appear to be less complex and more patient-friendly. Hydrogen peroxide has a mild effect on soft lenses.

Indications:

For the disinfection of hydrogel lenses.

316 OPHTHALMIC DRUG FACTS

Warnings:

Punctate Keratitis: Hydrogen peroxide will produce a mild-to-moderate punctate keratitis if not neutralized prior to instillation into the eye. To minimize this problem, many of the hydrogen peroxide solutions are currently packaged in bottles with red tips and warning labels on the bottles that direct the patient not to use the solution directly on the eye.

Discoloration: Use of an *otc* hydrogen peroxide not formulated for contact lens use may result in discoloration, and patient sensitivity because of colorants, incompatible stabilizers, and lack of salts necessary to provide satisfactory saline following neutralization.

otc	**AOSept** (Ciba Vision)	**Disinfecting Solution**: Buffered. 3% hydrogen peroxide, 0.85% NaCl, phosphoric acid, phosphates.	Thimerosal free. In 120, 237, 355, and 480 mL.
		AODISC Neutralizer: Platinum-coated tablet.	Tablet good for 100 uses or 3 months of daily use.[1]
otc	**Pure Eyes** (Ciba Vision)	**Disinfectant/Soaking Solution**: Buffered. 3% hydrogen peroxide, 0.85% NaCl, phosphonic acid, phosphates.	In 120 and 355 mL.
		Cleaner/Rinse Solution: Buffered, isotonic. NaCl, boric acid, sodium borate, sodium perborate (generating up to 0.006% hydrogen peroxide stabilized with phosphonic acid), surfactant.)	Thimerosal free. In 120 and 360 mL.
otc	**UltraCare** (Allergan)	**Disinfecting Solution**: Buffered. 3% hydrogen peroxide, sodium stannate, sodium nitrate, phosphates.	In 120 and 360 mL.
		Neutralizing Tablets: Catalase, hydroxypropyl methylcellulose, cyanocobalamin, buffering and tableting agents.	In 12s and 36s with cup.

[1] For use only with the *AOSept* system.

DISINFECTION, THERMAL (HEAT), SOFT LENSES

Actions:

Pharmacology: Heat disinfection avoids the use of preservatives and their corresponding potential for sensitivity. Heat is the most effective disinfection method, often killing organisms within 15 to 20 minutes compared with several hours with many chemical systems. Most of the units have temperatures reaching a maximum of 80° to 90°C.

Indications:

Heat disinfection is recommended when the other systems are not effective. Lens life is reduced because it heats deposits directly on the lens surface, resulting in discoloration. It is limited to lower water content lens materials.

Warnings:

Heat disinfection should not be used with Group 2 or Group 4 lenses.

CONTACT LENS CARE

Patient Information:

Recommended Chemical Disinfection Times for Soft Lenses			
System	Manufacturer	Disinfecting time (minimum)	Neutralization time (minimum)
AOSept	Ciba Vision	6 hours	6 hours
MiraSept	Alcon	10 minutes	10 minutes
Consept	Allergan	10 minutes	10 minutes
Pure Eyes	Ciba Vision	6 hours	None

PRESERVED SALINE SOLUTIONS, SOFT LENSES

otc	**Alcon Saline Especially for Sensitive Eyes** (Alcon)	**Solution:** Buffered, isotonic. Sorbic acid, EDTA. NaCl, borate buffer system.	Thimerosal free. In 355 mL.
otc	**ReNu Saline Solution** (Bausch & Lomb)	**Solution:** Buffered, isotonic. 0.00003% poly-aminopropyl biguanide, EDTA. Boric acid, NaCl.	Thimerosal free. In 355 mL.
otc	**Sensitive Eyes Plus Saline** (Bausch & Lomb)	**Solution:** Buffered, isotonic. 0.025% EDTA, 0.00003% polyaminopropyl biguanide. Boric acid, sodium borate, potassium chloride, NaCl.	In 118 and 355 mL.
otc	**Sensitive Eyes Saline** (Bausch & Lomb)	**Solution:** Buffered, isotonic. 0.1% sorbic acid, 0.025% EDTA. Boric acid, sodium borate, NaCl.	Thimerosal free. In 118, 237, and 355 mL.
otc	**SoftWear Saline for Sensitive Eyes** (Ciba Vision)	**Solution:** Isotonic. NaCl, boric acid, sodium borate, sodium perborate (generating up to 0.006% hydrogen peroxide stabilized with phosphonic acid).)	Thimerosal free. In 355 mL.
otc	**Sterile Preserved Saline Solution** (Bausch & Lomb)	**Solution:** Buffered, isotonic. 0.1% EDTA, 0.001% thimerosal. Boric acid, NaCl.	In 335 mL.

PRESERVATIVE FREE SALINE SOLUTIONS, SOFT LENSES

otc	**Blairex Sterile Saline** (Blairex)	**Solution:** Buffered, isotonic. NaCl, boric acid, sodium borate.	Preservative free. In 90, 240, and 360 mL aerosol.
otc	**Clear Conscience Saline Solution** (Clear Conscience)	**Solution:** Buffered, isotonic. NaCl, boric acid, sodium borate.	Preservative free. Thimerosal free. In 355 mL.
otc	**Lens Plus Sterile Saline** (Allergan)	**Solution:** Buffered, isotonic. NaCl, boric acid, nitrogen.	Preservative free. In 90, 240, 360, and 450 mL aerosol.
otc	**Saline** (Ciba Vision)	**Solution:** Buffered, isotonic. NaCl, boric acid.	Preservative free. In 237 and 355 mL aerosol.
otc	**Sensitive Eyes Preservative Free Sterile Saline Spray** (Bausch & Lomb)	**Solution:** Buffered, isotonic. 0.4% NaCl, boric acid, sodium borate.	Preservative free. In 355 mL aerosol.
otc	**Unisol 4** (Alcon)	**Solution:** Buffered, isotonic. NaCl, boric acid, sodium borate.	Preservative free. Thimerosal free. In 360 mL.
otc	**Unisol Plus** (Alcon)	**Solution:** Buffered, isotonic. NaCl, boric acid, sodium borate.	Preservative free. In 240 and 360 mL aerosol.

318   OPHTHALMIC DRUG FACTS

SURFACTANT CLEANING SOLUTIONS, SOFT LENSES

Actions:

Pharmacology: Similar to RGP lens solutions.

Indications:

Similar to RGP lens solutions.

Warnings:

Same as RGP lens solutions.

otc	**Daily Cleaner for Sensitive Eyes** (Ciba Vision)	**Solution**: 0.2% EDTA, 0.1% sorbic acid. Cocoamphocarboxyglycinate, sodium lauryl sulfate, hexylene glycol.	In 15 mL.
otc	**LC-65 Daily Contact Lens Cleaner** (Allergan)	**Solution**: Surface-active, buffered. Cocoamphocarboxyglycinate, sodium lauryl sulfate, hexylene glycol, NaCl, sodium phosphate, EDTA.	In 15 and 60 mL.
otc	**Lens Plus Daily Cleaner** (Allergan)	**Solution**: Surface-active, buffered. Cocoamphocarboxyglycinate, sodium lauryl sulfate, hexylene glycol, NaCl, sodium phosphate	Preservative free. In 15 and 30 mL.
otc	**MiraFlow Extra-Strength Daily Cleaner** (Ciba Vision)	**Solution**: 15.7% isopropyl alcohol, poloxamer 407, amphoteric 10.	Preservative free. Thimerosal free. In 12 and 25 mL.
otc	**Opti-Clean II Daily Cleaner Especially for Sensitive Eyes** (Alcon)	**Solution**: Buffered, isotonic. 0.1% EDTA, 0.001% polyquad. Polysorbate 21, polymeric cleaning agents.	Thimerosal free. In 15 and 30 mL.
otc	**Opti-Free Daily Cleaner** (Alcon)	**Solution**: Buffered, isotonic. 0.01% EDTA, 0.001% polyquad. Polysorbate 21, polymeric cleaning agents.	In 15 and 30 mL.
otc	**Opti-Free Supra Clens Daily Protein Remover** (Alcon)	**Solution**: Propylene glycol, sodium borate, highly purified porcine pancreatin enzymes.	Preservative free. In 1.5 and 5 mL.
otc	**Pliagel** (Alcon)	**Solution**: 0.5% EDTA, 0.25% sorbic acid. Poloxamer 407, potassium chloride, NaCl.	Thimerosal free. In 25 mL.
otc	**Sensitive Eyes Daily Cleaner** (Bausch & Lomb)	**Solution**: Buffered, isotonic. 0.5% EDTA, sorbic acid. Hydroxypropyl methylcellulose, poloxamine, sodium borate, NaCl.	In 20 mL.
otc	**Sensitive Eyes Saline/Cleaning** (Bausch & Lomb)	**Solution**: Buffered, isotonic. 0.15% sorbic acid, 0.1% EDTA. Boric acid, poloxamine, sodium borate, NaCl.	Thimerosal free. In 237 mL.
otc	**Sterile Daily Cleaner** (Bausch & Lomb)	**Solution**: Buffered, isotonic. 0.2% EDTA, 0.004% thimerosal. Sodium phosphates, NaCl, tyloxapol, hydroxymethylcelluslose, polyvinyl alcohol.	In 20 mL.

CONTACT LENS CARE

319

ENZYMATIC CLEANERS, SOFT LENSES

Actions:

Pharmacology: Similar to RGP lens solutions. As subtilisin is not deactivated quickly in hydrogen peroxide, it has been incorporated in several systems for use during hydrogen peroxide disinfection, decreasing the number of steps necessary for care and potentially increasing patient compliance. Likewise, commonly used chemical disinfection solutions (eg, *ReNu 1 Step*) combine enzymatic cleaning with disinfection.

Indications:

Similar to RGP lens solutions.

Warnings:

Same as RGP lens solutions.

otc	**Allergan Enzymatic** (Allergan)	**Tablets:** Papain, NaCl, sodium carbonate, sodium borate, EDTA. *To make solution for soaking, dilute in sterile saline.*	In 12s, 24s, 36s, and 48s.
otc	**Complete Weekly Enzymatic Cleaner** (Allergan)	**Tablets:** Subtilisin A. Effervescing, buffering, and tableting agents. *To make solution for soaking, dilute in sterile saline.*	In 8s.
otc	**Opti-Free Supra Clens Daily Protein Remover** (Alcon)	**Solution:** Propylene glycol, sodium borate, highly purified pork pancreatin enzymes.	Preservative free. In 1.5 and 5 mL.
otc	**Opti-Zyme Enzymatic Cleaner Especially for Sensitive Eyes** (Alcon)	**Tablets:** Highly purified pork pancreatin. *To make solution for soaking, dilute in preserved saline or sterile unpreserved saline solution.*	Preservative free. In 8s, 24s, 36s, and 56s.
otc	**ReNu 1 Step Enzymatic Cleaner** (Bausch & Lomb)	**Tablets:** Subtilisin, sodium carbonate, NaCl, boric acid.	In 8s and 16s.
otc	**ReNu Effervescent Enzymatic Cleaner** (Bausch & Lomb)	**Tablets:** Subtilisin, polyethelyne glycol, sodium carbonate, NaCl, tartaric acid. *For use with all disinfection regimens.*	In 10s, 20s, and 30s.
otc	**Sensitive Eyes Enzymatic Cleaner** (Bausch & Lomb)	**Tablets:** Subtilisin, polyethelyne glycol, sodium carbonate, NaCl, tartaric acid. *For use with all disinfection regimens.*	In 8s, 16s, and 40s.
otc	**Ultrazyme Enzymatic Cleaner** (Allergan)	**Tablets:** Subtilisin A. Effervescing, buffering, and tableting agents. *To make solution for soaking, dilute in 3% hydrogen peroxide disinfecting solution.*	In 5s, 10s, and 20s.
otc	**Unizyme Enzymatic Cleaner** (Ciba Vision)	**Tablets:** Subtilisin A. *For use with all Ciba Vision disinfection systems.*	In 12s.

[1] Developed for use with *Opti-Free Rinsing, Disinfecting and Storage Solution* and *Opti-Free Express Multi-Purpose Disinfecting Solution.* Its effectiveness has not been demonstrated with other products.

OPHTHALMIC DRUG FACTS

DISINFECTING/WETTING/SOAKING SOLUTIONS, SOFT LENSES

otc	**ReNu MultiPlus Multi-Purpose Solution** (Bausch & Lomb)	**Solution:** Isotonic. 0.0001% polyaminopropyl biguanide. Hydroxyalkylphosphonate, boric acid, EDTA, poloxamine, sodium borate, NaCl.	Thimerosal free. In 60, 118, 237, and 355 mL.

REWETTING SOLUTIONS, SOFT LENSES

Actions:

Pharmacology: Similar to RGP lens solutions.

Indications:

Similar to RGP lenses with the additional benefit of rehydrating the lens for additional comfort and increased wearing time.

Warnings:

None.

otc	**Clerz 2 Lubricating & Rewetting Drops** (Alcon)	**Solution:** Isotonic. NaCl, potassium chloride, sodium borate, EDTA, hydroxyethylcellulose, boric acid, sorbic acid, poloxamer 407.	Thimerosal free. In 15 mL.
otc	**Complete Lubricating and Rewetting Drops** (Allergan)	**Solution:** Buffered, isotonic. 0.0001% polyhexamethylene biguanide. NaCl, tromethamine, hydroxymethylcellulose, tyloxapol, EDTA.	Thimerosal free. In 15 mL.
otc	**Focus Lens Drops** (Ciba Vision)	**Solution:** Buffered, isotonic. 0.2% EDTA, 0.15% sorbic acid. NaCl, borate buffer, Oxy-Gentle, polyoxyethylene polyoxypropylene block copolymer.	Thimerosal free. In 5 and 15 mL.
otc	**Just Tears Lubricant Eye Drops** (Blairex)	**Solution:** Isotonic. 1.4% polyvinyl alcohol, EDTA, benzalkonium chloride. NaCl, potassium chloride.	In 15 mL.
otc	**Lens Drops** (Ciba Vision)	**Solution:** Buffered, isotonic. 0.2% EDTA, 0.15% sorbic acid. NaCl, borate buffer, carbamide, poloxamer 407.	Thimerosal free. In 15 mL.
otc	**Lens Plus Rewetting Drops** (Allergan)	**Solution:** Buffered, isotonic. NaCl, boric acid.	Preservative free. Thimerosal free. In 0.35 mL (30s).
otc)	**Opti-Free Rewetting Drops** (Alcon)	**Solution:** Buffered, isotonic. 0.05% EDTA, 0.001% polyquad. Citrate buffer, NaCl.	In 10 mL.
otc	**Opti-One Rewetting Drops** (Alcon)	**Solution:** Buffered, isotonic. 0.05% EDTA, 0.001% polyquad. Citrate buffer, NaCl.	In 10 mL.
otc	**Opti-Tears Soothing Drops** (Alcon)	**Solution:** Isotonic. 0.1% EDTA, 0.001% polyquad. Dextran, NaCl, potassium chloride, hydroxypropyl methylcellulose	Thimerosal free. In 15 mL.
otc	**ReNu Lubricating & Rewetting Drops** (Bausch & Lomb)	**Solution:** Isotonic. 0.15% sorbic acid, 0.1% EDTA. Boric acid, poloxamine, sodium borate, NaCl.	Thimerosal free. In 15 mL.

CONTACT LENS CARE

otc	**ReNu MultiPlus Lubricating & Rewetting Drops** (Bausch & Lomb)	**Solution:** 0.1% EDTA, 0.1% sorbic acid. Povidone, boric acid, potassium chloride, sodium borate, NaCl.	In 8 mL.
otc	**Sensitive Eyes Drops** (Bausch & Lomb)	**Solution:** Buffered. 0.1% sorbic acid, 0.025% EDTA. Boric acid, sodium borate, NaCl.	Thimerosal free. In 30 mL.

EXTEMPORANEOUS PREPARATIONS

Extemporaneous compounding of ophthalmic solutions may include the preparation of topical, periocular, or intraocular injections. Many topical ophthalmic solutions or suspensions are commercially available. However, certain topical ophthalmic solutions and all periocular and intraocular solutions are neither FDA-approved nor commercially available for ophthalmic administration. When these preparations are required, injectable sources are frequently used. In many cases, this may be limited to dilution of injectable products or the addition of injectable products to commercial ophthalmic preparations to increase their concentration or "fortify" them. These extemporaneously prepared products are considered the community standard based on clinical research and ethical practice, and, as such, may be required to effectively treat a patient with ophthalmic conditions.[1,2] Considerations for ophthalmic compounding must include topical (usually topical solutions), periocular (subconjunctival or sub-Tenon's; retrobulbar), or intraocular (intravitreal or intracameral) products.

GUIDELINES

Requirements for the preparation of topical ophthalmic preparations are published in the United States Pharmacopoeia.[3] The USP guidelines describe the requirements for the preparation of ophthalmic ointments, solutions, suspensions, and strips. Isotonicity, buffering, sterilization, preservation, and thickening agents are specifically addressed.

Because of concerns for possible eye infections, guidelines for the preparation of all sterile ophthalmic products were published by the American Society of Health-Systems Pharmacists (ASHP).[4] These guidelines state that all extemporaneous ophthalmic products be prepared in an approved and certified laminar airflow or biohazard hood. Proper aseptic technique is essential, as is required for any sterile product. Accuracy is stressed to prevent any miscalculation, which is especially a concern with preparation of intravitreal injections. The use of a 5 micron filter is recommended when a drug is reconstituted or if it is supplied in a glass ampule. When a drug product is not available in a sterile dosage form, a 0.22 micron filter should be used. The use of a preservative-free product is recommended when feasible. These guidelines are particularly helpful for health care personnel who are not familiar with preparing ophthalmic extemporaneous products. Information on > 50 ophthalmic medications including topical, subconjunctival, and intraocular formulations, is available in a "cookbook" format by Reynolds.[5] The uses, concentrations, dosing, and references also are included.

References found in the literature for the ocular administration of non-commercial ophthalmic products (eg, acetylcysteine, ceftazidime, disodium EDTA) only provide some assurance that the medication is tolerated in the eye without obvious ocular side

OPHTHALMIC DRUG FACTS

effects. Most of these references do not state which vehicles were used, expirations, or other essential information required to properly prepare the product.

STABILITY

Stability data must be based upon concerns for maintaining sterility rather than just the stability of the product itself. Obviously, if sterility cannot be maintained, then stability of the product is secondary. Little published information is available on stability dating of extemporaneously prepared topical ophthalmic solutions. Many institutions have extrapolated from published IV product stability, although this may not always be appropriate. Gentamicin- and tobramycin-fortified ophthalmic solutions are stable at 4° to 8°C for 3 months.[6] The stability of several antibiotics, including vancomycin, gentamicin, bacitracin, and cephalothin, in commercially available 0.5% hydroxypropyl methylcellulose artificial tear solution,[7] demonstrated no significant loss of potency at room temperature for 7 days. However, the use of different vehicles, antibiotic concentrations, storage conditions, and other factors may influence product stability. Frozen and refrigerated stability data may be useful if multiple bottles are prepared. Stability must be established if the product is dispensed for outpatient use or used in a hospital setting. Extemporaneously prepared ophthalmic solutions should be refrigerated after dispensing to reduce the risk of microbial growth or to ensure minimal loss of potency. A 7-day in-use storage life is acceptable for unpreserved eye drops containing alkaloids or antibiotics if they are stored in the refrigerator after opening.[8]

The stability of periocular or intraocular preparations is usually restricted to 6- to 24-hour expirations because information is limited and these expiration times are commonly used for other extemporaneously prepared injectable products.

Stability and sterility appear to be maintained with some preparations that are aseptically prepared, sealed, and frozen. Frozen stability of products such as periocular mitomycin,[9] intraocular ganciclovir,[10] and topical cefazolin[11] and vancomycin[11] has provided extended dating for these products.

STERILITY

Sterility must be maintained with any extemporaneously prepared ophthalmic product. The USP and ASHP recommend that sterile membrane filtration (0.22 micron filter) be used under aseptic conditions whenever possible.[3,4] Many institutions prepare extemporaneous ophthalmic products and employ a 0.22 micron filter for the final step to ensure sterilization. Some medications should not be filtered with a 0.22 micron filter. Amphotericin B, a colloidal suspension, should be filtered with nothing smaller than a 5 micron filter to prevent loss of drug. Suspensions and other formulations such as liposomal products should be researched to determine if membrane filtration is acceptable.

PH/BUFFERING

The pH of an extemporaneously prepared topical ophthalmic product is most often considered because of the concern for ocular irritation associated with eyedrops. The eye can tolerate a rather wide range of pH (between 3.5 and 10) for a single drop administration. If the pH is too high or too low, reflex tearing will dilute the drug concentration more quickly than if the pH is in the physiologic range of 7.4 for lacrimal fluid. Some medications require lower pH values to maintain longer shelf lives because they may be chemically unstable at higher pH levels. Buffering systems are not commonly employed in the current practice of preparing extemporaneous ophthalmic preprations. It is important that if a buffer system is used, it is close to pH 7.4, but does not hasten deterioration or precipitation of the drug.[3]

EXTEMPORANEOUS PREPARATIONS

The pH of the eyedrop may influence absorption of a drug into the intraocular fluids and tissues. Generally, the unionized form of a drug will penetrate the lipophilic corneal epithelium, the first significant barrier to intraocular penetration, better than a hydrophilic form will. The cornea contains tight epithelial and endothelial cell junctions that slow or prevent the passage of a drug through the cornea. A drug must penetrate the 3 layers of the cornea, including the epithelium (lipophilic barrier), stroma (water soluble), and endothelium (lipid soluble). Increasing the pH of a solution increases the amount of the unionized form, thereby increasing initial epithelial penetration of the drug.

ISOTONICITY

Isotonicity is not essential even for topical ophthalmic solutions. An acceptable range is from 0.7% to 2.0% (0.9% sodium chloride is considered isotonic). In fact, some ophthalmic products are produced as hypertonic (sodium chloride 5%) or hypotonic (*Hypotears*) solutions for their desired pharmacologic effects.

VEHICLES

Vehicles used for topical ophthalmic solutions vary and are usually either normal saline, water, various biocompatible polymers used in artifical tears, or, occasionally, balanced salt solution. Artificial tear polymer may provide comfort, prolonged contact time with the eye, the presence of a preservative system, and a neutral pH. However, potential problems include incompatibilities between the active or inactive ingredients and a reduction in preservative effectiveness due to dilution from the active drug. Some artificial tear preparations contain methylcellulose, which is an acceptable thickening agent to increase the viscosity and contact time of the ophthalmic solution.[3] Sterile water or normal saline is often used, but they contain no preservatives. The concern for potential contamination associated with the repeated administration of unpreserved solutions must be considered. If the active component has an initial low pH, the lower pH of water and normal saline may further contribute to irritation of the ophthalmic solution. Balanced salt solutions (bss) contain no preservatives, and potential incompatibilities with the various components of the bss should be considered.

Intraocular or periocular preparations most often use sterile water or normal saline as the preferred diluent. Use caution if balanced salt solutions are employed as vehicles because potential incompatibilities, especially with magnesium and calcium salts, may exist with the active ingredient or its inactive components. Balanced salt solution should not be used as a diluent for cromolyn sodium or tissue plasminogen activator.[5,12]

TOPICAL PREPARATIONS

Topical forms of administration include drops, ointments, gels, contact lenses, and collagen shields. The most common extemporaneously prepared product is the topical ophthalmic solution. Topical formulations deliver the drug to the site of action, which reduce the risk of systemic side effects, but do not totally alleviate them.

Extemporaneously prepared topical eye solutions are used most often in the treatment of bacterial keratitis. Until the approval of the fluoroquinolone antibiotics ciprofloxacin and ofloxacin for bacterial keratitis, standard regimens consisted of alternating an aminoglycoside (usually gentamicin- or tobramycin-fortified solutions) with a cephalosporin, most often cefazolin.[1,2,13,14] Some of the most common concentrations of antibiotic drops are gentamicin 13.6 mg/mL, tobramycin 13.6 mg/mL, cefazolin 50 mg/mL, and vancomycin 10 mg/mL.[15]

OPHTHALMIC DRUG FACTS

The aminoglycoside products (usually gentamicin or tobramycin) are fortified to a concentration of 9 to 14 mg/mL from the commerically available strength of 3 mg/mL. An injectable form of the active drug is added under aseptic conditions in a lamellar flow hood to an ophthalmic dropper bottle to "fortify" the commercial strength. Cefazolin ophthalmic solution 25 to 100 mg/mL is made from the injectable product and is reconstituted in water and further diluted in water, normal saline, or artificial tear solution.

Polyhexamethylene biguanide (PHMB 20%) is an environmental biocide for swimming pools. PHMB 0.02% is useful in *Acanthamoeba* keratitis as an extemporaneously prepared topical ophthalmic product.[17] Because the initial concentration is 20%, an intermediate dilution is suggested to ensure an accurate final concentration of 0.02%, because this is a 1000-fold difference.[16]

Ophthalmic ointments usually consist of a petrolatum and mineral oil base (added to reduce the temperature at which the ointment melts). Some ointments contain lanolin (emulsifier to incorporate water-soluble drugs into the ointment). Allergies to ophthalmic ointments are most often related to the incorporated lanolin. Most drugs are very stable in ointments and do not ionize. Ophthalmic ointments provide longer ocular contact time and comfort. However, contact time may not increase bioavailability because only the drug at the ointment-tear interface will be absorbed. Ointments also are associated with blurred vision and provide poor patient acceptance. Although ointments occasionally are prepared extemporaneously, this is uncommon because of the time required to prepare them, the rare instances of a clinical indication, and the special ophthalmic ointment tubes required.

Antibiotic-soaked collagen shields provide for prolonged topical drug levels. However, potential drug incompatibility problems, loss of the shield from the eye, requirements for rehydration with the antibiotic, and cost have limited their use.

PERIOCULAR

Periocular administration includes injections below the conjunctiva or Tenon's capsule. They are given either to prolong administration or to increase penetration of the drug into the eye. Advantages include increased local concentration of the drug, thereby avoiding potential systemic toxicity, and higher intraocular tissue concentrations. Because no FDA-approved formulations are available for periocular administration, injectable preparations are often used. In many cases, the concentration required is drawn directly from a commercial-strength vial. An example of this is gentamicin, which is given in a safe subconjunctival dose of 20 mg/0.5 mL. Direct use from the vial, or sometimes after a single dilution, is often employed with antibiotics, anesthetics, and corticosteroid preparations for use as subconjunctival or sub-Tenon's injections. A common peribulbar or retrobulbar anesthetic combination uses a 50:50 mixture of lidocaine and bupivacaine.

INTRAOCULAR

Intraocular injections are often used in serious eye infections and inflammatory conditions such as endophthalmitis, retinal necrosis, and cytomegalovirus retinitis. Intraocular injections provide immediate therapeutic drug levels. It is essential to ensure that the correct dose is prepared to prevent retinal toxicity. The half-life of the drug in the vitreous cavity is a consideration, especially if reinjection may be required. The volume of drug administered is usually in the 0.05 to 0.1 mL range. Proper injection technique is critical to prevent damage to any intraocular structures. Commonly used intraocular medications include vancomycin, ceftazidime, amikacin, ganciclovir, foscarnet, dexamethasone, and amphotericin B.[1,5]

EXTEMPORANEOUS PREPARATIONS

Intraocular doses are often in the microgram to milligram range. The proper dose must be established before the medication is prepared. In some instances, multiple dilutions are required to obtain an accurate concentration for intravitreal injection. Amphotericin B is administered as a 5 microgram injection and must be prepared from a commercial vial of 50 milligrams.[5] Amikacin is administered in a 400 mcg dose or less and must be diluted from a 500 or 100 mg (pediatric) vial.[5] Vancomycin is injected intravitreally in a dose of 1 mg after being diluted from a vial containing 500 mg. These concentrations may reflect a 10- or even 1000-fold dilution from the commercial-strength product. Careful calculation and validation from others is appropriate. Syringes must be able to measure low concentrations precisely. An adequate initial volume must be drawn up so that a reasonable volume can be transferred for further dilution.[4,5] To ensure no loss of drug in the needle hub of a tuberculin syringe, it is more accurate to deliver 0.3 mL from the 0.6 to 0.3 mL gradations on the syringe barrel than from the 0.3 mark to zero. To prevent any miscalculation, no air bubbles should be left in the syringe or needle when preparing the injection. It is prudent to add both drug and diluent to a single sterile vial to prevent any misclaculation in volume.[5] A larger volume of the final concentration of drug should be dispensed (eg, draw up 0.4 mL of a 1 mg/0.1 mL vancomycin) and labeled appropriately. The larger volume will allow for easy transfer of the final concentration of drug to another syringe, should this be required.

Richard G. Fiscella, RPh, MPH
University of Illinois

For More Information

Glasser DB and Baum J. Antibacterial Agents in Infections of the Eye, 2nd ed. Tabbara KF and Hyndiuk RA. Eds. Little, Brown and Company, Boston MA. 1996;207-31.

Liesegang TJ. Bacterial keratitis. *Infec Dis Clin NA* 1992;6:815-30.

United States Pharmacopoeia XXIII 1995;1945-46.

Reynolds LA. Guidelines for the preparation of sterile ophthalmic products. *Am J Hosp Pharm* 1991;48:2438-39.

Reynolds LA, Closson RG, eds. Extemporaneous Ophthalmic Preparations. Vancouver: Applied Therapeutics, Inc. 1993.

McBride HA, et al. Stability of gentamicin sulfate and tobramycin sulfate in extemporaneously prepared ophthalmic solutions at 8°C. *Am J Hosp Pharm* 1991;48:507-9.

Osborn E, et al. The stability of ten antibiotics in artificial tear solutions. *Am J Ophthalmol* 1976;82:775-80.

Oldham GB, Andrews V. The control of microbial contamination in unpreserved eye drops. (in press BJO 1996).

Fiscella RG, et al. Stability of mitomycin for ophthalmic use. *Am J Hosp Pharm* 1992;49:2440.

Fiscella RG, Aramwit P. Ganciclovir for intravitreal injection. *Am J Health-Syst Pharm* 1995;52:422.

Trissel LA. Handbook on Injectable Drugs 8th ed. American Society of Hospital Pharmacists Incorporated 1994.

Ward C and Weck S. Dilution and storage of recombinant tissue plasminogen activator (Activase) in balanced salt solutions. *Am J Ophthalmol* 1990;109:98-99.

Parks DJ, et al. Comparison of topical ciprofloxacin to conventional antibiotic therapy in the treatment of ulcerative keratitis. *Am J Ophthalmol* 1993;115:471-77.

O'Brien TP, et al. Efficacy of ofloxacin vs cefazolin and tobramycin in the therapy for bacterial keratitis. *Arch Ophthalmol* 1995;113:1257-65.

Fiscella RG. Extemporaneously compounded ophthalmic antibiotic solutions: survey of usage and costs and pharmacotherapeutic considerations. (submitted to AJHP).

Yee E, et al. Topical polyhexamethylene biguanide (pool cleaner) for treatment of *Ananthamoeba* keratitis. *Am J Hosp Pharm* 1993;50:2522-23.

EXTEMPORANEOUS PREPARATIONS

OCULAR DOSAGE FORM *Drug Class*	Commercial Strength	Ophthalmic Strength	Dilution Directions	Special Instructions	Comments
TOPICAL					
Antibiotics					
Gentamicin (or Tobramycin)	40 mg/mL (injection) and 3 mg/mL (ophth soln)	9 to 14 mg/mL	Add 2 mL of injectable to 5 mL bottle (7 mL or 13.6 mg/mL)		Use same bottle eyedrops came in
Cefazolin	1 gram (vial-recon)	25 to 100 mg/mL aseye drop	Recon vial with 3 mL water, qs to 10 mL with water - transfer to ophthalmic bottle	Artificial tear used to qs	Frozen stability appears to be good for ≥ 28 days - concerns are to ensure sterility when frozen
Vancomycin	0.5 gram (vial-recon)	10 mg/mL	Recon with 10 mL sterile water, transfer to ophthalmic bottle		Frozen stability good for 28 days / Must ensure sterility when frozen / Unbuffered pH is in 4 to 4.5 range
Local anesthetics					
Proparacaine	2 mL / 15 mL	0.5%	No dilution necessary		Store at 8° to 24°C (46° to 75°F)
Other					
PHMB	20% solution	0.02%	Dilution with sterile water is best	First dilute an intermediate solution of *0.5% PHMB*, then further dilute to 0.02% with sterile water	Stability is very good - 30 days / Intermediate dilution is more accurate
PERIOCULAR					
Antibiotics					
Gentamicin	40 mg/mL vial	20 mg/0.5 mL	No dilution required		
Cefazolin	1 gram vial (recon)	100 mg/ 0.5 mL	Recon with sterile water		
Corticosteroids					
Dexamethasone	4 mg/mL or 10 mg/mL	2 mg/0.5 mL / 5 mg/0.5 mL	No dilution required	Given sub-conjunctivally	Short half life - 24 to 48 hours
Triamcinolone acetonide	40 mg/mL	20 mg/0.5 mL	No dilution required	Given sub-Tenon's	Long half life - may last weeks to months
Antimetabolites					
Mitomycin	5 mg vial (recon)	0.2-0.4 mg/mL	Dilute with sterile water	Solution soaked into sponge	Frozen stability in 0.2 to 0.4 mg range is good for 60 days[9]

OCULAR DOSAGE FORM / Drug Class	Commercial Strength	Ophthalmic Strength	Dilution Directions	Special Instructions	Comments
INTRAOCULAR					
Antibiotics					
Vancomycin	500 mg (recon)	1 mg/0.05 to 0.1 mL	Recon with 10 mL normal saline	Take 2 mL of reconstituted solution add sterile vial; add 8 mL of sterile water (final conc. = 1 mg/0.1 mL)	Double check dilution; filter
Amikacin	100 mg/2 mL vial	400 mcg/0.05 to 0.1 mL	Dilute with sterile normal saline (NS)	Take 1 mL of amikacin, add 11.5 mL saline in vial (final conc. = 400 mcg/0.1 mL)	Double check dilution
Ceftazidime	1 > vial (recon)	2 mg/0.05 to 0.1 mL	Dilute with sterile water	Add 9.4 mL of water to > 1 ceftazidime vial. Transfer 2 mL of solution to vial, add 8 mL of NS (final conc. = 2 mg/0.1 mL)	Double check dilution
Antivirals					
Ganciclovir	500 mg vial (recon)	200 to 2000 mcg/ 0.05 to 0.1 mL	Dilute with sterile water	Recon with 2.5 mL NS; transfer 0.1 mL to sterile vial, add 9.9 mL NS *(final conc. = 200 mcg/0.1 mL)* or transfer 1 mL and add 9 mL NS *(final conc. = 2000 mcg/0.1 mL)*	Refrigerate for storage
Foscarnet	Solution 24 mg/mL	1200 to 2400 mcg/0.05 to 0.1 mL	Use directly from vial		
Others					
Tissue plasminogen activator (tPA) (alteplase)	20 mg vial	6.25 to 25 mcg/ 0.1 mL	Dilute 20 mg vial with 20 mL sterile water as per directions; further dilute 1 mL of above with 3 mL of NS (250 mcg/mL)		Frozen stability good for ≥ 1 year

SYSTEMIC DRUGS AFFECTING THE EYE

The eye is highly susceptible to toxic substances because of its rich blood supply, multiple tissue types, and relatively small size. Many systemically administered drugs have the potential to cause adverse ocular effects, and nearly all ocular structures are vulnerable. This section considers the most common drugs that are documented to cause ocular toxicity and summarizes the salient features of the ocular effects.

DRUGS AFFECTING THE CORNEA AND LENS

Antimalarial Drugs

Quinacrine, chloroquine, and hydroxychloroquine can cause changes in the cornea. In the early stages, diffuse punctate deposits appear in the corneal epithelium; later, the deposits aggregate into curved lines that converge and coalesce just below the central cornea. These opacities take on a whorl-like configuration. Less than half of patients affected by corneal changes have visual symptoms consisting of halos around lights, glare, and photophobia. Visual acuity usually remains unchanged. Once drug therapy is discontinued, both subjective symptoms and objective corneal signs disappear.

Chlorpromazine

Chlorpromazine is the only phenothiazine that causes changes in the cornea and lens. Lenticular pigmentation can vary from fine, dot-like opacities on the anterior lens surface to a central, lightly pigmented, pearl-like, opaque mass surrounded by smaller clumps of pigment. Corneal pigmentary changes almost invariably occur only in patients who have concomitant lens opacities. Corneal pigmentation occurs at the level of the endothelium and Descemet's membrane, primarily in the interpalpebral fissure area. These ocular changes rarely reduce visual acuity, but patients may occasionally report glare, halos around lights, or hazy vision. The pigmentary deposits are generally irreversible even when drug therapy is reduced or discontinued.

Systemic Drugs Affecting The Eye		
Systemic Drug	**Examples**	**Structure/Function Affected**
Alcohol	alcohol	Extraocular muscles
Amiodarone	*Cordarone*	Cornea and lens
Antianxiety Agents	chlordiazepoxide (eg, *Librium*)	Extraocular muscles Causes cycloplegia

OPHTHALMIC DRUG FACTS

Systemic Drugs Affecting The Eye		
Systemic Drug	**Examples**	**Structure/Function Affected**
Anticholinergics	atropine, scopolamine	Tear secretion Pupil (mydriasis) Causes cycloplegia
Antidepressants	amitriptyline (eg, *Elavil*)	Extraocular muscles Causes cycloplegia
Antihistamines	chlorpheniramine (eg, *Chlor-Trimeton*) diphenhydramine (eg, *Benadryl*)	Tear secretion Extraocular muscles Pupil (mydriasis) Causes cycloplegia
Antimalarials	chloroquine (eg, *Aralen Phosphate*) hydroxychloroquine (eg, *Plaquenil Sulfate*) quinacrine (eg, *Atabrine HCl*)	Cornea, lids, retina
Barbiturates	phenobarbital	Extraocular muscles
β-blockers	atenolol (eg, *Tenormin*)	Tear secretion Reduces intraocular pressure
Carbonic Anhydrase Inhibitors	acetazolamide (eg, *Diamox*)	Causes myopia
CNS Stimulants	amphetamines (eg, *Dexedrine*), cocaine, methylphenidate (eg, *Ritalin*)	Pupil (mydriasis) Lowers intraocular pressure
Chloramphenicol	*Chloromycetin*	Optic nerve
Chlorpromazine	*Thorazine*	Cornea and lens, lids Extraocular muscles
Cocaine	crack cocaine	Cornea and conjunctiva
Corticosteroids	prednisone cortisol	Lens Elevates intraocular pressure
Digitalis Glycosides	digoxin (eg, *Lanoxin*)	Retina
Diuretics	hydrochlorothiazide (eg, *HydroDIURIL*)	Causes myopia
Ethambutol	*Myambutol*	Optic nerve
Gold Salts	auranofin (*Ridaura*) gold sodium thiomalate (*Aurolate*)	Cornea and lens Conjunctiva and lids Extraocular muscles
Indomethacin	*Indocin*	Cornea, retina
Isotretinoin	*Accutane*	Conjunctiva and lids Tear secretion Retina
Minocycline	*Dynacin, Minocin*	Sclera, blue-gray or brownish Papilledema
Opiates	morphine, codeine, heroin	Pupil (miosis)
Phenytoin	*Dilantin*	Extraocular muscles
Psoralens	methoxsalen (*Oxsoralen*)	Cornea and lens
Quinine	*Quinamm*	Retina
Salicylates	aspirin (eg, *Bayer*)	Extraocular muscles
Sildenafil	*Viagra*	Retina, vision color disturbances
Sulfonamides	sulfisoxazole (*Gantrisin*)	Causes myopia
Tamoxifen	*Nolvadex*	Retina
Tetracycline	*Sumycin*	Conjunctiva and lens
Thioridazine	*Mellaril*	Retina
Vigabatrin	*Sabril*	Symptomatic or asymptomatic field loss

SYSTEMIC DRUGS AFFECTING THE EYE

Indomethacin

The incidence of corneal toxicity associated with indomethacin therapy is 11% to 16%. The corneal lesions appear as either fine stromal, speckled opacities or have a whorl-like distribution resembling that of chloroquine keratopathy. These changes diminish or disappear within 6 months after discontinuing indomethacin. No definite relationship has been established between dosage of drug and corneal changes.

Photosensitizing Drugs

Photosensitizing drugs are compounds that absorb optical radiation and undergo a photochemical reaction, resulting in chemical modifications of tissue. The psoralen compounds are classic examples of photosensitizing drugs and are widely used by dermatologists to treat psoriasis and vitiligo. This treatment, commonly referred to as PUVA therapy, involves administering methoxsalen (*Oxsoralen*) or related compounds, followed by exposure to UV radiation. Cataract formation is well documented in patients undergoing PUVA therapy.

Gold Salts

Following prolonged administration, gold salts can be deposited in various tissues of the body, a condition known as chrysiasis. Ocular chrysiasis can involve the conjunctiva, cornea, and lens. Corneal chrysiasis consists of numerous gold deposits that appear as yellowish-brown, violet, or red particles distributed irregularly in the stroma. The deposition of gold usually spares the peripheral 1 to 3 mm and superior ¼ to ½ of the cornea, and the deposits tend to localize to the posterior stroma. Lenticular chrysiasis appears as fine dust-like, yellowish, glistening deposits in the anterior capsule or anterior subcapsular region.

Corticosteroids

Systemic steroids can produce posterior subcapsular (PSC) cataracts that are clinically indistinguishable from complicated cataracts and cataracts caused by exposure to ionizing radiation. They often cannot be distinguished from age-related PSC cataracts. Even if the steroid dosage is reduced or discontinued, the cataract usually remains unchanged. Visual impairment is rare in patients with steroid-induced PSC cataracts. Most patients retain visual acuity of 20/40 or better, but patients may report light sensitivity, frank photophobia, reading difficulty, or glare. Inhaled steroids may be associated with increased risk of cataract.

Amiodarone

Cases of optic neuropathy or optic neuritis, usually resulting in visual impairment, have occurred in patients treated with amiodarone. In some cases, visual impairment has progressed to permanent blindness. Optic neuropathy or neuritis may occur at any time following initiation of therapy. A causal relationship to the drug has not been clearly established. If symptoms of visual impairment appear, prompt ophthalmic examination is recommended. Appearance of optic neuropathy or neuritis calls for reevaluation of therapy. Regular ophthalmic examination, including fundoscopy and split lamp examination, is recommended during administration of amiodarone. Amiodarone causes a distinctive keratopathy early in the course of treatment. The onset may be as early as 6 days following initiation of treatment, but it more commonly appears after 1 to 3 months of therapy. Virtually all patients will demonstrate corneal changes after 3 months of treatment. The corneal deposits are bilateral and are initially similar to the horizontal configuration of a Hudson-Stahli line, but eventually assume the configuration of a whorl-like opacity in the corneal epithelium. Once amiodarone therapy is discontinued, the keratopathy gradually resolves within 6 to 18 months. Lenticular opacities generally cause no visual symptoms, but moderate-to-severe keratopathy can lead to complaints of blurred vision, glare, and halos around lights or light sensitivity. Visual acuity is usually normal.

DRUGS AFFECTING THE CONJUNCTIVA AND LIDS

Isotretinoin

Ocular complications of isotretinoin (*Accutane*) include blepharoconjunctivitis, dry eye symptoms, contact lens intolerance, and subepithelial corneal opacities. There appears to be a dose-dependent relationship between isotretinoin therapy and blepharoconjunctivitis.

Chlorpromazine

Discoloration of the conjunctiva, sclera, and exposed skin has been reported with phenothiazine therapy. The discoloration is usually slate blue. Melanin-like granules have been observed in the superficial dermis.

Minocycline

Reports of blue, blue-gray, dark blue, or brownish sclera. This is an indication to stop the drug because these have been associated with irreversible papilledema, possibly more frequently than tetracycline because of minocycline's greater lipid solubility. May aggravate sicca or cause irritation in contact lens wearers. Subconjunctival drug concentration or yellow stain of preexisting calcium concentrations.

Tetracyclines

Conjunctival deposits similar to those seen in epinephrine-treated glaucoma patients have been reported in patients treated with oral tetracycline. These deposits appear as dark-brown to black granules in the palpebral conjunctiva. When observed under ultraviolet light, the brown pigment concentrations give a yellow fluorescence characteristic of tetracycline.

DRUGS THAT DECREASE AQUEOUS TEAR SECRETION

Anticholinergics

Dryness of mucous membranes is a common side effect of anticholinergic drugs because atropine and related agents inhibit glandular secretion in a dose-dependent manner.

Antihistamines

H_1 antihistamines have varying degrees of atropine-like actions, including the ability to alter tear film integrity. Both aqueous and mucin production may decrease with use of systemic antihistamines.

SYSTEMIC DRUGS AFFECTING THE EYE

Isotretinoin

Dry eye symptoms are commonly reported with use of isotretinoin. The incidence has been estimated to be as high as 20%, and ≈ 8% of patients experience contact lens intolerance.

Beta Blockers

Reduced tear secretion is a reported side effect of oral β-blockers. Most of the reported cases have occurred with practolol (not available in the US), but other β-blockers have also been implicated in patients with dry eye syndrome.

DRUGS CAUSING MYDRIASIS

The iris is an excellent indicator of autonomic activity because of the delicate balance between adrenergic and cholinergic innervation to the iris dilator and sphincter muscles, respectively. Adrenergic and cholinergic agents can thus easily influence pupil size and activity.

Anticholinergics

Drugs with pronounced anticholinergic action, such as *atropine* or related compounds, can cause significant mydriasis. Systemic administration of ≥ 2 mg of atropine can cause pupillary dilation and cycloplegia. Both mydriasis and reduced pupillary light response can occur when transdermal scopolamine (*Transderm Scōp*) is used for ≥ 3 days. This usually occurs through direct contamination of the eye by rubbing with fingers following application of the patch.

Central Nervous System Stimulants

CNS stimulants, such as amphetamines, methylphenidate, and cocaine, can cause mydriasis. Likewise, CNS depressants, such as phenobarbital and antianxiety agents, can dilate the pupil through their action on the adrenergic division of the autonomic nervous system.

DRUGS CAUSING MIOSIS

Opiates (eg, heroin, morphine, codeine) characteristically constrict the pupil. Systemically administered anticholinesterase agents can also cause miosis.

DRUGS AFFECTING EXTRAOCULAR MUSCLES

Drugs that affect the autonomic nervous system or central vestibular system or cause extrapyramidal effects may cause nystagmus, diplopia, extraocular muscle palsy, or oculogyric crisis. Nystagmus can be caused by intoxication with salicylates, phenytoin, antihistamines, gold salts, and barbiturates. Diplopia has been associated with phenothiazines, antianxiety agents, and antidepressants. Alcohol can impair both smooth pursuits and saccades.

DRUGS CAUSING MYOPIA

Systemically administered sulfonamides can induce transient myopia. The myopia is acute in onset and subsides within days or weeks following withdrawal of the medication. Diuretics and carbonic anhydrase inhibitors may also cause myopia. Variable glaucoma control in diabetes can produce intermittant myopia.

DRUGS CAUSING CYCLOPLEGIA

Drugs with mild anticholinergic properties (eg, antianxiety agents, antihistamines, tricyclic antidepressants) and agents with strong anticholinergic effects (eg, atropine, scopolamine), can dilate the pupil and cause dry eye symptoms, but the cycloplegic effects are less commonly encountered in clinical practice. The drugs most commonly associated with clinical cycloplegia include chloroquine and phenothiazines.

DRUGS AFFECTING INTRAOCULAR PRESSURE

Drugs known to be capable of dilating the pupil can cause acute or subacute angle-closure glaucoma if the anterior chamber angle is narrow. Steroids are widely known to elevate intraocular pressure in the presence of open angles. Other drugs, such as β-blockers, also can reduce intraocular pressure.

DRUGS AFFECTING THE RETINA

Chloroquine and Hydroxychloroquine

Chloroquine maculopathy consists of a granular hyperpigmentation surrounded by a zone of depigmentation, which is surrounded by another ring of pigment. This clinical picture can vary in intensity, but is characteristic of chloroquine retinopathy and is referred to as a "bull's eye" lesion. Variations of pigmentary disturbances can occur, and some patients may show retinal changes resembling retinitis pigmentosa.

Thioridazine

Thioridazine can cause significant retinal toxicity, leading to reduced visual acuity, color vision changes, and disturbances of dark adaptation. These symptoms usually occur 30 to 90 days after initiation of treatment. Fundus appearance is often normal during the early stages, but within several weeks or months a pigmentary retinopathy develops, characterized by clumps of pigment developing first in the periphery and then progressing toward the posterior pole.

Quinine

Acute vision loss is common in quinine toxicity (eg, overdose due to attempted suicide) and frequently consists of a clinical presentation of no light perception along with dilated and nonreactive pupils. In the early stages, visual fields usually demonstrate concentric contraction. Improvement of the visual fields may require days or months, but the field loss can sometimes become permanent.

Talc

Medication tablets intended for oral use contain inert filler materials, such as talc (magnesium silicate), cornstarch, cotton fibers, and other substances. Chronic drug abusers may prepare a suspension of medication for injection by dissolving a crushed tablet of cocaine, methylphenidate, codeine, or other narcotic in water. The solution is then boiled and filtered through a crude cigarette or cotton filter prior to injection. The talc particles eventually embolize to the retinal circulation and produce a characteristic form of retinopathy. Multiple, tiny, yellow-white, glistening particles are scat-

SYSTEMIC DRUGS AFFECTING THE EYE

tered throughout the posterior pole and are more numerous in the capillary bed and small arterioles of the perimacular area. Retinal neovascularization can also occur.

Digitalis Glycosides

Digitoxin and digoxin can cause changes in color vision and impairment of vision. Various visual phenomena often precede cardiac abnormalities as the earliest symptoms of digitoxin intoxication. A common symptom is snowy vision, wherein objects appear to be covered with frost or snow.

Indomethacin

Indomethacin can induce pigmentary changes of the macula and other areas of the retina. The lesions usually consist of discrete pigment scattering and fine areas of depigmentation around the macula.

Tamoxifen

Tamoxifen can cause white or yellow refractile opacities in the macular and paramacular area, with or without macular edema. The patient can experience reduced visual acuity associated with the macular lesions, and the visual fields can demonstrate abnormalities.

Isotretinoin

Isotretinoin therapy in dosages of 1 mg/kg body weight daily can impair dark adaptation, with or without excessive glare sensitivity. Once therapy is discontinued, both the abnormal dark adaptation and abnormal electroretinogram (ERG) usually resolve within several months.

Sildenafil

Sildenafil (*Viagra*) can cause retinal dysfunction and affect vision function for > 5 hours. Visual disturbances include bluish color tinge, light sensitivity, and blurred vision. There is no safety information on the administration of sildenafil to patients with retinitis pigmentosa; administer with caution to these patients.

Vigabatrin

Vigabatrin can cause symptomatic or asymptomatic field loss, mainly bilateral concentric peripheral constriction with variable degree of visual field defects. Cases of tunnel vision have occurred.

DRUGS AFFECTING THE OPTIC NERVE

Amiodarone

Optic neuropathy occurs in $\approx$ 2% of patients taking this drug. The optic nerve appearance is characterized by disc swelling with or without parapapillary disc hemorrhages.

Ethambutol

Ethambutol can cause ocular symptoms of reduced visual acuity, color vision changes, and visual field loss. Signs of ocular toxicity can appear several weeks following initial therapy, but the onset of ocular complications usually occurs several months after treatment is begun. The primary ocular manifestation of ethambutol toxicity is retrobulbar neuritis.

Chloramphenicol

Chloramphenicol causes both optic neuritis and retrobulbar neuritis. There is severe bilateral reduction of visual acuity accompanied by dense central scotomas. The optic discs are usually edematous and hyperemic, the retinal veins are engorged and tortuous, and hemorrhages are often seen. Optic atrophy is a late complication.

Jimmy D. Bartlett OD, DOS
University of Alabama at Birmingham

For More Information

Bartlett JD, Jaanus SD, eds. Clinical Ocular Pharmacology, ed. 4. Boston: Butterworth-Heinemann, 2001.

Bartlett JD. Ophthalmic toxicity by systemic drugs. In: Chiou GCH, ed. Ophthalmic Toxicology, ed 2. Philadelphia: Taylor and Francis, Inc. 1999;Chap 6.

Fraunfelder FT. Drug Induced ocular side effects and drug interactions, ed. 4. Philadelphia: Lea & Febiger, 1995.

Fraunfelder FT, Meyer SM. The national registry of drug-induced ocular side effects. *J Toxicol Cutaneous Ocul Toxicol*1982;1:65.

Grant WM. Toxicology of the Eye, ed. 4. Springfield, IL: Charles C. Thomas, 1993.

Koneru PB, et al. Oculotoxicities of systemically administered drugs. *J Ocul Toxicol* 1986;2:385.

Systemic Medications Used for Ocular Conditions

Topical, peribulbar, or intraocular drug administration may not be effective routes of administration for treatment of all eye diseases. Systemic medication is often required to achieve effective concentrations of drug in and around the ocular tissues. Included in this chapter are the more common indications and systemic medications employed for the treatment of these ocular conditions. Dosages may vary depending upon patient response, new recommendations, and guidelines. Some conditions require concurrent treatment by other routes of administration (eg, topical drops, subconjunctival or intravitreal injections).

ANTIMICROBIAL AGENTS

Antimicrobial agents may be given by topical, intraocular, peribulbar, and systemic routes of administration. Systemic antimicrobial agents are used for anterior segment, posterior segment or orbital infections, often in conjunction with topical treatment. Duration of treatment may vary, although generally 7 to 14 days is adequate in most cases. The etiology of the various conditions may vary, but the more prevalent causes are listed.

340 — OPHTHALMIC DRUG FACTS

Antibacterials				
Condition	Etiology	Antibiotic	Dose	Comment
Blepharitis/ meibomian gland/ acne rosacea	*Staphylococcal* species	Tetracycline	250 to 500 mg orally every 6 hours. May be reduced to 250 mg daily in some cases.	Not for antibacterial effect. Reduces free fatty acid byproducts. Tetracycline is contraindicated in pregnancy and in children < 10 years of age. Treat for ≥ 1 month for meibomian gland dysfunction.
		Doxycycline	50 to 100 mg 1 to 2 times/day	
Internal hordeolum	*Staphylococcal* species	Dicloxacillin	250 mg orally every 6 hours	Use with caution in penicillin allergy.
		Cephalexin	250 to 500 mg orally every 6 hours	Use with caution in penicillin allergy.
Acute dacryocystitis	*Staphylococcal* sp., *pneumoniae* *H. influenzae*	Dicloxacillin	250 mg orally every 6 hours	Use with caution in penicillin allergy.
		Cephalexin	250 to 500 mg orally every 6 hours	Use with caution in penicillin allergy.
		Amoxicillin/ Clavulanate (*Augmentin*)	125 to 250 mg orally every 8 hours	Amoxicillin/clavulanate is recommended in children. (*H. influenzae*)
Conjunctivitis	*Gonococcal*[1] (ophthalmic)	Ceftriaxone		
		neonatal	25 to 50 mg/kg, up to 125 mg IV or IM	AAO practice standards require daily injections for 7 days.
		adult	1 gram IV or IM daily	May treat up to 5 days.
		Cefixime (*Suprax*)	400 mg orally for 1 dose	Ciprofloxacin 500 mg or ofloxacin 400 mg is also indicated as single-dose treatment.
	Chlamydial[1] (adult inclusion)	Doxycycline	100 mg orally twice daily	Treat for ≥ 3 weeks.
		Tetracycline	500 mg orally 3 times daily	Treat for ≥ 3 weeks.
		Erythromycin	500 mg orally 4 times daily	Treat for ≥ 3 weeks.
		Ofloxacin (*Floxin*)	300 mg orally twice daily	Treat for 7 days.
		Azithromycin (*Zithromax*)	1 gram orally once daily	Azithromycin may require only single dose.
	(neonatal inclusion)	Erythromycin	50 mg/kg/day orally in 4 divided doses	Treat for 14 days.
	H. influenza	Amoxicillin	125 to 250 mg orally every 8 hours	Often used in conjunction with topical therapy.
Keratitis	*Pseudomonas* (various others possible)	Gentamicin	3 m/kg every 8 hours (request peak& trough serum levels)	Use if pending scleral involvement. Antibiotic selection depends upon organism isolated.
Lid trauma/ oculoplastics procedures	*Staphylococcus, Streptococcus, H. influenzae,* etc.	Cephalexin	250 to 500 mg orally every 6 hours	Prophylaxis
		Dicloxacillin	250 to 500 mg orally every 6 hours	
		Amoxicillin/ Clavulanate (*Augmentin*)	125 to 500 mg orally every 8 hours	Suggest amoxicillin/ clavulanate if *H. influenzae* is suspected (more often in children).
Preseptal cellulitis	*Streptococcus, H. influenzae, Staphylococcus,* etc.	Amoxicillin/ Clavulanate	250 to 875 mg orally 2 to 3 times daily	Oral antibiotics may be sufficient.

SYSTEMIC MEDICATIONS USED FOR OCULAR CONDITIONS

341

Antibacterials				
Condition	**Etiology**	**Antibiotic**	**Dose**	**Comment**
Orbital cellulitis	*Streptococcus, H. influenzae, Staphylococcus,* etc.	Ceftriaxone and antistaphylococcal penicillins (*Nafcillin*)	1 > IV every 12 hours 1 to 2 > IV every 4 to 6 hours	IV therapy is required.
Endophthalmitis/ penetrating eye injury prophylaxis	*Staphylococcus, Streptococcus Bacillus,* etc.	Aminoglycoside and cefazolin	Gentamicin 3 mg/kg every 8 hours and cefazolin 1 g every 8 hours	Not all clinicians use systemic therapy.
Retinitis	*Toxoplasmosis*	Sulfadiazine and	1 > orally every 6 hours	Watch for sulfa hypersensitivity. Treat for 3 to 6 weeks.
		Pyrimethamine (*Daraprim* and)	25 mg orally 1 to 2 times/day (loading dose 75 mg)	May need folinic acid to prevent bone marrow depression; treat for 3 to 6 weeks.
		Clindamycin (optional)	300 mg orally every 6 hours	Treat for 3 to 6 weeks; pseudomembranous colitis is a risk.
Neurosyphilis	*Treponema pallidum*	Aqueous crystalline penicillin G	12 MU/day IV for 10 days	Caution if allergies; in HIV up to 24 MU/day for 14 to 21 days. CNS toxicity in doses > 20 MU/day.
		Ceftriaxone	1 > daily IV or IM for 14 days	

[1] Recommend concurrent treatment for gonorrhea and chlamydia.

Antivirals				
Condition	**Etiology**	**Antiviral**	**Dose**	**Comment**
Keratitis/ keratoconjunctivitis	Herpes zoster	Acyclovir (*Zovirax*)	600 to 800 orally 5 times daily for 7 to 10 days	Best if used within 72 hours of onset.
		Valacyclovir (*Valtrex*)	1000 mg orally 3 times daily for 7 days	Best if used within 72 hours of onset.
		Famciclovir (*Famivr*)	500 mg orally 3 times daily for 7 days	Best if used within 72 hours of onset.
Cytomegalovirus (CMV) Retinitis		Ganciclovir	IV-induction - 5 mg/kg every 12 hours for 14 to 21 days; maintenance 5 mg/kg every day or 6 mg/kg 5 days/week	Bone marrow suppression; granulocytopenia, thrombocytopenia. Dosing may vary with renal impairment.
			Oral capsule - 1000 mg 3 times daily	Maintenance
		Foscarnet (*Foscavir*)	IV-induction - 60 mg/kg every day, maintenance - 90 to 120 mg/kg every day	Renal toxicity, adjust for dose. Other side effects include headache, nausea, vomiting.
		Cidofovir (*Vistide*)	IV-5 mg/kg once per week for 2 weeks then 5 mg/kg every 2 weeks	IV saline and oral probenecid given before and after each dose; dosage reduction required with increased serum creatinine.
Varicella or Herpes Simplex (ARN; PORN)		Acyclovir (*Zovirax*)	IV - 14 mg/kg every 8 hours (or 1500 mg/m^2)	Adequate hydration is essential.

OPHTHALMIC DRUG FACTS

Antifungals[1]				
Condition	Etiology	Antifungals[1]	Dose	Comment
Endophthalmitis	Candida, Aspergillus, Fusarium, etc.	Itraconazole (Sporanox)	200 to 400 mg orally twice a day	Monitor liver function tests (LFTs).
		Ketoconazole (Vizoral)	200 mg orally every 6 to 8 hours	Monitor LFTs.
		Amphotericin B	0.5 to 0.8 mg/kg/day IV	More effective in endogenous type. Systemic toxicity (eg, hypokalemia, chills, nausea, vomiting) Liposomal preparation causes fewer side effects.
		Fluconazole (Diflucan)	100 to 200 mg orally 1 to 2 times/day (or IV)	Well tolerated, minimal side effects. Antifungal spectrum limited.
		Flucytosine (Ancobon)	50 to 150 mg/kg/day orally in 4 doses	Not used alone because of potential resistance.

[1] Rifampin 600 mg/day has been added to regimen to supplement antifungal activity. Various protocols and combinations have been used. Most have not been studied adequately to recommend one regimen or antifungal agent over another. Some clinicians may add systemic antifungal agents to supplement treatment of fungal keratitis.

ANALGESICS

Various types of systemic analgesics may be used for pain. Nonnarcotic analgesics may be sufficient for minor eye pain. Acetaminophen and NSAIDs (eg, ibuprofen, aspirin, naproxen) are also commonly used. Narcotic-containing medications such as acetaminophen with codeine (*Tylenol #3*) or acetaminophen with hydrocodone (*Vicodin*) may be required for more severe pain. Pain will vary significantly among individuals. Therefore, careful assessment is required by the clinician to determine the appropriate amount of pain relief the patient may require.

Narcotic Analgesics				
Condition	Etiology	Analgesic	Dose	Comment
Keratitis	PRK/RK Corneal abrasions	Acetaminophen with codeine 30 mg (narcotic)	1 to 2 tablets every 4 to 6 hours	Short-term control of severe eye pain. May cause drowsiness, nausea, or constipation.
		Acetaminophen with hydrocodone 5 to 7.5 mg	1 to 2 tablets every 4 to 6 hours	Short-term control of severe eye pain. May cause drowsiness, nausea, or constipation.

Non-Narcotic Analgesics				
Condition	Etiology	Analgesic	Dose	Comment
Keratitis	Epithelial defect General eye pain	Acetaminophen 500 mg	1 to 2 tablets every 4 to 6 hours	For mild eye pain
		Ketorolac (Toradol) 10 mg	1 tablet every 4 to 6 hours (40 mg/day maximum)	Not to exceed 5 days combined IM/IV and PO GI bleeding.
		Ibuprofen 200 mg (otc)	1 to 2 tablets every 4 to 6 hours	Take with food. Some bleeding risk.
		Tramadol (Ultram) 50 mg	1 to 2 tablets every 6 hours (400 mg/day maximum)	Drowsiness; potential for abuse.

SYSTEMIC MEDICATIONS USED FOR OCULAR CONDITIONS

ANTIHISTAMINES

The systemic administration of antihistamines for signs or symptoms of seasonal allergies may benefit patients with ocular symptoms. Patients may not require topical medication for treatment of conjunctivitis if systemic antihistamines control or alleviate both systemic and ocular symptoms. Some patients do not wish to take systemic antihistamines; therefore, local treatment with various topical agents may be preferred. Other patients receiving systemic antihistamines may require supplemental therapy with topical medication to achieve adequate control of ocular symptoms.

Non-sedating antihistamines			
Condition	Etiology	Antihistamine	Dose
Conjunctivitis	Seasonal allergic	Loratadine (*Claritin*)	10 mg every day
		Cetirazine (*Zyrtec*)	10 mg every day
		Fexofenadine (*Allegra*)[1]	60 mg twice daily

[1] Non-sedating antihistamines may interact with erythromycin, antifungals, phenytoin, or cyclosporine. May cause cardiac toxicity (torsades de pointes).

Sedating antihistamines				
Condition	Etiology	Antihistamine	Dose	Comment
Conjunctivitis	Seasonal allergic	Chlorpheniramine	4 to 12 mg every 4 to 12 hours	Sedation may be a problem
		Diphenhydramine	25 to 50 mg every 4 to 6 hours	
		Many others		Sedation

ANTI-INFLAMMATORY AGENTS

Systemic corticosteroids have been used in many ocular conditions' is not limited to the conditions below, because systemic NSAIDs probably do not penetrate the eye in sufficient levels to provide good intraocular anti-inflammatory effect and have somewhat limited application. Generally, however, immunosuppressive agents are reserved for more severe or unresponsive conditions.

Corticosteroids				
Condition	Etiology	Corticosteroid	Dose	Comment
Scleritis	Autoimmune vascular-collagen disease (eg, arthritis, SLE, Wegener) Other etiologies include infectious, metabolic, or granulomatous diseases	Prednisone	Variable - 20 to 100 mg/day	Watch for side effects, including rebound inflammation, psychosis, electrolyte disturbance, peptic ulcer aggravation, hyperglycemia, asceptic necrosis, hypertension, pancreatitis. Informed consent requires review with patient.
Hyphema	Trauma Red blood cells	Prednisone	20 mg twice daily (adult)	Decreasing dose in children.
Keratitis	Viral/bacterial	Prednisone	20 to 60 mg/day	If infection is not under control or if topical steroids cannot be used (ie, with an epithelial defect).
Vitritis	Post-op membrane	Prednisone	20 to 100 mg/day	Short course under 2 weeks; taper dose to prevent rebound inflammation.

OPHTHALMIC DRUG FACTS

Corticosteroids				
Condition	**Etiology**	**Corticosteroid**	**Dose**	**Comment**
Retinitis	Toxoplasmosis	Prednisone	20 to 100 mg/day	Used if impending macular involvement or severe posterior segment inflammation.
Optic neuropathy	Traumatic	Methylprednisolone	30 mg/kg loading dose then, starting 2 hours later, 15 mg/kg every 6 hours, usually for a maximum of 3 to 5 days	Megadose steroid Watch for side effects (hyperglycemia, steroid psychosis, aggravation of peptic ulcer, rebound inflammation,electrolyte imbalance).
Neuritis	Demyelinizing Optic	Methylprednisolone	250 mg every 6 hours for 3 days IV followed by oral prednisone 1 mg/kg/day for 11 days	Same as megadose

Nonsteroidal Anti-inflammatory Drugs (NSAIDs)				
Condition	**Etiology**	**NSAID**	**Dose**	**Comment**
Conjunctivitis	Vernal	Aspirin 325 mg	650 mg 3 times daily	May give additional relief with topical mast cell stabilizers or steroids.
Scleritis	Diffuse or nodular; necrotizing	Indomethacin	75 to 150 mg/day	Take with food; combination with prednisone 60 to 80 mg/day is more effectivethan either alone.
		Ibuprofen	400-800 mg/day 3 to 4 times per day (2400 mg max)	Take with food
		Naproxen	250 to 500 mg 2 to 3 times per day	Take with food
Myositis	Idiopathic orbital	Indomethacin	25 to 50 mg 3 times/ day	Not used often

IMMUNOSUPPRESSIVE AGENTS

Many of the immunosuppressive agents listed below have been used in treating other autoimmune-related diseases in addition to those listed. Most are reserved for cases unresponsive to initial therapy because of concerns for increased systemic toxicity and vigilant monitoring that is required. Doses may vary because extensive clinical studies are lacking.

Immunosuppressive Agents				
Condition	**Etiology**	**Agent**	**Dose**	**Comment**
Uveitis	Unknown Autoimmune	Azothioprine[1]	1 to 2.5 mg/kg/day orally (50 mg 3 times daily)	Bone marrow depression, nausea, vomiting
		Bromocriptine	Variable	Headache, nausea, vomiting, fatigue, dizziness
		Cyclosporine A[1] (eg, *Neoral*)	4 to 5 mg/kg/day orally (variable)	Nephrotoxicity, hypertension, gingival hyperplasia, hypertrichosis, etc
		Methotrexate	12.5 to 15 mg/week	Watch for bone marrow depression, nausea, vomiting, pneumonitis

SYSTEMIC MEDICATIONS USED FOR OCULAR CONDITIONS 345

Immunosuppressive Agents				
Condition	**Etiology**	**Agent**	**Dose**	**Comment**
Cicatricia pemphigoid	Unknown	Dapsone	25 mg/day orally for week 1, increase to 50 mg/day variable dosing	Hemolytic anemia, nausea, vomiting, anorexia, methemoglobinemia
		Azathioprine (*Imuran*)	1 to 2 mg/kg/day orally	Bone marrow depression, nausea, vomiting Often combined with corticosteroids
		Cyclophosphamide[1] (eg, *Cytoxan*)	2 to 3 mg/kg/day orally	Hemorrhagic cystitis, nausea, vomiting, alopecia, thrombocytopenia
Behçet syndrome	Unknown	Chlorambucil (*Leukeran*)	Up to 2.5 mg orally 4 times daily	Bone marrow depression, mutagenicity; start with low dose, increase slowly
		Colchicine	1 to 1.5 mg/day orally	Nausea, vomiting, diarrhea

[1] Also used in Behçet syndrome.

AMINOCAPROIC ACID

Aminocaproic acid (*Amicar*) is an antifibrinolytic agent used orally for the prevention of secondary rebleeds in traumatic hyphemas. Corticosteroids may also be effective, cost less, and exhibit fewer side effects than aminocaproic acid.

Aminocaproic Acid				
Condition	**Etiology**	**Drug**	**Dose**	**Comment**
Hyphema	Traumatic	Aminocaproic acid (*Amicar*)	50 mg/kg orally every 4 hours for 5 days; not to exceed 5 > every 4 hours (max 30 g/day)	Treat for 5 days Nausea, vomiting, hypotension

OCULAR HYPOTENSIVE AGENTS

Systemic ocular hypotensive agents are some of the most effective agents for decreasing intraocular pressure (IOP). Carbonic anhydrase inhibitors effectively decrease IOP, but are associated with various systemic side effects. Hyperosmotic agents are especially effective in reducing very elevated IOPs, although the underlying cause must be corrected to prevent rebound increase in IOP. Hyperosmotic agents are generally indicated for short-term control of IOP because their effects last for 6 to 8 hours.

Carbonic Anhydrase Inhibitors				
Condition	**Etiology**	**CAI**	**Dose**	**Comment**
Glaucoma	Open-angle	Acetazolamide	125 to 500 mg orally every 6 to 12 hours	Systemic side effects include GI intolerance, paresthesias, hypokalemia, CNS (drowsiness, lethargy, depression), renal stones, sulfa hypersensitivity, etc.
		Methazolamide	25 to 50 mg orally 2 to 3 times daily	Same as acetazolamide, more CNS, fewer GI effects.
	Acute	Acetazolamide	500 mg injectable IV	Systemic side effects include GI intolerance, parasthesias, hypokalemia, CNS (drowsiness, lethargy, depression), renal stones, sulfa hypersensitivity, etc.

OPHTHALMIC DRUG FACTS

Hyperosmotic Agents				
Condition	Etiology	Osmotic Agent	Dose	Comment
Glaucoma	Acute Preoperative (to lower IOP)	Glycerin 50 to 75% (*Osmoglyn*)	1 to 1.5 g/kg orally	May cause hyperglycemia in diabetics Sweet taste may cause nausea and vomiting
		Isosorbide 45% (*Ismotic*)	1.5 to 2 g/kg orally	Causes less nausea and vomiting than glycerin
		Mannitol IV 15 to 25% (*Osmitrol*)	1.5 to 2 g/kg IV	Watch crystal formation; use with in-line IV filter, keep warm Infuse over 30 minutes Watch for electrolyte disturbances, thirst, diuresis, potential cardiovascular overload

VITAMINS/MINERALS

Various vitamins and minerals have established roles in the treatment of ophthalmic conditions. Others are not well documented.

Vitamin/ Minerals				
Condition	Etiology	Vitamin/Mineral	Dose	Comment
Dry eye/keratitis	Vitamin A deficiency	Vitamin A	50,000 U every day	Fat soluble vitamin, toxicity includes dry mucous membranes, increased eye irritation.
Optic Neuritis	Nutritional or toxic	Vitamin B_{12} hydroxycobalamin	1000 U IM daily, reduce dose to weekly then monthly	Cyanocobalamin may not be as effective.
	Drug toxicity (INH)	Pyridoxine (B_6)	50 mg/day	Often given concurrently with INH
Macular degeneration	Deficiency of antioxidant vitamins (eg, E, C, A) Zinc Selenium Copper	*Ocuvite, Icaps Plus-* various mfr.	1 tablet 1 to 2 times daily	Causative agent not well established; recent evidence has suggested beta-carotene may not be beneficial.

For More Information

Olin BR, Hebel SK, eds. Drug Facts & Comparisons. Facts & Comparisons. St. Louis: 1997.

Tabbara KF, Hyyndiuk RA, eds. Infections of the Eye, ed 2. Boston: Little, Brown and Company, 1996.

Bartlett JD, Jaanus SD, eds. Clinical Ocular Pharmacology, ed 4. Boston: Butterworth-Heinemann, 2001.

Sanford JP, Gilbert DN, Sande MA, eds. Guide to Antimicrobial Therapy. Dallas: Antimicrobial Therapy Inc., 1995.

Preferred Practice Pattern Series, American Academy of Ophthalmology, San Francisco CA.

Optometric Clinical Practice Guidelines, American Optometric Association, St. Louis MO.

DRUGS WITH OFF-LABELED OPHTHALMIC USES

For many years, the drug package insert was interpreted as a legal standard for drug use. However, the legal implications of the package insert have been challenged, and in some cases, various courts have recognized that drugs may be used for clinical indications other than those specified in the package insert. It is possible for prescribed dosage schedules to differ from those specified in the package insert if such a schedule is consistent with sound scientific rationale and medical practice.

Because it has been recognized that the package insert may not contain the most recent information about a drug, it is now generally agreed that the clinician should be free to use a drug for an indication not in the package insert if 2 conditions have been met:

1. Such use is part of the rational practice of medicine intended for the benefit of the patient;

2. Documented evidence exists for use of a drug in the manner prescribed.

When using an approved drug for an unlabeled purpose, the patient should be informed regarding the nature of the intended therapy, and the practitioner is advised to obtain the patient's written permission (informed consent) before beginning treatment. Since drug-related side effects are a significant cause of malpractice litigations, it is essential that patients understand the risks of potential side effects. In determining what constitutes sound medical practice in malpractice litigations, the package insert is admissible into evidence, but it does not establish conclusively the standards of acceptable practice or that departure from the directions contained in the package insert constitutes negligence. One of the best protections against unfavorable malpractice verdicts is to prescribe medications in the best interests of the patient according to rational standards of practice.

The drugs listed in the following table have been approved by the Food and Drug Administration (FDA), but not for the ophthalmic purposes listed. Each agent, however, has been documented to be useful for the diagnosis or therapy of certain ocular conditions.

OPHTHALMIC DRUG FACTS

Drugs With Unlabeled Ophthalmic Uses		
Generic (*Trade*)	Labeled Indication	Unlabeled Ophthalmic Use
Acetylcysteine (*Mucomyst*)	Mucolytic agent in bronchopulmonary conditions	Topical mucolytic treatment of vernal, giant papillary conjunctivitis, filamentary keratitis
Acyclovir (*Zovirax*)	Treatment of varicella-zoster and genital herpes simplex	Treatment of epithelial HSV keratitis
Aminocaproic acid (*Amicar*)	Antifibrinolytic agent for the treatment of excessive bleeding	Oral treatment of traumatic hyphema
Aspirin (eg, *Bayer*)	Anti-inflammatory, analgesic, antipyretic agent	Oral treatment of vernal conjunctivitis
Diclofenac sodium (*Voltaren*)	Treatment of postoperative cataract inflammation; photophobia associated with incisional refractive surgery, and pain associated with radial keratotomy	Anti-inflammatory treatment following argon laser trabeculoplasty, treatment of seasonal allergic conjunctivitis
Fluorescein sodium (eg, *Fluorescite*)	Topical or IV diagnostic ophthalmic dye	Oral fluorography for diagnosis of retinal vascular diseases
Ketorolac tromethamine (*Acular*)	Treatment of seasonal allergic conjunctivitis and post-cataract surgery inflammation	Treatment of pain associated with corneal trauma
Lodoxamide (*Alomide*)	Treatment of vernal keratoconjunctivitis	Treatment of seasonal allergic conjunctivitis
Polyhexamethylene biguanide	Swimming pool and contact lens disinfectant	Treatment of *Acanthamoeba* keratitis
Sodium hyaluronate (*Amvisc*) Chondroitin sulfate (*Viscoat*)	Viscoelastic agents in intraocular surgery	Topical treatment of severe dry eye disorders
Suprofen (*Profenal*)	Prevention of intraoperative miosis during cataract extraction	Topical treatment of contact lens-associated GPC

ACETYLCYSTEINE

Acetylcysteine (*Mucomyst*) has been approved for use as a mucolytic agent in acute and chronic bronchopulmonary conditions. The agent is administered by nebulization for its local effect on the bronchopulmonary tree. The product contains disodium edetate and sodium hydroxide and, therefore, has a significant odor accompanying its clinical use. When used on the eye, acetylcysteine dissolves mucous threads and decreases tear viscosity. The drug is commonly prepared for topical ocular use by diluting the commercial preparation to 2% to 5% in artificial tears or physiologic saline.

ACYCLOVIR

Acyclovir *(Zovirax)* has been approved for treatment of genital herpes simplex (HSV). During initial episodes of the disease, oral acyclovir can decrease the duration of viral shedding and healing time of the genital lesions, decrease the severity of symptoms, and reduce the development of new lesions. Acyclovir ointment is also approved for treatment of initial genital herpes, and acyclovir IV seems to be effective for severe initial episodes of the disease. Acyclovir is also the treatment of choice for biopsy-proven herpes simplex encephalitis. For HSV keratitis, 3% acyclovir ointment may be useful to treat epithelial involvement. Although acyclovir is effective in treating HSV epithelial keratitis, there is no clear superiority of the drug compared with other commercially available antiviral agents.

AMINOCAPROIC ACID

Aminocaproic acid *(Amicar)* is an antifibrinolytic agent approved for treatment of excessive bleeding from systemic hyperfibrinolysis and urinary fibrinolysis. The drug

DRUGS WITH OFF-LABELED OPHTHALMIC USES

may also be useful for the treatment of some patients with traumatic hyphema. Some studies have shown the drug to be effective in reducing the rate of rebleeding from ≈ 30% to 3% or 4%. Dosage is 100 mg/kg body weight every 4 hours to a maximum dose of 30 g/day. It may be possible to administer one-half of this dosage to reduce side effects while maintaining efficacy. It has been established that the drug is ineffective in children.

ASPIRIN

The efficacy of salicylates in the treatment of ocular inflammation has been infrequently studied in human models, but several reports have suggested that aspirin may be valuable for intractable cases of vernal conjunctivitis. Patients who remain symptomatic following treatment with cromolyn sodium, steroids, or a combination of agents may demonstrate improvement in signs and symptoms when aspirin is added to the therapeutic regimen.

DICLOFENAC SODIUM

Diclofenac sodium (*Voltaren*) is a topically applied nonsteroidal anti-inflammatory agent that is currently approved for treatment of inflammation following cataract surgery. The drug is probably effective because of its antiprostaglandin mechanism. In a recent study, the anti-inflammatory effect of diclofenac was evaluated following argon laser trabeculoplasty (ALT). Diclofenac or placebo drops were given once before and after trabeculoplasty and then 4 times daily for 4 days. The increase of anterior chamber flare was completely inhibited by topical diclofenac. Therefore, 0.1% diclofenac may represent an effective anti-inflammatory therapy following ALT. Studies have also demonstrated the safety and efficacy of topical diclofenac for treatment of seasonal allergic conjunctivitis and pain associated with corneal refractive surgery. Diclofenac is helpful in recurrent erosion pain, after PRK or PTK (use steroids and antibiotic in the presence of an epithelial defect).

FLUORESCEIN SODIUM

Fluorescein sodium (eg, *Fluorescite*) is approved for topical and IV use (see Ophthalmic Dyes chapter). Oral fluorography was reintroduced in 1979, allowing fluorescein studies without the potential systemic effects attributable to IV fluorescein. Various studies using oral fluorography have established this technique as a viable alternative for the diagnosis of certain retinal vascular diseases. The procedure is especially useful for conditions in which late dye leakage is expected. Oral fluorography is performed using either bulk powder fluorescein sodium USP or the commercially available vials of 10% injectable fluorescein sodium. The dosage typically used is 1000 to 1500 mg of fluorescein sodium mixed with a citrus drink and allowed to cool in crushed ice.

LIQUID PERFLUOROCARBONS

Liquid perfluorocarbons are heavier-than-water liquids that are used to push the retina against the back of the eye with the patient in the supine position. They are clear, have low viscosity and low surface tension, and are immiscible with water. Their refractive indices vary; some are so close to aqueous that it is hard to see the interface between the perfluorocarbon and the aqueous. With others, the refractive index is significantly different from that of aqueous, and a clear meniscus is visible between the perfluorocarbon and the physiologic intraocular fluids or BSS. Some liquid perfluorocarbons are intended for intraoperative use only but others have been left in the eyes for prolonged periods of time.

They are ideally suited for unrolling the flap of a giant retinal tear. After vitrectomy, the perfluorocarbon can be injected by hand through a cannula whose tip is positioned posterior to, or under, the flap of the giant tear. As the perfluorocarbon flows into the eye, it will settle on the back of the retina, pushing it against the posterior choroid. Subretinal fluid will be displaced anteriorly and flow into the central vitreous cavity through the giant retinal tear as the perfluorocarbon is injected. Because of its low viscosity, the perfluorocarbon liquid may flow into the subretinal space if it is brought anterior to the edge of the tear. Commonly, a partial fill is used to partially unroll the tear, further vitrectomy is done to relieve traction on the anterior edge of the tear, and then more perfluorocarbon is added to further flatten the retina. Endolaser can be given through the perfluorocarbon. Gas is then infused into the eye through the pars plana infusion port as the perfluorocarbon is aspirated. Perfluorocarbons have vapor pressures that vary from < 1 to > 57. The residues of those with high vapor pressures do not need to be rinsed out because they quickly vaporize into the intraocular gas. If the vapor pressure is low, however, the inside of the retina should be rinsed with about 0.5 ml of BSS to remove residual perfluorocarbons. This rinse is then aspirated off the posterior retina.

Perfluorocarbons are also heavier than intraocular lenses. Therefore, they can be used to float a displaced intraocular lens off the posterior retina, probably making it safer and easier to reposition or remove. The injection of a perfluorocarbon may be especially helpful when there is a concomitant retinal detachment as the perfluorocarbons will simultaneously push the retina against the back of the eye, holding it away from the intraocular instruments, and lift the intraocular lens anteriorly.

Perfluorocarbons can be used to push the retina posteriorly in detachments complicated by fibrovascular tissue proliferation (eg, proliferative diabetic retinopathy) or by preretinal fibrous membranes (eg, massive periretinal proliferation). This can make the membranes easier to visualize and dissect in some cases. However, because of their low surface tension, the perfluorocarbon liquids will quickly flow through any posterior retinal breaks into the subretinal space if there is residual traction present around the breaks. An additional posterior retinotomy may then be made to remove the perfluorocarbon.

Some perfluorocarbons have been left in the eyes to provide prolonged tamponade of the inferior retina. Eventually the perfluorocarbon liquid must be removed in a second operation.

BIGUANIDE

Chlorhexidine, a biguanide compound (Zeneca Pharmaceuticals), is an antiseptic that is used to treat open wounds, gingivitis, and skin infections. It has been used by some clinicians to treat *Acanthamoeba* keratitis, usually in combination with propamidine isethionate drops 0.1%. Chlorhexidine 0.02% eyedrops are not commercially available and have to be extemporaneously compounded from a stock solution. Chlorhexidine 0.02% has been effective for treatment of *Acanthamoeba* keratitis that is unresponsive to polyhexamethylene biguanide (PHMB) 0.02%. Debate exists as to which compound, chlorhexidine or PHMB, is more effective for the treatment of *Acanthamoeba* keratitis.

Polyhexamethylene biguanide (PHMB) is a polymeric environmental disinfectant commonly used for disinfecting swimming pools and, more recently, as a contact lens disinfectant. This agent has a broad spectrum of activity, effective against both gram-positive and gram-negative bacteria. There have been recent reports of PHMB effectiveness in treatment of *Acanthamoeba* keratitis when conventional therapy has failed. When topical therapy employing propamidine and neomycin is ineffective,

DRUGS WITH OFF-LABELED OPHTHALMIC USES

treatment with topical PHMB may be successful. The formulation can be prepared, under sterile conditions, from the stock 20% solution and diluted 1:1000 for administration as a 0.02% solution.

VISCOELASTIC AGENTS

Sodium hyaluronate (*Amvisc*) and chondroitin sulfate (*Viscoat*), are approved as vitreous replacement substances and for use during intraocular surgery to protect the corneal endothelium. When prepared as a 0.1% topical solution in saline, sodium hyaluronate may be beneficial for patients with severe dry eye syndromes. The beneficial effects of sodium hyaluronate have been attributed to its viscoelastic properties, which lubricate and protect the ocular surface. Most patients achieve control of symptoms with topical instillation up to 4 times daily.

SUPROFEN

When used as a 1% solution, topically applied suprofen (*Profenal*), a propionic acid derivative, has been shown to be superior to placebo in the treatment of contact lens-associated giant papillary conjunctivitis (GPC). In a randomized, double-masked comparison, suprofen provided a greater reduction of signs and symptoms such as papillae and mucous strands.

Jimmy D. Bartlett OD, DOS
University of Alabama at Birmingham

For More Information

Absolon MJ, Brown S. Acetylcysteine in keratoconjunctivitis sicca. *Br J Ophthalmol* 1968;52:310.

Camacho H, Bajaire B, Mejia LF. Silicone oil in the management of giant retinal tears. *Ann Ophthalmol* 1992;24:45.

Cerqueti PM, et al. Lodoxamide treatment of allergic conjunctivitis. *Int Arch Allergy Appl Immunol* 1994;105:185.

Collum LMT, et al. Randomized double-blind trial of acyclovir and idoxuridine in dendritic corneal ulceration. *Br J Ophthalmol* 1980;64:766.

DeLuise VP, Peterson WS. The use of topical Healon tears in the management of refractory dry-eye syndrome. *Ann Ophthalmol*1984;1:823.

Donnenfeld ED, et al. Controlled evaluation of a bandage contact lens and a topical nonsteroidal anti-inflammatory drug in treating traumatic corneal abrasions. *Ophthalmology* 1995;102:979.

Eller AW, et al. A survey of intraocular silicone oil use in the United States. *Ophthalmology* 1992;99:1174.

Herbort CP, et al. Anti-inflammatory effect of diclofenac drops after argon laser trabeculoplasty. *Arch Ophthalmol*1993;111:481.

Hung SO, et al. Oral acyclovir in the management of dendritic herpetic corneal ulceration. *Br J Ophthalmol* 1984;68:398.

Irwin R. Practical aspects of oral fluorography. *J Ophthal Photog* 1981;4:16.

Jackson WB, et al. Treatment of herpes simplex keratitis: Comparison of acyclovir and vidarabine. *Can J Ophthalmol* 1984;19:107.

Kelley JS, Kincaid M. Retinal fluorography using oral fluorescein. *Arch Ophthalmol* 1979;97:2331.

Kraft SP, et al. Traumatic hyphema in children. Treatment with epsilon-aminocaproic acid. *Ophthalmology* 1987;94:1232.

Kutner B, et al. Aminocaproic acid reduces the risk of secondary hemorrhage in patients with traumatic hyphema. *Arch Ophthalmol* 1987;105:206.

Larkin DFP, et al. Treatment of *Acanthamoeba*keratitis with polyhexamethylene biguanide. *Ophthalmology* 1992;99:185.

Limberg MB, et al. Topical application of hyaluronic acid and chondroitin sulfate in treatment of dry eyes. *Am J Ophthalmol*1987;103:194.

McGetrick JJ, et al. Aminocaproic acid decreases secondary hemorrhage after traumatic hyphema. *Arch Ophthalmol* 1983;101:1031.

Mengher LS, et al. Effect of sodium hyaluronate (0.1%) on break-up time (NIBUT) in patients with dry eyes. *Br J Ophthalmol*1986;70:442.

Meyer E, et al. Efficacy of antiprostaglandin therapy in vernal conjunctivitis. *Br J Ophthalmol* 1987;71:497.

Mindel JS, Goldstein JI. Non-approved use of Food and Drug Administration approved drugs. *Am J Ophthalmol* 1979;88:626.

Noble MJ, Cheng H. Oral fluorescein and cystoid macular edema: Detection in aphakic and pseudophakic eyes. *Br J Ophthalmol*1984;68:221.

Palmer DJ, et al. A comparison of two dose regimens of epsilon aminocaproic acid in the prevention and management of secondary traumatic hyphemas. *Ophthalmology* 1986;93:102.

Potter JW, et al. Oral fluorography. *J Am Optom Assoc* 1985;56:784.

Roth SH. Drug use, the package insert, and the practice of medicine. *Arch Intern Med* 1982;142:871.

Stuart JC, Linn JG. Dilute sodium hyaluronate (Healon) in the treatment of ocular surface disorders. *Ann Ophthalmol*1985;17:190.

Wood TS, et al. Suprofen treatment of contact lens associated GPC. *Ophthalmology* 1988;96:822.

ORPHAN AND INVESTIGATIONAL DRUGS

In addition to the Food and Drug Administration (FDA) approved drugs and the drugs with unlabeled ophthalmic uses (see the Drugs with Off-labeled Ophthalmic Uses chapter), 2 other groups of drugs are of interest to eye care practitioners: Investigational New Drugs (INDs) and Orphan Drugs. INDs are drugs which are not approved by the FDA, but are being investigated by a pharmaceutical company or sponsor. Orphan drugs are drugs made available by manufacturers for the treatment of rare diseases.

ORPHAN DRUGS

The term "orphan drug" first appeared in the medical literature in a 1968 editorial. It was used to disclaim nonapproved substances as drugs and included compounds such as lithium carbonate, d-xylose, and sodium fluoride. These products were frequently labeled "for chemical purposes, not for drug use," "for research use only, not for clinical use," and "for manufacturing use only." The term "orphan drug" has since been applied to drugs and devices used in the treatment or diagnosis of rare diseases.

The FDA established the Office of Orphan Products Development in 1982. These products consist of drugs, biologicals (eg, vaccines), medical devices, and foods for the diagnosis, treatment, or prevention of rare diseases.

Government Incentives To Assist In Orphan Drug Development
♦ Developers of orphan drugs have 7 years of exclusive licensing, during which time the product may not be marketed by another company in the US without the sponsor's permission.
♦ Developers may claim up to 63% of the cost of clinical investigations as a tax credit.
♦ The FDA can grant up to $70,000 in support of a sponsor's orphan drug clinical research. The Orphan Drug Act authorizes $4,000,000 per year for these research grants.
♦ The FDA can assist sponsors of orphan drugs in the development of investigational guidelines and protocols.
♦ When appropriate, the FDA can modify approval requirements for specific orphan drugs (eg, modify the size of study populations).
♦ The FDA can assign to orphan drugs a high review priority. The review phase (time from a new drug application submission to approval) for 9 orphan drugs receiving approval in 1985 and 1986 was 2.7 years.

Tatro, DS. Orphan drugs. *Drug Newsletter* 1988 Apr;7(4):26.

Ophthalmic drugs established by the FDA as Orphan Drugs are listed in the following table.

OPHTHALMIC DRUG FACTS

Orphan Drugs		
Drug Generic (*Trade*)	**Indication**	**Manufacturer/Sponsor**
9-cis-retinoic acid	Prevention of retinal detachment caused by proliferative vitreoetinopathy.	Allergan, Inc. P.O. Box 19534 Irvine, CA 92612
Al-RSA	Treatment of autoimmune uveitis.	AutoImmune, Inc. 128 Spring St. Lexington, MA 02173
Aminocaproic acid (*Caprogel*)	For the topical treatment of traumatic hyphema of the eye.	Eastern Virginia Medical School P.O. Box 1980 Norfolk, VA 23501
Botulinum toxin type A (*Botox*)	Treatment of strabismus associated with dystonia in adults (patients ≥ 12 years of age)	Allergan, Inc. P.O. Box 19534 Irvine, CA 92612
Botulinum toxin type F (*Dysport*)	Treatment of essential blepharospasm.	Ipsen Limited
Brimonidine (*Aplhagan*)	Treatment of anterior ischemic optic neuropathy.	Allergan, Inc. P.O. Box 19534 Irvine, CA 92612
Cromolyn sodium 4% ophthalmic solution (*Opticrom 4% ophthalmic solution*)	Treatment of vernal keratoconjuctivitis.	Fisons Corp. P.O. Box 1710 Rochester, NY 14603
Dexamethasone	For use in posterior segment drug delivery system in the treatment of idiopathic intermediate uveitis.	Oculex Pharmaceuticals, Inc. 601 W. California St. Sunnyvale, CA 94086
Dextran 70 (*Dehydrex*)	Treatment of recurrent corneal erosion unresponsive to conventional therapy.	Holles Laboratories, Inc. 30 Forest Notch Cohasset, MA 02025
Flucinolone	Treatment of uveitis involving the posterior segment of the eye.	Bausch & Lomb Eye Care P.O. Box 450 Rochester, NY 14604
Gangliosides as sodium salts (*Cronassial*)	Treatment of retinitis pigmentosa.	Fidia Pharmaceutical Corp. 2000 K St., NW Suite 700 Washington, DC 20006
Levocabastine HCl ophthalmic suspension 0.05%	Treatment of vernal keratoconjunctivitis.	Iolab Pharmaceuticals 500 Iolab Dr. Claremont, CA 91711
Transforming growth factor-beta 2	Treatment of full thickness macular holes.	Celtrix Pharmaceuticals, Inc. 3055 Patrick Henry Dr. Santa Clara, CA 95054
Tretinoin	Treatment of squamous metaplasia of the ocular surface epithelia (conjunctiva or cornea) with mucous deficiency and keratinization.	Hannan Ophthalmic Marketing Services, Inc. 163 Meetinghouse Rd. Duxbury, MA 02332

The Orphan Drug Act has provided an environment for the development of products for rare diseases and should continue to facilitate this process. In 1984, the Orphan Drug Act was amended to define a rare disease or condition as that which (a) affects < 200,000 persons or (b) affects > 200,000 persons and for which the manufacturing company has no reasonable prospect of recovering research and development costs from sales within the US. Occasionally, a drug which is already commercially available may achieve orphan status for an indication that does not involve a large patient population. The incentives provided by both the Orphan Drug Act and other federal initiatives make it possible for commercial manufacturers to produce drugs for FDA approval at minimal costs. Individuals with rare diseases can be assured that efforts will continue to be made to find treatments.

Published information about orphan drugs is made available by various agencies. These sources can be contacted to obtain information about the acquisition or availability of an orphan drug product.

ORPHAN AND INVESTIGATIONAL DRUGS

Information Sources For Rare Diseases And Orphan Drug Treatment		
Organization	**Information**	**Telephone**
National Organization for Rare Disorders (NORD) P.O. Box 8923 New Fairfield, CT 06812-8923	Information on rare diseases and their treatment.	(203) 746-6518
Federal Register. Dockets Management Branch (HFA-305) Food and Drug Administration Room 4-62 5600 Fishers Lane Rockville, MD 20857	List of orphan drugs and biologicals, designated uses, sponsor's name and address. Available under Docket #84N-0102.	not available
Office of Orphan Products Development (HF-35) Food and Drug Administration 5600 Fishers Lane Rockville, MD 20857	Technical information on orphan drug development, product availability, research grants, and drug sponsorship.	(301) 443-2043

Tatro, DS. Orphan Drugs. *Drug Newsletter* 1988 Apr;7(4):26.

INVESTIGATIONAL NEW DRUGS

The FDA is responsible for determining if a new drug is safe and effective before it is approved for marketing. During the IND process, scientific and statistical information about the drug is gathered. The FDA cannot release information pertaining to formulas, manufacturing processes or the indentity of patients involved in clinical trials. However, the Freedom of Information Act does allow release of specially prepared information which does not contain trade or confidential information.

New Drug Development		
Stage	**Description**	**Duration**
Preclinical Trials	Research and development, initial drug synthesis and animal testing.	1 to 3 years (average 18 months)
IND filing	Allows interstate transport and human testing.	30 days
Clinical Trials		2 to 10 years (average 5 years)
Phase I:	Drug safety, tolerance, pharmacokinetics are determined in 20 to 100 normal adult males.	Several months
Phase II:	Given to 100 to 200 people with the disease to determine effectiveness and dose response.	Up to 2 years
Phase III:	Assessment of safety and efficacy in 800 to 1000 patients. Studies include drug interactions, and use in the elderly and in liver and kidney disease.	1 to 4 years
NDA review	NDA submitted to FDA for approval to market.	2 months to 7 years (average: 12 months)
Post-market surveillance	Adverse reaction reporting, survey/samples, and inspections.	Ongoing

A practitioner may obtain a Treatment IND allowing the use of IND drugs in a controlled situation. There are 2 ways to obtain a Treatment IND: 1) Contact the drug sponsor or 2) contact the FDA directly.

The sponsor usually provides a practitioner with technical information about the drug and a description of the approved treatment protocol. When the sponsor is unwilling to provide the treatment protocol, an individual may contact the FDA. The practitioner must meet all of the FDA's requirements for a Treatment IND. The FDA must respond to the request for a Treatment IND within 30 days of the application.

Investigational Drugs

Drug Name Generic (Trade)	Developmental Stage	Class/Use	Manufacturer/ Sponsor
Adaprolol maleate	Phase II	For treatment of glaucoma using Site-Active targeted delivery system	Pharmos
Adenosine regulating agents	Research	ARAs for ophthalmic indications	Allergan
ADL 2-1294	Phase I	Peripheral opiate anti-hyperalgesic for the treatment of inflammatory pain associated with corneal abrasions, surgical and laser keratectomies and keratoconjunctivitis	Adolor
AGN-192151 (*AGN-191151*)	Phase II	Hypotensive lipid/treatment for glaucoma, once-daily formulation	Allergan
Alpha-1 antichymotrypsin (*LEX001*)	Research	Treatment of inflammatory diseases of the eye	Sparta Pharm
Aminocaproic acid (*Caprogel*)	Phase III, orphan designation Licensed from Virginia Center for Innovative Technology	Treatment of traumatic hyphema caused by blunt, nonpernetrating trauma, topical gel formulation	Orphan Medical
Anecortave acetate	Phase II	Treatment of age-related macular degeneration, injection	Alcon (Nestle S.A.)
Anti-glaucoma agent	Preclinicals (IND planned for mid-1999)	Site-specific drug formulation for treatment of glaucoma	Selectus Pharm
Bactericidal/ permeability- increasing protein (*BPI-21*) (*I-PREX*)	Preclinicals (Pre-IND filing)	Topical ophthalmic formulation of BPI-21/ anti-infective and anti-angiogenic, treatment of corneal injury, corneal ulcer, associated infection, and corneal transplantation	XOMA
Batimastat (*BB-94/ISV-120*)	Phase IIb	Prevention of postsurgical recurrence of pyterygium using DuraSite delivery	InSite Vision/ British Biotech
BCX-34	Preclinicals	Purine nucleoside phosphorylase (PNP) enzyme inhibitor, treatment of T-cell mediated disorders of the eye, ophthalmic formulation	BioCryst Pharm
Brimonidine (*AGN-190342*)	Phase III	For optic nerve survival in glaucoma	Allergan/Pfizer
Brimonidine	Phase III	Alpha-2 agonist/neuroprotectant for optic nerve survival in glaucoma	Allergan
Cell adhesion molecule (CAM) inhibitors	Research	Treatment of ophthamologic infectious diseases	Chiron
Cell adhesion molecule (CAM) inhibitors	Research	Treatment of ophthamologic infectious diseases	Roche Bioscience (Roche Holding Ltd.)
Chondroitinase	Phase I	Treatment of patients undergoing vitrectomy, orphan indication	Bausch & Lomb Surgical
Cidofovir (*Vistide*)	Phase II development discontinued 2000 Licensed from Gilead	Broad-spectrum antiviral for treatment of a variety of ophthalmic viruses, including adenovirus, eye drop formulation	Bausch & Lomb Surgical
Ciliary neurotrophic factor (*Axokine*)	Preclinicals	Second generation chimeric neuroophic factor/treatment for macular degeneration and retinitis pigmentosa	Regeneron Pharm
Clostridium botulinum toxin type A (*Dysport*)	Phase III	Treatment of ocular muscle disorders including blepharospasm	Speywood Pharm

ORPHAN AND INVESTIGATIONAL DRUGS

Investigational Drugs			
Drug Name Generic (*Trade*)	**Developmental Stage**	**Class/Use**	**Manufacturer/ Sponsor**
Clostridium botulinum toxin type A (*Dysport*)	Undisclosed	Treatment of ocular muscle disorders including torticollis	Speywood Pharm
Clostridium botulinum toxin type F	Undisclosed	Treatment of essential blepharospasm, spasmodic torticollis	Speywood Pharm
CNS-1237	Preclinicals	CNS-1237 series, glutamate release blockers/neuroprotectant for retinal degeneration, and Parkinson disease	Cambridge Neuro Science
CNS-5065	Preclinicals	CNS-5065 series/glutamate inhibitors, neuroprotectant focal and global cerebral ischemia, spinal cord injury, retinal regeneration and Parkinson disease	Cambridge Neuro Science
Collagenase	Clinicals	Purified collagenase/treatment of glaucoma, controlled release to the eye, using patented delivery device	Bausch & Lomb Pharm Division BioSpecifics Technologies
Corneaplasty	Phase I/II	Refractive correction	Advanced Coreal Sysems
Curdlan Sulfate	Phase I/II	Beta-(1-3) glucan sulfated polysaccharide cellular therapy for HIV and cytomegalovirus (CMV) infections)	Ajinomoto
Cyclosporine (*Restasis*)	NDA Submitted 3/99	Treatment of moderate to severe dry eye	Allergan/ Novartis
Cysteamine hydrochloride	Phase III	Treatment of corneal cystine crystal accumulation in cystinosis patients, orphan indication	Sigma-Tau Pharm (Sigma-Tau S.p.A.)
Daclizumab monoclonal antibody (*Zenapax*)	Phase I/II	Humanized SMART Anti-Tac monoclonal antibody (MAb) directed at the alpha chain of the human IL-2 receptor (CD25) as immunosuppressant for treatment of uveitis	Protein Design Labs
Dehydrex (*Dehydrex*)	Phase III, orphan designation	Treatment of recurrent corneal erosion	Holles Labs
Dexanabinol (*HU-211*)	Phase II	Treatment of glaucoma and optic neuropathies	Pharmos
Diclofenac	Phase I	Treatment of post-surgical inflammation following cataract extraction, using Ocufit SR pohthalmic drug delivery syterm	Escalon Medical
Diclofenac (*ISV-205*)	Phase IIb completed	Anti-glaucoma agent for protection of the trabecular meshwork and prevention of disease progression, using DuraSite extended-release eye-drop based delivery system	InSite Vision
Dronabinol (*Marinol*)	Phase II	Treatment of glaucoma	Unimed Pharm
Eliprodil	Phase I	Treatment of glaucoma	Alcon (Nestle S.A.)
Engineered cells, ophthalmic diseases	Research	Treatment of ophthalmic diseases, using engineered cells releasing neurotrophic factors, anti-inflammatories, or anti-angiogenics	Cytotherapeu-tics
Enzyme-based iodine technology, eye diseases	Research	Ophthalmic products based on Symbollon enzyme-based iodine technology/treatment of infective eye diseases	Bausch & Lomb Pharm Division/ Symbollon Corporation
Epinastine	Development	Treatment of ocular allergy	Allergan/ Boehringer Ingelheim

OPHTHALMIC DRUG FACTS

Investigational Drugs			
Drug Name Generic (*Trade*)	**Developmental Stage**	**Class/Use**	**Manufacturer/ Sponsor**
Fetal liver kinase-1 receptor/tyrosin kinase antagonist, ophthalmic use	Research	FIK-1 angiogenesis inhibitor, ophthalmic use in treatment of neovascular diseases such as severe diabetic retinopathy and age-related macular degeneration	Allergan
Fibroblast growth factor (mitotoxin conjugate)	Research	Proprietary mitotoxin conjugate of fibroblast growth factor (FGF) linked to saporin/topical glaucoma therapies	Selective Genetics/ Pharmacia& Upjohn
Fibroblast growth factor (mitotoxin conjugate)	Preclinicals	Proprietary mitotoxin conjugate of fibroblast growth factor (FGF) linked to saporin/prevention of lens clouding following cataract surgery	Selective Genetics/ Pharmacia& Upjohn
FIK-1 RTK antagonist	Research	Ophthalmic use in treatment of neovascular diseases such as severe diabetic retinopathy and age-related macular degeneration	Sugen/Allergan
Fomivirsen (*ISIS-2922*)	NDA Submitted 4/98	Monotherapy and in combination with oral ganciclovir, rapid and prolonged control of cytomegalovirus (CMV) retinitis in AIDS patients, intravitreal inj. formulation	Ciba Vision Ophthalmics (Novartis AG)
Foscarnet sodium/ ddl (*Foscavir*) *trisodium phosphonoformate/ dideoxyinosine*	Phase II/III	Treatment of cytomegalovirus (CMV) retinitis	Astra USA
GEM-132	Phase II	Treatment for CMV retinitis, intravitreal and IV formulations	Hybridon
Gene therapy, retinal detachment	Preclinicals	Treatment for traction retinal detachment.	Genetic Therapy (Novartis AG)
Glutamate ion channel blockers, glaucoma)	Preclinicals	Glutamate ion channel blockers (including N-methyl-D-aspartate NDMA ion channel blockers), sodium channel blockers, and combination blockers for treatment of glaucoma and other ophthalmic diseases	Allergan/ Cambridge NeuroScience
GM 6001 (*Galardin MMPI*)	Phase III	Matrix metalloproteinase (proteoglycanase) inhibitor/synthetic therapeutic for treatment of corneal ulcers, topical formulation, orphan indication	Ligand Pharm
Hormone growth hormone (hGH) receptor antagonist (*Trovert*)	Phase II	Treatment of diabetic retinopathy	Senus Drug Pharm/ Genentech
Hyaluronidase (*Keratase*)	Phase IIb	Treatment of corneal opacification	Ista Pharm
Hyaluronidase (*Vitrase*)	Phase III, fast-track designation 10/98	Treatment of severe vitreous hemorrage	Ista Pharm
Hylan A (*Hylashield 24*)	Clinicals	Corneal and conjunctival visoprotector for mild conditions, solution formulation	Biomatrix
Hylan A (*Hylasol*)	Clinicals	Ophthalmic viscosurgery	Biomatrix
Hylan A (*HsS*)	Clinicals	Ophthalmic surgical viscoprotection solution formulation	Biomatrix
Hypericin (aromatic polycyclic dione) (APD-1) (*VIMRxyn*)	Preclinicals	Treatment of cytomegalovirus (CMV) retinitis	VIMRx Pharm
INS 365	IND Ready	Treatment of ocular surface diseases such as dry eye	Inspire Pharm

ORPHAN AND INVESTIGATIONAL DRUGS

Investigational Drugs			
Drug Name Generic (*Trade*)	Developmental Stage	Class/Use	Manufacturer/ Sponsor
Insulin-like growth factor (IGF)/BP3 complex (*SomatoKine*)	Phase III	Treatment of surgical/traumatic wounds and ophthalmic diseases	Celtrix Pharm
Ioperamide/ peripheral mu agonist opioid ADL 2-1294	Phase II	Treatment of ophthalmic pain associated with corneal abrasions, surgical and laser keratectomies and keratoconjunctivitis, topical ophthalmic formulation	Adolor
ISIS-13312	Phase I	Second generation antisense compound for treatment of cytomegalovirus (CMV) retinitis	ISIS Pharm
Isopropyl unoprostone (*Rescula*)	Phase III	Treatment of glaucoma	Ciba Vision Ophthalmics (Novartis AG)
ISV-900)	Research	Genetic diagnostic and prognostic for glaucoma	InSite Vision
Levobunolol HCl (*BetaSite*)	Phase III completed (NDA submission planned)	Treatment of glaucoma, using DuraSite sustained release eye drop delivery	Insite Vision
Lexipafant (BB-882) (*Zacutex*)	Phase II	Treatment for allergic conjunctivitis using DuraSite delivery formulation	British Biotech plc/InSite Vision
Lisinopril (*Zestril Diabetes*)	NDA filed	Treatment of diabetic retinopathy and high-dose congestive heart failure	Zeneca Pharm (Zeneca Inc.)
LGD-1550)	Phase I/IIa	Retinoid X receptors/selective retinoid-retinoic acid receptor, treatment of eye disease, oral formulation	Ligand Pharm
Loteprednol etabonate/ tobramycin (*Lotemax*)	Phase II completed	Combination site-active anti-inflammatory and antibiotic/therapy for seasonal allergic conjunctivitis and post-cataract surgery inflammation	Bausch & Lomb Pharm Division
Memantine	Phase III	Neuroprotective compound to limit damage caused by increased IOP in glaucoma	Allergan
Monoclonal antibody (MAb), anti-VEGF	Preclinicals	Humanized MAb/protein directed against vascular endothelial growth factor (VEGF) to block blood vessel growth, treatment for certain ophthalmic disorders)	Genentech
Motexafin lutetium (*Optrin*)	Phase II	Photodynamic therapy for age-related macular degeneration, injection formulation	Alcon/ Pharmacyclics
N-acetylcysteine (NAC) (*Fluimucil*)	Phase II	Treatment of severe dry eye syndrome	Zambon
Nedocromil Sodium (*Tilavist*)	Phase III	NSAID for treatment of allegic conjunctivitis, ophthamlic solution	Allergan
Neurotrophic factors	Research	Treatment of neurodegenerative and other diseases, including ocular diseases	Glaxo Wellcome/ Regeneron Pharm
NRT technology, degenerative retinal disease	Research	Unnamed new drugs based on proprietary NRT technology for treatment of degenerative retinal disorders and other diseases involving oxidative stress	Centaur Pharm
OcuNex	Research	Treatment of dry eye syndrome and promotion of healing after eye injuries, infections, or eye surgery	Telios Pharm
Oligonucleotide antisense compounds	Preclinicals	Compounds to inhibit vascular endothelial growth factor (VEGF) in retinopathies, psoriasis and cancers, topical, intravitreal, and IV formulations)	Hybridon

Investigational Drugs			
Drug Name Generic (*Trade*)	**Developmental Stage**	**Class/Use**	**Manufacturer/ Sponsor**
Pegvisomant	Phase II	Human growth hormone receptor antagonist for treatment of diabetic retinopathy	Sensus Drug Development (Pharmacia Corp.)
Phospholipids	Phase I	Encapsulated water-insoluble pharmaceutical agents in phospholipids, using Insoluble Drug Delivery (IDD) technology, parenteral, oral, and ophthalmic uses)	RTP Pharm
Pilocarpine	Phase II completed	Treatment of glaucoma, using Submicron Emulsion (SME) delivery system)	Pharmos
Pilocarpine (*PilaSite*)	Phase III completed	Treatment of chronic glaucoma, using DuraSite sustained-release eye drop delivery system	Bausch & Lomb/InSite Vision
Piroxicam	Phase III	NSAID for treatment of cataracts, ophthalmic formulation	Akorn/Pfizer
Povidone liodine	IND filing planned for 1999	2.5% povidone-iodine/prophylaxis of ophthalmic neonatorum	Escalon Medical
Prinomastat matrix metalloproteinase inhibitor AG-3340 MMPI	Phase II	Treatment of age-related macular degeneration, oral formulation	Agouron Pharm (Pfizer, Inc.)
Procaterol	Phase II	Treatment of allergic conjunctivitis	Otskua American Pharm
Proparacaine (*ProSite*)	Phase II completed	Topical anesthetic/adjunct in ophthalmic surgery, using DuraSite sustained-release delivery system	InSite Vision
Retinal pigment epithelial cells	Preclinicals	Porcine retinal pigment epithelial cells for implantation/treatment of age-related macular degeneration	Diacrin
Retinamide	Phase I/II	Retinoid/oral treatment of myelodysplastic syndromes (MDS), orphan indication)	Sparta Pharm
RMP-7 (*Cereport*)	Phase II	Bradykinin analogue for drug delivery to the eye/receptor mediated permeabilizer (RMP) delivery technology for ocular indications)	Alza
Rostaporfin (*SnET2*) **tin ethyl etiopurpurin** (*Photopoint*)	Phase III (2001 NDA filing planned); fast-track status	Treatment of complications of advanced age-related macular (wet) degeneration	Pharmacia/ Miravant Medical Technologies
Sevirumab (MSL-109); monoclonal antibody (MAb); anti- CMV (*Protovir*)	Undisclosed	Treatment for cytomegalovirus (CMV) infection in AIDS patients (retinitis)	Protein Design Labs/Sandoz Pharm
Sulfacetamide (*Sodium Sulamyd*)	sNDA submitted	Antibacterial agent, ophthalmic solution and ointment formulations	Schering-Plough
Tazarotene (*Tazorac*)	Phase II (trials planned)	Receptor-selective retinoid/treatment of photodamage, cream formulation	Allergan
Thalidomide BMS-205935	Phase II	Antiangiogenic therapy for treatment of age-related macular degeneration	EntreMed
Tirilazad mesylate (*Freedox IV Solution*)	Preclinicals	Antioxidant with non-systemic ophthalmic applications, using DuraSite delivery system	InSite Vision/ Pharmacia & Upjohn
Tin ethyl etiopurpurin (*SnET2*) (*Purlytin*)	Preclinicals	Photodynamic therapy (PDT) for treatment of ophthalmic diseases	Pharmacia & Upjohn

ORPHAN AND INVESTIGATIONAL DRUGS

Investigational Drugs			
Drug Name Generic (*Trade*)	**Developmental Stage**	**Class/Use**	**Manufacturer/ Sponsor**
Tryptase inhibitor, conjunctivitis	Research	Second generation tryptase inhibitor/ treatment of allergic conjunctivitis	AXYS Pharm/Bayer AG
Valganciclovir (*Cymeval*)	Phase III	Antiviral agent/treatment for CMV retinitis	Hoffman-La Roche (Roche Holding Ltd.)
Vascular edothelial growth factor)	Research	VEGF receptor for ophthalmic disease	Agouron Pharm
Verapamil HCl (*CalOptic*)	Phase III (NDA filing planned	Treatment for ocular hypertension and other symptoms of glaucoma	Cooper Vision Pharm
Vitrase	Phase III, fast track designation 10/98	Treatment of vitreous hemorrhage	Advanced Corneal Systems
XMP-200	Preclinicals	Dimeric bactericidal/permeabilty increasing protein (BPI) for treatment of ophthalmic conditions	XOMA
Zenarestat (*FK-366*)	Phase III Discontinued 10/00 because of potential kidney toxicity	Treatment of nerve damage caused by diabetes, including diabetic neruopathy	Fujisawa/Pfizer
Zopolrestat (*Alond*)	Phase III	Treatment of retinopathy	Pfizer

AMERICAN OPTOMETRIC ASSOCIATION GUIDELINES

The following sections are excerpted from the American Optometric Association *Clinical Practice Guidelines* for management of conjunctivitis, open-angle glaucoma, and acute anterior uveitis. Clinicians should not rely on these guidelines alone for patient care and management but should refer also to other sources for more detailed discussion of patient care information. These guidelines are copyrighted by the American Optometric Association and reprinted courtesy of that organization.

\multicolumn{8}{c	}{Frequency and Composition of Evaluation and Management Visits for Conjunctivitis}
Type of Patient	Frequency of Followup	History	Visual Acuity	Slit Lamp Biomicroscopy	Ophthalmoscopy	Management Plan
Allergic conjunctivitis	Mild—every 5-7 days Moderate—every 3-5 days Severe—every 1-3 days	Yes	Yes	Yes	As indicated	Identify/remove allergen Use of nonpreserved lubricants, cold compresses, topical pharmaceuticals, systemic antihistamines Educate patient
Bacterial conjunctivitis	Mild—every 5-7 days Moderate—every 3-5 days Severe—every 1-3 days	Yes	Yes	Yes	As indicated	Identify organism and specific antimicrobial agent Hyperacute form: obtain smears and cultures, do saline lavage Use of topical or systemic antibiotics Refer for evaluation and treatment of underlying systemic condition Educate patient
Viral conjunctivitis	Mild—every 5-7 days Moderate—every 3-5 days Severe—every 1-3 days	Yes	Yes	Yes	As indicated	Use of cold compresses, lubricants, ocular decongestants Herpes simplex: use of antiviral agent Herpes zoster: use of topical antibiotic/steroid combinations Educate patient
Chlamydial conjunctivitis	Mild—every 5-7 days Moderate—every 3-5 days Severe—every 1-3 days	Yes	Yes	Yes	As indicated	Use of systemic antibiotics Refer for evaluation and treatment of underlying systemic condition Educate patient

OPHTHALMIC DRUG FACTS

Frequency and Composition of Evaluation and Management Visits for Open-Angle Glaucoma							
Type of Patient	Frequency of Examination	Tonometry	Gonioscopy	ON/NFL Assessment	Stereoscopic ON and FNL Photography	Perimetry*	Management Plan
New glaucoma patient or new glaucoma suspect	Weekly or biweekly to achieve target pressure	Multiple readings may be necessary to establish baseline	Standard classification and drawing at initial visit	Dilate; optic nerve drawing at initial visit	As part of initial glaucoma evaluation	Repeat to establish baseline	Prepare problem list with treatment plan
Glaucoma suspect	6-12 months, depending on level of risk	Multiple readings may be necessary to establish baseline	Annual	Dilate every other visit	Every 2 years	Annual	Review
Stable – mild stage	4-6 months	Every visit	Annual	Dilate every other visit	Annual	Annual	Review
Stable – moderate stage	2-4 months	Every visit	Annual	Dilate every other visit	Annual	6 months	Review
Stable – severe state	1-3 months	Every visit	6 months	Dilate every other visit	Annual	3-4 months	Review
Unstable – IOP poorly controlled; ON or VF progressing	Weekly or biweekly until stability is established	Every visit	Initial visit and each time other clinical findings warrant a reassessment	Dilate at initial visit and each time other clinical findings warrant reassessment	Annual or each time ON or NFL changes	4-6 weeks or as needed to establish new baseline	Formulate new plan until stable
Recently established stability	1-3 months	Every visit; reestablish baseline	Depends on severity of the glaucoma	Dilate every interim visit	Annual or each time ON or NFL changes	Depends on severity of the disease	Review

* Threshold automated perimetry is recommended.

AMERICAN OPTOMETRIC ASSOCIATION CLINICAL PRACTICE GUIDELINES 365

Acute Anterior Uveitis: Treatment and Follow-up*

1. Mild uveitis (Optional depending on symptoms)
   a. Cyclopentolate, 1% (3 times daily) or homatropine, 5% (2 to 3 times daily)
   b. Prednisolone, 1% (2 to 4 times daily)[a]
   c. Oral aspirin or ibuprofen, 2 tablets (every 4 hours)[b]
   d. Consider beta blockers if IOP is elevated
   e. Reevaluate in 4 to 7 days (or prn if worsening)

2. Refer to primary care physician for systemic evaluation (when indicated)

3. Moderate uveitis
   a. Homatropine 5% (4 times daily) or scopolamine, 0.25% (twice daily)
   b. Prednisolone 1% (4 times daily)[a]
   c. Oral aspirin or ibuprofen, 2 tablets (every 4 hours)[b]
   d. Consider beta blockers if IOP is elevated
   e. Dark glasses
   f. Advise patient carefully (eg, pain, course, compliance)
   g. Reevaluate in 2 to 4 days (or prn)

4. Severe uveitis
   a. Atropine 1% (2 to 3 times daily) or homatropine, 5% (every 4 hours)
   b. Prednisolone 1% (every 2 to 4 hours)[a]
   c. Oral aspirin or ibuprofen, 2 tablets (every 3 to 4 hours)[b]
   d. Consider beta blockers if IOP is elevated
   e. Dark glasses
   f. Advise patient carefully
   g. Reevaluate in 1 to 2 days

[a] Shake steroid suspensions well before using. May use dexamethasone or fluoromethalone steroid ointments at bedtime.
[b] Contraindicated in the presence of concurrent hyphema.

*Adapted from Catania LJ. Primary care of the anterior segment, 2nd ed. Norwalk, CT: Appleton & Lange, 1995;372.

EXCIPIENT GLOSSARY

Acetic acid: Buffering (acidifying), tonicity agent.

Acetone sodium bisulfite: Antioxidant (0.01% to 1%).

Acetoxyphenylmercury, see Phenylmercuric acetate.

Acetylcysteine: Mucolytic; corneal vulnerary; antioxidant.

Alcohol (ethanol, ethyl alcohol): Solvent; preservative.

Alkyl ether sulfate, see Sodium lauryl sulfate.

Aluminum tristearate: Astringent.

Amphoteric 10: Wetting, solubilizing, emulsifying agent.

Anhydrous lanolin, see Lanolin anhydrous.

Anhydrous liquid lanolin: Absorbent ointment base.

Anhydrous sodium carbonate, see Sodium carbonate.

Antibacterial: Kills, suppresses bacteria growth.

Antifungal: Kills, suppresses fungus growth.

Antimicrobial: Kills, suppresses microorganism growth.

Antioxidants: Prevents, delays deterioration of products by oxygen.

Ascorbic acid (vitamin C): Antioxidant (0.01% to 0.1%).

Astringent: Topical agent that causes contraction of tissues or arresting of secretions.

Bacqucil, see Polyhexamethylene biguanide.

Bacteriostatic: Inhibits bacteria growth or reproduction.

Baking soda, see Sodium bicarbonate.

Benzalkonium chloride: Antimicrobial preservative (0.05% to 0.02%) (0.01% most common). Most effective at pH 8.

Benzene ethanol, see Phenylethyl alcohol.

Benzethonium chloride: Antimicrobial preservative. Maximum concentration for direct instillation into eye is 1:10,000 (0.01%).

Benzoate of soda, see Sodium benzoate.

Benzyl alcohol: Antimicrobial preservative at concentrations less than 2%. Solvent at concentrations of greater than 5%. Also used as local anesthetic, antiseptic.

Benzyl carbinol, see Phenylethyl alcohol.

Boric acid: Tonicity, antiseptic, buffering agent at 2%.

Bovine catalase, see Catalase.

Buffering agents: Stabilize pH of solutions against changes produced by introduction of acids or bases.

Camphor: Counterirritant; local anesthetic; topical cream. Not for use in the eye.

Carbamide: Antibacterial.

Carbomer 934P: Suspending, emulsifying agent in suspensions and gels.

Carbopol 940, see Carbomer 934P.

Carboxymethylcellulose sodium: Viscosity-increasing, suspending agent.

Catalase (bovine catalase): Enzymes that promote reactions involving decomposition of hydrogen peroxide to water and oxygen.

Cationic cellulose derivative polymer: Wetting agent.

Cellulose methyl ether, see Methylcellulose.

Cetanol, see Cetyl alcohol.

Cetyl alcohol (cetanol, palmityl alcohol): Used in ointment as a stiffening, emulsifying agent.

Cetylpyridinium chloride: Antimicrobial preservative; disinfectant.

Chlorhexidine: Antibacterial; antiseptic.

Chlorhexidine gluconate: Preservative in concentrations of 0.01%. Disinfection of contact lenses in concentrations of 0.002% to 0.006%.

Chlorobutanol: Antimicrobial preservative (0.15% to 0.5%). Should be used in solutions pH 5 to 5.5.

Chlorobutanol anhydrase, see Chlorobutanol.

Cholesterol: Emulsifying, solubilizing agent in ointments.

Citnatin, see Sodium citrate.

Citric acid (2-hydroxy-1,2,3-propane-tricarboxylic acid): Sequestering, buffering (acidifying), antioxidant agent.

Citrosodine, see Sodium citrate.

CMC, see Carboxymethylcellulose sodium.

Demulcent: Soothes and relieves irritated, inflamed, or abraded areas.

Dextran 40: Tonicity, demulcent, wetting agent.

Dextran 70: Viscosity-increasing, tonicity, demulcent, wetting agent.

Dextrose: Tonicity agent.

Dibasic sodium phosphate, see Disodium hydrogen phosphate.

Disinfectant: Destroys or inhibits growth or activity of pathogenic microorganisms.

Disodium hydrogen phosphate, see Sodium phosphate.

Disodium hydrogen phosphate dihydrate: Buffering agent.

Disodium laureth sulfosuccinate: Wetting agent.

Edetate disodium, see EDTA.

Edetates, see EDTA.

Edetic acid, see EDTA.

EDTA (edetates, edetate disodium, edetic acid, ethylenediamine-tetraacetic acid): Enhances activity of preservatives (0.1%); antioxidant synergist; antibacterial. Chelating agent which sequesters trace metal ions necessary for autooxidation reactions and microbial growth (0.005% to 0.1%).

Emulsifying agent: Stabilizes an emulsion.

Emulsion: Preparation of one liquid distributed in small globules throughout the body of a second immiscible liquid.

Ethanol, see Alcohol.

Ethoxylated polyoxypropylene glycol: Surfactant.

Ethyl alcohol, see Alcohol.

Ethylenediaminetetraacetic acid, see EDTA.

Eucalyptol: Antiseptic.

Fatty acid amide: Surfactant.

Fungicide: Destroys fungus.

Gelatin: Viscosity-increasing, emulsifying, suspending agent.

Gelatin A, see Gelatin.

Germicide: Kills microorganisms.

Glycerin: Viscosity-increasing, tonicity agent; lubricant; preservative; solvent.

Glycerol monostearate: Emulsifying, solubilizing agent.

Glycerol stearate, see Glyceryl monostearate.

Glyceryl monostearate (glycerol monostearate, glycerol stearate): Emulsifying, solubilizing, thickening agent.

Glycols, see Propylene glycol.

Hamamelis water: Astringent.

Humectant: Moistening agent.

Hydrochloric acid: Acidifying agent.

Hydrogen peroxide: Disinfectant.

Hydroxyethyl cellulose: Viscosity-increasing, suspending agent.

Hydroxypropyl methylcellulose (methyl hydroxypropylcellulose, methylcellulose propylene glycol ether): Viscosity-increasing, demulcent, suspending agent.

Hydroxypropyl methylcellulose 2906, see Hydroxypropyl methylcellulose.

Hydroxypropyl methylcellulose 2910, see Hydroxypropyl methylcellulose.

Hypertonicity agent, see Tonicity agent.

Isopropanol, see Isopropyl alcohol.

Isopropyl alcohol (isopropanol): Solvent; disinfectant.

Lactose: Diluent.

Lanolin: Ointment base; emulsion.

Lanolin alcohol: Paraffin-base substance containing 6% alcohol used in preparation of water-in-oil creams and ointments; emulsifying, solubilizing agent.

Lanolin anhydrous: Used in preparation of absorbent ointment base.

Lanolin oil: Emulsifying, suspending agent.

Laureth-23: Surfactant, emulsifying, solubilizing, wetting agent.

Lauryl sulfate salt of imidazoline, see Sodium lauryl sulfate.

Light mineral oil, see Mineral oil.

Liquid paraffin, see Mineral oil.

Liquid petrolatum, see Mineral oil.

Magnesium chloride: Electrolyte.

Magnesium chloride hexahydrate, see Magnesium chloride.

Manita, see Mannitol.

Manna sugar, see Mannitol.

Mannite, see Mannitol.

Mannitol (manita, manna sugar, mannite): Tonicity agent.

Menthol: Counterirritant; local analgesic. Not for use in the eye.

Mercurial preservatives, see Thimerosal.

Mercurothiolate, see Thimerosal.

Merphenyl nitrate, see Phenylmercuric nitrate.

Methylcellulose (cellulose methyl ether): Viscosity-increasing, wetting, soaking, suspending agent.

Methylcellulose propylene glycol ether, see Hydroxypropyl methylcellulose.

Methyl glycol, see Propylene glycol.

Methyl hydroxypropylcellulose, see Hydroxypropyl methylcellulose.

EXCIPIENT GLOSSARY

Methylparaben, see Parabens.

Methyl/propylparaben, see Parabens.

Microclens polymeric: Cleaner.

Mineral oil (liquid paraffin, liquid petrolatum): Vehicle; emollient; solvent.

Monosodium phosphate, see Sodium phosphate.

Mucolytic agent: Destroys, liquifies, or dissolves mucus.

Octoxynol 40: Detergent; emulsifying, dispersing agent.

Octylphenoxypolyethoxyethanol: Surfactant.

Palmityl alcohol, see Cetyl alcohol.

Parabens: Parahydroxybenzoic acid esters mixtures sometimes used as antimicrobial preservative. Found unacceptable by the FDA as ophthalmic solution preservatives.

PEG, see Polyethylene glycol.

PEG-15 tallow polyamine, see Polyethylene glycol.

PEG-78 glyceryl monococoate, see Polyethylene glycol.

PEG-80 glyceryl cocoate, see Polyethylene glycol.

PEG-80 sorbitan laurate, see Polyethylene glycol

PEG-90M, see Polyethylene glycol.

PEG-150 distearate, see Polyethylene glycol.

PEG-200 glyceryl monotallowate, see Polyethylene glycol.

PEG 300, see Polyethylene glycol.

PEG 400, see Polyethylene glycol.

PEG 8000, see Polyethylene glycol.

Petrolatum: Emollient, ointment base.

Petroleum jelly, see Petrolatum.

Phenethyl alcohol, see Phenylethyl alcohol.

Phenol: Germicide; preservative.

Phenylethanol, see Phenylethyl alcohol.

Phenylethyl alcohol (benzene ethanol, benzyl carbinol, phenethyl alcohol, phenylethanol): Antimicrobial preservative (0.25% to 0.5%).

Phenylmercuric acetate (acetoxyphenylmercury): Mercurial antimicrobial preservative (0.002% to 0.004%).

Phenylmercuric borate (phenylmercuriborate, phenomerborum): Antimicrobial preservative; antiseptic agent (0.002% to 0.004%).

Phenylmercuric nitrate (merphenyl nitrate): Mercurial antiseptic; antimicrobial preservative (0.002% to 0.004%).

Phosphonic acid, see Phosphoric acid.

Phosphoric acid: Buffering (acidifying), tonicity agent; solvent.

Poloxalene: Surfactant.

Poloxamer: Solubilizing, wetting, gelling, emulsifying, viscosity-increasing agent; ointment base.

Poloxamer 185, see Poloxamer.

Poloxamer 188, see Poloxamer.

Poloxamer 282, see Poloxamer.

Poloxamer 407, see Poloxamer.

Polycarbophil: Vehicle which increases bioavailability by prolonging medication release.

Polyethylene base, see Polyethylene glycol.

Polyethylene glycol (PEG, polyoxyethylene glycol): Viscosity-increasing, gelling, solubilizing, suspending agent; water-soluble ointment base; solvent.

Polyethylene glycol 400, see Polyethylene glycol.

Polyhema (polyhydroxyethylmethacrylate): Ingredient used in drug matrices.

Polyhexamethylene biguanide (bacqucil): Disinfectant.

Polyhydroxyethylmethacrylate, see Polyhema.

Polyoxyethylene glycol, see Polyethylene glycol.

Polyoxyethylene polyoxpropylene: Emulsifying, wetting, solubilizing agent; defoamer; detergent; lubricant.

Polyoxyl 35 castor oil: Emulsifying, solubilizing, wetting agent; surfactant.

Polyoxyl 40 stearate: Surfactant; emulsifier.

Polyquaternium-1: Disinfection agent used in contact lens care systems.

Polysorbate 20: Wetting, solubilizing agent; emulsifying surfactant.

Polysorbate 60: Wetting, solubilizing agent; emulsifying surfactant.

Polysorbate 80: Viscosity-increasing, wetting, solubilizing agent; emulsifying surfactant.

Polyvidone, see Povidone.

Polyvinyl alcohol (PVA): Suspending, viscosity-increasing agent; emulsifier; lubricant; protectant.

Polyvinylpyrrolidone, see Povidone.

Potassium bicarbonate: Buffering, tonicity agent.

Potassium borate: Buffering, tonicity agent.

Potassium carbonate: Buffering (alkalinizing), tonicity agent.

Potassium chloride: Tonicity agent.

Potassium citrate: Buffering, tonicity agent.

Potassium phosphate: Buffering, tonicity agent.

Potassium sorbate: Antimicrobial preservative.

Potassium tetraborate: Buffering, tonicity agent.

Povidone (polyvidone, polyvinylpyrrolidone, PVP): Suspending, dispersing, viscosity-increasing agent.

OPHTHALMIC DRUG FACTS

Preservatives: Prevents or inhibits microorganism growth.

Propylene glycol (1,2-propanediol, propane-1,2-diol, methyl glycol): Viscosity-increasing, tonicity, suspending agent; humectant; solvent; preservative.

Propylene oxide: Lubricant; surfactant; oil demulsifier; solvent.

Propylparaben, see Parabens.

PVA, see Polyvinyl alcohol.

PVP, see Povidone.

Quaternium-15: Emulsifying agent; detergent-germicide; surfactant.

Retinol palmitate: Antioxidant.

Silica gel: Stabilizing, suspending agent.

Sodium acetate: Tonicity, buffering agent.

Sodium acetate trihydrate, see Sodium acetate.

Sodium acid carbonate, see Sodium bicarbonate.

Sodium benzoate (benzoate of soda): Antifungal; bacteriostatic preservative (0.1%).

Sodium bicarbonate (baking soda, sodium acid carbonate, sodium hydrogen carbonate): Buffering, tonicity, alkalinizing agent.

Sodium biphosphate: Buffering, tonicity agent.

Sodium bisulfite: Antioxidant (0.01% to 0.3%), stabilizing agent.

Sodium borate: Buffering, alkalinizing agent.

Sodium carbonate: Buffering, tonicity, alkalinizing agent.

Sodium cellulose glycolate, see Carboxymethylcellulose sodium.

Sodium chloride: Tonicity agent.

Sodium citrate (citnatin, citrosodine, trisodium citrate): Buffering, tonicity, alkalinizing agent. Buffer (0.3% to 2%).

Sodium citrate dihydrate, see Sodium citrate.

Sodium CMC, see Carboxymethylcellulose sodium.

Sodium dihydrogen phosphate hydrate, see Sodium phosphate.

Sodium ethylmercurothiosalicylate, see Thimerosal.

Sodium hydrogen carbonate, see Sodium bicarbonate.

Sodium hydroxide: Buffering, tonicity, alkalinizing agent.

Sodium lactate: Emulsifying agent.

Sodium lauryl sulfate: Emulsifying, solubilizing, wetting agent; detergent; surfactant.

Sodium metabisulfite: Antioxidant (0.01% to 0.3%).

Sodium perborate: Antiseptic.

Sodium phosphate: Buffering, tonicity agent.

Sodium phosphate, dibasic, see Disodium hydrogen phosphate.

Sodium phosphate, monobasic, see Disodium hydrogen phosphate.

Sodium propionate: Preservative; antifungal.

Sodium thiosulfate: Antioxidant; antifungal.

Solvent: Vehicle or substance that dissolves another substance.

Sorbic acid (2,4-hexadienoic acid, 2-propenylacrylic acid): Antimicrobial; preservative (0.05% to 0.2%). Frequently used in combination with other antimicrobials.

Sorbitol: Vehicle; humectant; viscosity-increasing agent.

Stearic acid (octadecanoic acid, cetylacetic acid, stearophanic acid): Solidifying, emulsifying, solubilizing agent.

Sulfasuccinate: Emulsifying, wetting, dispersing agent.

Tartaric acid: Buffering, acidifying agent.

Thimerosal (mercurial preservatives, mercurothiolate, sodium ethylmercurothiosalicylate, thiomersalate): Mercurial antiseptic, antimicrobial preservative (0.005% to 0.02%).

Thiomersalate, see Thimerosal.

Thiourea: Antioxidant.

Titanium dioxide: UV absorbent; scatters UV light at 290 to 700nm.

Tonicity agent: Enables ophthalmic solutions to be isotonic with natural tears.

Tri-quaternary cocoa-based phospholipid: Buffering agent.

Tris (hydroxymethyl) amino methane, see Tromethamine.

Trisodium citrate, see Sodium citrate.

Tromethamine (tris [hydroxymethyl] aminomethane): Emulsifying, buffering agent.

Tween 21, see Polysorbate 80.

Tyloxapol: Wetting, solubilizing, emulsifying agent.

Viscosity-increasing agent: Prolongs contact time of product with eye, increasing drug absorption and activity.

Vitamin C, see Ascorbic acid.

Wetting agent: Reduces surface tension of eye.

White petrolatum, see Petrolatum.

Zinc sulfate: Weak antiseptic; recommended concentrations of 0.05% to 0.25%.

Manufacturers and Distributors Index

00074
Abbott Laboratories
100 Abbott Park Rd.
Abbott Park IL 60064-3500
800-441-4987
www.abbott.com

Advanced Vision Research
7 Alfred St., Ste. 330
Woburn MA 01801
781-932-8327
800-579-8327
www.theratears.com

17478
Akorn, Inc.
2500 Millbrook Dr.
Buffalo Grove IL 60089
800-535-7155
www.akorn.com

00065, 00998
Alcon Laboratories, Inc.
6201 S. Freeway
Fort Worth TX 76134
800-451-3937
www.alconlabs.com

00023, 11980
Allergan, Inc.
2525 DuPont Dr.
Irvine CA 92715
714-246-4500
800-433-8871
www.allergan.com

17314
Alza Corp.
1900 Charleston Rd.
Mt. View CA 94039
650-564-5000
800-634-8977
www.alza.com

89709, 90605
Amcon Laboratories
40 N. Rock Hill Rd.
St. Louis MO 63119
314-961-5758
800-255-6161
www.amcon-labs.com

00517
American Regent
1 Luitpold Dr.
Shirley NY 11967
800-645-1706
www.luitpold.com

00003, 00015
Apothecon, Inc.
(Bristol-Myers Squibb)
P.O. Box 4500
Princeton NJ 08543-4500
609-897-2000
800-321-1335
www.apothecon.com

00186
AstraZeneca
   Pharmaceuticals LP
1800 Concord Pike
Wilmington DE 19850
800-236-9933
800-237-8898
www.astrazeneca-us.com

00264
B. Braun Medical
2525 McGaw Ave.
Irvine CA 92614
949-660-2000
800-227-2862
www.bbraunusa.com

10119
**Bausch & Lomb North
   American Vision Care**
1400 N. Goodman St.
P.O. Box 450
Rochester NY 14692-0450
716-338-6000
800-553-5340
www.bausch.com

24208, 57782
**Bausch & Lomb
   Pharmaceuticals**
8500 Hidden River Pkwy.
Tampa FL 33637
813-975-7770
800-323-0000
www.bausch.com

Bausch & Lomb Surgical
555 W. Arrow Hwy.
Claremont CA 91711
909-624-2020
800-531-2020
www.blsurgical.com

Baxter Healthcare
1 Baxter Pkwy.
DF4-1W
Deerfield IL 60015
847-948-4770
800-422-9837
www.baxter.com

12843, 16500
**Bayer Consumer Care
   Division**
P.O. Box 340
Elkhart IN 46515
800-348-2240
www.bayercare.com

31280
BD (Becton Dickinson & Co.)
1 Becton Dr.
Franklin Lakes NJ 07417
201-847-6800
888-237-2762
www.bd.com

55390
Bedford Laboratories
300 Northfield Rd.
Bedford OH 44146
440-232-3320
800-562-4797

50486
Blairex Labs, Inc.
P.O. Box 2127
Columbus IN 47202-2127
812-378-1864
800-252-4739
www.blairex.com

Burroughs Wellcome Co.
See GlaxoWellcome

OPHTHALMIC DRUG FACTS

Celltech
755 Jefferson Rd.
Rochester NY 14623-0000
800-234-5535

00436
Century Pharmaceuticals, Inc.
10377 Hague Rd.
Indianapolis IN 46256-3399
317-849-4210

Chiron Vision
See Bausch & Lomb Surgical

00346
Ciba Vision Corporation
11460 Johns Creek Pkwy.
Duluth GA 30097
800-845-6585
www.cibavision.com

Clintec Nutrition
3 Pkway. N. Ste. 500
Deerfield IL 60015
847-948-2000
800-422-2571
www.baxter.com

54799
Cynacon/OCuSOFT
5311 Ave. N.
Richmond TX 77471
281-342-3350
800-233-5469
www.ocusoft.com

55994
Dakryon Pharmaceuticals
See Medco Pharmaceuticals

10310
Del Laboratories, Inc.
178 EAB Plaza
Uniondale NY 11556
516-844-2020
800-952-5080
www.dellabs.com

00777
Dista Products Co.
See Eli Lilly and Co.

00168
E. Fougera Co.
60 Baylis Rd.
Melville NY 11747
516-454-6996
800-645-9833
www.fougera.com

Eagle Vision, Inc.
6263 Poplar Ave., Ste. 650
Memphis TN 38119
901-682-9400
800-222-7584
www.eaglevis.com

00002, 59075
Eli Lilly and Co.
Lilly Corp. Center
Indianapolis IN 46285
317-276-2000
800-545-5979
www.elililly.com

00641
Elkins-Sinn, Inc.
See Wyeth-Ayerst

Escalon Medical Corp.
351 E. Conestoga Rd., Plz. Level
Wayne PA 19087
610-688-6830
800-433-8197
www.escalonmed.com

Falcon Ophthalmics, Inc.
6201 S. Freeway
Fort Worth TX 76134
817-551-8710
800-343-2133
www.alconlabs.com

Fisons Corp.
See Celltech

00258, 00456, 00535
Forest Pharmaceuticals, Inc.
13600 Shoreline
St. Louis MO 63045
314-493-7000
800-678-1605
www.forestpharm.com

10432
Freeda Vitamins, Inc.
36 E. 41st St.
New York NY 10017-6203
212-685-4980
800-777-3737
www.imall.com/stores/freeda

00469, 57317
Fujisawa Healthcare, Inc.
3 Pkwy. N. Center
Deerfield IL 60015-2548
847-317-8800
800-888-7704
www.fujisawa.com

00781
Geneva Pharmaceuticals, Inc.
2599 W. Midway Blvd.
P.O. Box 469
Broomfield CO 80038-0469
800-525-8747
800-622-9191
www.genevarx.com

GlaxoSmithKline
5 Moore Dr.
P.O. Box 13398
Research Triangle Park NC 27709
888-825-5249
www.gsk.com

GlaxoSmithKline
1 Franklin Plaza
Philadelphia PA 19102
888-825-5249
www.gsk.com

GlaxoSmithKline Consumer Healthcare
P.O. Box 1467
Pittsburgh PA 15230
www.gsk.com

00081, 00173
GlaxoWellcome, Inc.
see GlaxoSmithKline

00182
Goldline Laboratories, Inc.
See Ivax Pharmaceuticals

Henry Schein, Inc.
135 Duryea Rd., Mail Route 150
Melville NY 11747
516-843-5500
800-472-4346
www.henryschein.com

00839
H.L. Moore Drug Exchange, Inc.
See Moore Medical Corp.

47992
Holles Laboratories, Inc.
30 Forest Notch
Cohasset MA 02025-1198
800-356-4015

00548
I.M.S., Ltd.
See Celltech

00814
Interstate Drug Exchange
See Henry Schein, Inc.

Iolab Pharmaceuticals
See Ciba Vision Corporation

Ivax Pharmaceuticals, Inc.
4400 Biscayne Blvd.
Miami FL 33178
305-575-4100
800-327-4114

00137
Johnson & Johnson
1 Johnson & Johnson Plz.
New Brunswick NJ 08933
732-524-0400
www.jnj.com

KabiVitrum, Inc.
See Pharmacia

00588
Keene Pharmaceuticals, Inc.
303 S. Mockingwood
Keene TX 76059-0007
817-645-8083
800-541-0530

MANUFACTURERS AND DISTRIBUTORS INDEX 373

La Haye Laboratories, Inc.
2205 152nd Ave. N.E.
Redmond WA 98052
425-644-2020
800-344-2020
www.lahaye.com

Lacrimedics, Inc.
P.O. Box 1209
Eastbound WA 98245
360-376-7095
800-367-8327
www.lacrimedics.com

10651
Lavoptik, Inc.
661 Western Ave.
St. Paul MN 55103
612-489-1351

00005, 53124
**Lederle Professional Medical
    Services**
401 N. Middletown Rd.
Pearl River NY 10965-1299
914-732-5000
800-999-9384

23558
Lee Pharmaceuticals
1434 Santa Anita Blvd.
South Elmonte CA 91733
626-442-3141
800-950-5337
www.leepharma.com

00904
Major Pharmaceuticals
31778 Enterprise Dr.
Livonia MI 48150
734-525-8700
800-688-9696

Marlin Industries
P.O. Box 560
Grover City CA 93483-0560
805-473-2743
800-423-5926

00259
Mayrand, Inc.
See Merz Pharmaceuticals

00264
McGaw, Inc.
See B. Braun Medical

Medco Pharmaceuticals
2015 Hwy. 190 Bypass
Covington LA 70433
800-793-8740

00585
Medeva Pharmaceuticals
See Celltech

00348, 75137
Medtech Laboratories, Inc.
3510 N. Lake Creek
P.O. Box 1108
Jackson WY 83011-1108
307-739-8208
800-443-4908

Menicon USA
333 W. Pontiac Way
Clovis CA 93612
800-636-4266
www.menicon.com

00006
Merck & Co.
P.O. Box 4
West Point PA 19486
800-672-6372
www.merck.com

Merz Pharmaceuticals
4215 Tudor Ln.
Greensboro NC 27410
336-856-2003
800-334-0514
www.merzusa.com

00682, 46672
Mikart, Inc.
1750 Chattahoochee Ave.
Atlanta GA 30318
404-351-4510
www.mikart.com

Moore Medical Corp.
389 John Downey Dr.
P.O. Box 1500
New Britian CT 06050
860-826-3600
800-444-8765
www.mooremedical.com

53489
**Mutual Pharmaceutical, Inc.
(United Research
    Laboratories)**
1100 Orthodox St.
Philadelphia PA 19124
215-288-6500
800-523-3684
www.urlmutual.com

Novartis Consumer Health
560 Morris Ave.
Summit NJ 07901
908-598-7600
800-548-3708
www.us.novartis.com

Novartis Ophthalmics, Inc.
11460 Johns Creek Parkway
Duluth GA 30097-1556
866-393-6336

00028, 00067, 00083, 58887
**Novartis Pharmaceuticals
    Corp.**
59 Route 10
East Hanover NJ 07936
973-781-8300
888-669-6682
www.pharma.us.novartis.com

00362
**Novocol
(Septodont, Inc.)**
P.O. Box 11926
Wilmington DE 19850
302-328-1102
800-872-8305
www.septodontinc.com

NutraMax Laboratories, Inc.
2208 Lakeside Blvd.
Edgewood MD 21040
410-776-4000
800-925-5187
www.nutramaxlabs.com

51944
Ocumed, Inc.
119 Harrison Ave.
Roseland NJ 07068
973-226-2330

OCuSOFT
See Cynacon/OCuSOFT

Optikem International, Inc.
2172 S. Jason St.
Denver CO 80223
303-936-1137

52238
Optopics Laboratories, Corp.
40 Main St.
P.O. Box 210
Fairton NJ 08320
856-451-9350

59148
**Otsuka America
    Pharmaceutical, Inc.**
2440 Research Blvd., Ste. 250
Rockville MD 20850
301-990-0030
800-562-3974
www.otsuka.com

00071
**Parke-Davis
(Warner-Lambert)**
201 Tabor Rd.
Morris Plains NJ 07950
800-223-0432
www.parke-davis.com

00349
Parmed Pharmaceuticals, Inc.
4220 Hyde Park Blvd.
Niagara Falls NY 14305
716-284-5666
800-727-6331
www.parmed.com

00418
Pasadena Research Labs
See Taylor Pharmaceuticals

PBH Wesley Jessen
See Wesley Jessen

OPHTHALMIC DRUG FACTS

00927
Pfeiffer Co.
71 University Ave.
P.O. Box 4447
Atlanta GA 30315
404-614-0255
800-342-6450

00069, 00663, 74300
**Pfizer US Pharmaceutical
 Group**
235 E. 42nd St.
New York NY 10017-5755
800-438-1985
www.pfizer.com

00013, 00016
Pharmacia Corp.
700 Portage Rd.
Kalamazoo MI 49001-6529
616-833-4000
800-253-8600
www.pnu.com

Pharmafair
See Bausch & Lomb
 Pharmaceuticals

Pharmics, Inc.
2350 S. Redwood Rd.
Salt Lake City UT 84119
801-972-4138
800-456-4138
www.pharmics.com

00077
Pilkington Barnes Hind
See Wesley Jessen

47144
Polymer Technology Corp.
100 Research Dr.
Wilmington MA 01887
978-658-6111
800-885-1241
www.polymer.com

00603
Qualitest Pharmaceuticals
1236 Jordan Rd.
Huntsville AL 35811
256-859-4011
800-444-4011

00686
Raway Pharmacal, Inc.
15 Granit Rd.
Accord NY 12404-0047
914-626-8133

54092
**Roberts Pharmaceutical
 Corp.**
4 Industrial Way West
Eatontown NJ 07724
732-389-1182
800-828-2088
www.robertspharm.com

00004, 00033, 00140, 18393,
42987
Roche Pharmaceuticals
340 Kingsland St.
Nutley NJ 07110-1199
973-235-5000
800-526-6367
www.rocheusa.com

00049
Roerig
See Pfizer US Pharmaceutical
 Group

00074
**Ross Products Division,
 Abbott Labs**
625 Cleveland
Columbus OH 43215
800-227-5767
www.abbott.com

00536
Rugby Labs, Inc.
2170 Satellite Blvd., Ste. 300
Duluth GA 30097
678-584-5678
800-645-2158

00024
Sanofi-Synthelabo, Inc.
90 Park Ave.
New York NY 10016
212-551-4000
800-223-1062
www.sanofi-synthelabous.com

00364, 00591
Schein Pharmaceutical, Inc.
100 Campus Dr.
Florham Park NJ 07932
800-356-5790
www.schein-rx.com

00274, 00032
Scherer Laboratories, Inc.
2301 Ohio Dr., Ste. 234
Plano TX 75093
972-612-6225
800-449-8290

00085, 11017, 41000, 41100
**Schering-Plough HealthCare
 Products**
3 Oak Way
Berkeley Heights NJ
 07922-0603
908-679-1784
800-842-4090
www.schering-plough.com

00766
**SmithKline Beecham
 Consumer Healthcare**
see GlaxoSmithKline
 Consumer Healthcare

00007, 00029, 00108, 00128
**SmithKline Beecham
 Pharmaceuticals**
see GlaxoSmithKline

Sola/Barnes-Hind
See Wesley Jessen

51318
Stellar Pharmacal Corp.
1990 N.W. 44th St.
Pompano Beach FL
 33064-1278
954-971-9704
800-845-7827
www.starpharm.com

00402
**Steris Laboratories, Inc.
(Schein)**
620 N. 51st Ave.
Phoenix AZ 85043
602-278-1400
800-692-9995

57706
Storz Ophthalmics
See Bausch & Lomb Surgical

00033, 18393, 42987
Syntex Laboratories
See Roche Pharmaceuticals

00418
Taylor Pharmaceuticals
942 Calle Negocio, Ste. 150
San Clemente CA 92674-5136
969-492-4030
800-223-9851

00677
**United Research
 Laboratories**
1100 Orthodox St.
Philadelpha PA 19124
215-288-6500
800-523-3684
www.urlmutual.com

00009
Upjohn Co.
See Pharmacia & Upjohn

54891
Vision Pharmaceuticals, Inc.
P.O. Box 400
Mitchell SD 57301-0400
605-996-3356
800-325-6789
www.visionpharm.com

00619
Walker Laboratories
4200 Laclede Ave.
St. Louis MO 63108
314-533-9600
800-325-8080
www.1800homeopathy.com

00047, 52544, 51875, 55515
Watson Laboratories, Inc.
311 Bonnie Circle Dr.
Corona CA 91720
909-270-1400
800-272-5525
www.watsonpharm.com

MANUFACTURERS AND DISTRIBUTORS INDEX

Wesley Jessen
333 E. Howard
Des Plains IL 60018
800-854-2790
www.wesley-jessen.com

00008, 00031
Wyeth-Ayerst
555 Lancaster Ave.
St. Davids PA 19807
610-902-1200
800-666-7248
www.ahp.com/wyeth

00172, 00182
Zenith Goldline
   Pharmaceuticals
see Ivax Pharmaceuticals

Chapter Summaries

The following tables are provided as a quick-look product guide. The tables cover Chapter 2 (Ophthalmic Dyes) through Chapter 12 (Nonsurgical Adjuncts) and contain a summary of product information including: generic name, trade name, manufacturer(s), ingredient(s), strength(s), doseform(s), and how supplied. For complete information about a particular product, please consult the index for the appropriate page number.

Ophthalmic Dyes

Generic Name Trade Name	Doseform/ Strength	How Supplied
Fluorescein Sodium		
Ak-Fluor, Rx (Akorn)	**Injection**: 10%	In 5 mL amps and vials.
Fluorescite, Rx (Alcon)	**Injection**: 10%	In 5 mL amps with syringes.
AK-Fluor, Rx (Akorn)	**Injection**: 25%	In 2 mL amps and vials.
Fluorescite, Rx (Alcon)	**Injection**: 25%	In 2 mL amps.
Fluorescein Sodium, Rx (Alcon)	**Solution**: 2%	In 1, 2, and 15 mL.
Ful-Glo, Rx (Akorn)	**Strips**: 0.6 mg	In 300s.
Fluorets, Rx (Akorn)	**Strips**: 1 mg	In 100s.
Fluorexon		
Fluoresoft, otc (Holles)	**Solution**: 0.35%	In 0.5 mL pipettes (12s).
Indocyanine Green		
Cardio-Green (CG), Rx (Becton-Dickinson)	**Powder for Injection**: 25 mg, 50 mg	In 10 mL amps of aqueous solvent (2s).
Lissamine Green		
Lissamine Green, otc (Cyanacon/Ocusoft)	**Strips**: 1.5 mg	100 sterile strips per carton.
Rose Bengal		
Rosets, otc (Akorn)	**Strips**: 1.3 mg/strip	In 100s.

Local Anesthetics, Injectable

Generic Name Trade Name	Doseform/ Strength	How Supplied
Lidocaine HCl and Lidocaine Combinations		
Xylocaine MPF, Rx (Astra)	**Injection**: 4%	In 5 mL amps and 5 mL disp. syringe with laryngotracheal cannula.
Xylocaine, Rx (Astra)	**Injection**: 0.5% with 1:200,000 epinephrine	In 50 mL multiple-dose vials.[1]
Xylocaine, Rx (Astra)	**Injection**: 1% with 1:100,000 epinephrine	In 10, 20, and 50 mL multiple-dose vials.[1]

Local Anesthetics, Injectable

Generic Name Trade Name	Doseform/ Strength	How Supplied
Xylocaine MPF, Rx (Astra)	**Injection**: 1% with 1:200,000 epinephrine	In 30 mL ampules, and 5, 10, and 30 mL single-dose vials.[2]
Xylocaine MPF, Rx (Astra)	**Injection**: 1.5% with 1:200,000 epinephrine	In 5 and 30 mL ampules, and 5, 10, and 30 mL single-dose vials.[2]
Xylocaine , Rx (Astra)	**Injection**: 2% with 1:100,000 epinephrine	In 10, 20, and 50 mL multiple-dose vials.[1]
Xylocaine MPF , Rx (Astra)	**Injection**: 2% with 1:200,000 epinephrine	In 20 mL ampules, and 5, 10, and 20 mL single-dose vials.[2]
Mepivacaine HCl		
Polocaine, Rx (Astra)	**Injection**: 1%	In 50 mL vials.
Polocaine MPF, Rx (Astra)	**Injection**: 1%	In 30 mL vials.
Polocaine MPF, Rx (Astra)	**Injection**: 1.5%	In 30 mL vials.
Polocaine, Rx (Astra)	**Injection**: 2%	In 50 mL vials.
Polocaine MPF, Rx (Astra)	**Injection**: 2%	In 20 mL vials.
Bupivacaine HCl and Bupiva-caine Combinations		
Bupivacaine HCl, Rx (Abbott)	**Injection**: 0.75%	In 20 mL amps and 20 mL *Abboject*.
Sensorcaine MPF, Rx (Astra)	**Injection**: 0.75%	In 30 mL amps and 10 and 30 mL vials.
Sensorcaine MPF, Rx (Astra)	**Injection**: 0.75% with 1:200,000 epinephrine	In 30 mL amps and 10 and 30 mL vials.[2]
Etidocaine HCl		
Duranest MPF, Rx (Astra)	**Injection**: 1%	In 30 mL single-dose vials.
Duranest MPF, Rx (Astra)	**Injection**: 1% with 1:200,000 epinephrine	In 30 mL single-dose vials.[2]
Duranest MPF, Rx (Astra)	**Injection**: 1.5% with 1:200,000 epinephrine	In 20 mL amps.[2]

[1] With methylparaben.
[2] With sodium metabisulfite.

Local Anesthetics, Topical

Generic Name Trade Name	Doseform/ Strength	How Supplied
Tetracaine HCl		
Tetracaine HCl, Rx (Various, eg, Alcon, Bausch & Lomb, Novartis, Schein)	**Solution**: 0.5%	In 1, 2, and 15 mL.
AK-T-Caine PF, Rx (Akorn)	**Solution**: 0.5%	In 15 mL.
Proparacaine HCl		
Proparacaine HCl, Rx (Various, eg, Bausch & Lomb, Falcon)	**Solution**: 0.5%	In 2 and 15 mL, and UD 1 mL.
AK-TAINE, Rx (Akorn)	**Solution**: 0.5%	In 15 mL.[1,2]
Alcaine, Rx (Alcon)	**Solution**: 0.5%	In 15 mL Drop-Tainers.[3,4]
Ophthetic, Rx (Allergan)	**Solution**: 0.5%	In 15 mL.[1,2]
Miscellaneous Local Anesthetic Combinations		
Fluoracaine, Rx (Akorn)	**Solution**: 0.5% propara- caine HCl and 0.25% fluorescein sodium	In 5 mL.[1,5]
Fluress, Rx (Akorn)	**Solution**: 0.4% benoxi- nate HCl and 0.25% fluorescein sodium	In 5 mL with dropper.[6]

[1] Refrigerate.
[2] With 0.01% benzalkonium Cl, glycerin, and sodium Cl.
[3] With glycerin and 0.01% benzalkonium Cl.
[4] Refrigerate after opening.
[5] With glycerin, povidone, polysorbate 80, and 0.01% thimerosal.
[6] With povidone, boric acid, and 1% chlorobutanol.

Mydriatics

Generic Name Trade Name	Doseform/ Strength	How Supplied
Phenylephrine HCl		
Phenylephrine HCl, Rx (Various, eg, Bausch & Lomb, Falcon)	**Solution**: 2.5%	In 2, 5, and 15 mL.
AK-Dilate, Rx (Akorn)	**Solution**: 2.5%	In 2 and 15 mL.[1]
Mydfrin 2.5%, Rx (Alcon)	**Solution**: 2.5%	In 3 and 5 mL Drop-Tainers.[2]
Neo-Synephrine, Rx (Sanofi-Synthelabo)	**Solution**: 2.5%	In 15 mL.[3]
Phenyleprhine HCl, Rx (Various, eg, Novartis)	**Solution**: 10%	In 1, 2, and 5 mL.

CHAPTER SUMMARIES

Mydriatics

Generic Name Trade Name	Doseform/ Strength	How Supplied
AK-Dilate, Rx (Akorn)	**Solution**: 10%	In 2 and 5 mL.[1]
Neo-Synephrine, Rx (Sanofi-Synthelabo)	**Solution**: 10%	In 5 mL.[4]
Neo-Synephrine Viscous, Rx (Sanofi-Synthelabo)	**Solution**: 10%	In 5 mL.[5]

[1] With benzalkonium chloride.
[2] With 0.01% benzalkonium chloride, EDTA, and sodium bisulfite.
[3] With 1:7500 benzalkonium choride.
[4] With 1:10,000 benzalkonium chloride and methylcellulose.
[5] With 1:10,000 benzalkonium chloride.

Cycloplegic Mydriatics

Generic Name Trade Name	Doseform/ Strength	How Supplied
Atropine Sulfate		
Atropine Sulfate Ophthalmic, Rx (Various, eg, Bausch & Lomb, Foug- era)	**Ointment**: 1%	In 3.5 and UD 1 g.
Isopto Atropine, Rx (Alcon)	**Solution**: 0.5%	In 5 mL Drop-Tainers.[1]
Atropine Sulfate, Rx (Various, eg, Alcon, Bausch & Lomb, Fougera, Ivax)	**Solution**: 1%	In 2, 5, and 15 mL and UD 1 mL.
Atropine Care, Rx (Akorn)	**Solution**: 1%	In 2, 5, and 15 mL.[2]
Atropisol, Rx (Novartis)	**Solution**: 1%	In 2, 5, and 15 mL and 1 mL Dropperettes.[3]
Isopto Atropine, Rx (Alcon)	**Solution**: 1%	In 5 and 15 mL Drop-Tainers.[1]
Homatropine HBr		
Isopto Homatropine, Rx (Alcon)	**Solution**: 2%	In 5 and 15 mL Drop-Tainers.[4]
Homatropine HBr, Rx (Various, eg, Alcon, Ciba Vision)	**Solution**: 5%	In 1, 2, and 5 mL.
AK-Homatropine, Rx (Akorn)	**Solution**: 5%	In 5 mL.
Isopto Homatropine, Rx (Alcon)	**Solution**: 5%	In 5 and 15 mL Drop-Tainers.[5]
Scopolamine HBr **(Hyoscine HBr))**		
Isopto Hyoscine, Rx (Alcon)	**Solution**: 0.25%	In 5 and 15 mL Drop-Tainers.[6]

OPHTHALMIC DRUG FACTS

Cycloplegic Mydriatics

Generic Name Trade Name	Doseform/ Strength	How Supplied
Cyclopentolate HCl		
Cyclogyl, Rx (Alcon)	**Solution**: 0.5%	In 2, 5, and 15 mL Drop-Tainers.[3]
Cyclopentolate HCl, Rx (Various, eg, Bausch & Lomb)	**Solution**: 1%	In 2, 5, and 15 mL.
AK-Pentolate, Rx (Akorn)	**Solution**: 1%	In 2, 5, and 15 mL.[3]
Cyclogyl, Rx (Alcon)	**Solution**: 1%	In 2, 5, and 15 mL.[3]
AK-Pentolate, Rx (Akorn)	**Solution**: 2%	In 2, 5, and 15 mL white opaque dropper bottles.
Cyclogyl, Rx (Alcon)	**Solution**: 2%	In 2, 5, and 15 mL Drop-Tainers.[3]
Tropicamide		
Tropicamide, Rx (Various, eg, Bausch & Lomb, Falcon)	**Solution**: 0.5%	In 2 and 15 mL.
Mydriacyl, Rx (Alcon)	**Solution**: 0.5%	In 15 mL Drop-Tainers.[7]
Tropicacyl, Rx (Akorn)	**Solution**: 0.5%	In 2 and 15 mL.
Tropicamide, *Rx* (Various, eg, Falcon)	**Solution**: 1%	In 3 and 15 mL.
Mydriacyl, Rx (Alcon)	**Solution**: 1%	In 3 and 15 mL Drop-Tainers.[7]
Tropicacyl, Rx (Akorn)	**Solution**: 1%	In 2 and 15 mL.[8]

[1] With 0.01% benzalkonium chloride, 0.5% hydroxypropyl methylcellulose, and boric acid.
[2] With 0.01% benzalkonium chloride, hydroxypropyl methylcellulose, and boric acid.
[3] With benzalkonium chloride, EDTA, and boric acid.
[4] With 0.01% benzalkonium chloride, 0.5% hydroxypropyl methylcellulose, and polysorbate 80.
[5] With 0.005% benzethonium chloride and 0.5% hydroxypropyl methylcellulose.
[6] With 0.01% benzalkonium chloride and 0.5% hydroxypropyl methylcellulose.
[7] With 0.01% benzalkonium chloride and EDTA.
[8] With 0.1% benzalkonium chloride and EDTA.

Mydriatic Combinations

Trade Name	Doseform/Strength	How Supplied
Cyclomydril, Rx (Alcon)	**Solution**: 0.2% cyclopentolate HCl and 1% phenylephrine HCl	In 2 and 5 mL Drop-Tainers.[1]
Murocoll-2, Rx (Bausch & Lomb)	**Drops**: 0.3% scopolamine HBr and 10% phenylephrine HCl	In 5 mL.[2]

[1] With 0.01% benzalkonium chloride, EDTA, and boric acid.
[2] With 0.01% benzalkonium chloride, sodium metabisulfite, and EDTA.

CHAPTER SUMMARIES 383

Antiallergy and Decongestants

Generic Name Trade Name	Doseform/ Strength	How Supplied
Naphazoline HCl		
20/20 EyeDrops, otc (S.S.S.)	**Solution**: 0.012%	In 15 mL.[1]
Allergy Drops, otc (Bausch & Lomb)	**Solution**: 0.012%	In 15 mL.[2]
Clear Eyes, otc (Ross)	**Solution**: 0.012%	In 15 and 30 mL.[3]
Clear Eyes ACR, otc (Ross)	**Solution**: 0.012%	In 15 and 30 mL.[4]
Naphcon, otc (Alcon)	**Solution**: 0.012%	In 15 mL. [5]
VasoClear, otc (Novartis)	**Solution**: 0.02%	In 15 mL.[6]
VasoClear A, otc (Novartis)	**Solution**: 0.02%	In 15 mL.[7]
Allergy Drops Maximum *Strength, otc* (Bausch & Lomb)	**Solution**: 0.03%	In 15 mL.[8]
Naphazoline HCl, Rx (Various, eg, , Ivax, Major, Qualitest)	**Solution**: 0.1%	In 15 mL.
AK-Con, Rx (Akorn)	**Solution**: 0.1%	In 15 mL.[5]
Albalon, Rx (Allergan)	**Solution**: 0.1%	In 15 mL.[9]
Nafazair, Rx (Bausch & Lomb)	**Solution**: 0.1%	In 15 mL.[5]
Naphcon Forte, Rx (Alcon)	**Solution**: 0.1%	In 15 mL Drop-Tainers.[5]
Vasocon Regular, Rx (Novartis)	**Solution**: 0.1%	In 15 mL.[10]
Oxymetazoline		
OcuClear, otc (Schering-Plough)	**Solution**: 0.025%	In 30 mL.[11]
Visine L.R., otc (Pfizer)	**Solution**: 0.025%	In 15 and 30 mL.[11]
Phenylephrine HCl		
AK-Nefrin, otc (Akorn)	**Solution**: 0.12%	In 15 mL.[12]
Prefrin Liquifilm, otc (Allergan)	**Solution**: 0.12%	In 20 mL.[13]
Relief, otc (Allergan)	**Solution**: 0.12%	Preservative free. In UD 0.3 mL.[14]
Zincfrin Solution, otc (Alcon)	**Solution**: 0.12%	In 15 mL Drop-Tainers.[15]

OPHTHALMIC DRUG FACTS

Antiallergy and Decongestants

Generic Name Trade Name	Doseform/ Strength	How Supplied
Tetrahydrozoline HCl		
Tetrahydrozoline HCl, otc (Various, eg, Rugby)	**Solution**: 0.05%	In 15 and 30 mL.
Collyrium Fresh, otc (Wyeth-Ayerst)	**Solution**: 0.05%	In 15 mL.[16]
Eyesine, otc (Akorn)	**Solution**: 0.05%	In 15 mL.[5]
Geneye, otc (Ivax)	**Solution**: 0.05%	In 15 and 22.5 mL.[5]
Murine Tears Plus, otc (Ross)	**Solution**: 0.05%	In 15 and 30 mL.[17]
Optigene 3, otc (Pfeiffer)	**Solution**: 0.05%	In 15 mL.[5]
Tetrasine, otc (Optopics)	**Solution**: 0.05%	In 15 and 22.5 mL.[18]
Tetrasine Extra, otc (Optopics)	**Solution**: 0.05%	In 15 mL.[19]
Visine, otc (Pfizer)	**Solution**: 0.05%	In 15, 22.5, and 30 mL.[5]
Visine A.C., otc (Pfizer)	**Solution**: 0.05%	In 15 mL.[20]
Visine Advanced Relief, otc (Pfizer)	**Solution**: 0.05%	In 15 and 30 mL.[21]

[1] With 0.01% benzalkonium chloride, 0.4% glycerin, 0.25% zinc sulfate, and EDTA.
[2] With 0.2% PEG-300 and 0.01% benzalkonium chloride.
[3] With benzalkonium chloride, EDTA, 0.2% glycerin, and boric acid.
[4] With benzalkonium chloride, EDTA, 0.25% zinc sulfate, and 0.2% glycerin.
[5] With 0.01% benzalkonium chloride and EDTA.
[6] With 0.01% benzalkonium chloride, 0.25% polyvinyl alcohol, 1% PEG-400, and EDTA.
[7] With 0.005% benzalkonium chloride, EDTA, 0.25% zinc sulfate, 0.25% polyvinyl alcohol, and 1% PEG-400.
[8] With 0.01% benzalkonium chloride, 0.5% hydroxypropyl methylcellulose, and EDTA.
[9] With 0.004% benzalkonium chloride, EDTA, and 1.4% polyvinyl alcohol.
[10] With benzalkonium chloride, polyvinyl alcohol, EDTA, and PEG-800.
[11] With 0.01% benzalkonium chloride and 0.1% EDTA.
[12] With 0.005% benzalkonium chloride, 1.4% polyvinyl alcohol, and EDTA.
[13] With 1.4% polyvinyl alcohol, 0.004% benzalkonium chloride, and EDTA.
[14] With 1.4 polyvinyl alcohol, EDTA.
[15] With 0.01% benzalkonium chloride, polysorbate 80, and 0.25% zinc sulfate.
[16] With 0.01% benzalkonium chloride, 0.1% EDTA, and 1% glycerin.
[17] With benzalkonium chloride, EDTA, 1.4% polyvinyl alcohol, and 0.6% povidone.
[18] With benzalkonium chloride and EDTA.
[19] With 1% polyethylene glycol 400, benzalkonium chloride, and EDTA.
[20] With 0.01% benzalkonium chloride, EDTA, and 0.25% zinc sulfate.
[21] With benzalkonium chloride, 1% polyethylene glycol 400, 1% povidone, 0.1% dextran 70, and EDTA.

CHAPTER SUMMARIES

Antihistamines

Generic Name Trade Name	Doseform/ Strength	How Supplied
Azelastine HCl		
Optivar, Rx (Muro Pharmaceutical)	**Solution:** 0.05%	In 10 mL containers with a LDPE dropper tip.[1]
Emedastine Difumarate		
Emadine, Rx (Alcon)	**Ophthalmic** **suspension:** 0.05%	In 5 mL opaque, plastic dispenser.[2]
Ketotifen Fumarate		
Zaditor, Rx (Ciba Vision)	**Solution:** 0.25 mg/mL (0.345 mg/mL ketotifen fumarate)	In 5 mL.[3]
Levocabastine HCl		
Livostin, Rx (Novartis)	**Suspension:** 0.05%	In 2.5, 5, and 10 mL dropper bottles.[4]
Olopatadine HCL		
Patanol, Rx (Alcon)	**Solution:** 0.1%[5]	In 5 mL Drop-Tainers.

[1] With 0.125 mg benzalkonium chloride, EDTA, hydroxypropylmethylcellulose, sorbitol solution, and sodium hydroxide.
[2] With 0.01% benzalkonium, tromethamine, sodium chloride, hydroxypropyl methylcellulose, and hydrochloric acid/sodium hydroxide.
[3] With 0.01% benzalkonium chloride, glycerol, and sodium hydroxide/hydrochloric acid.
[4] With 0.15 mg benzalkonium chloride, propylene glycol, and EDTA.
[5] With 0.01% benzalkonium chloride.

Corticosteroids

Generic Name Trade Name	Doseform/ Strength	How Supplied
Dexamethasone		
Dexamethasone Sodium *Phosphate, Rx* (Various, eg, Bausch & Lomb, Rugby, Schein)	**Solution:** 0.01% dexa- methasone phosphate (as sodium phosphate)	In 5 mL.
AK-Dex, Rx (Akorn)	**Solution:** 0.01% dexa- methasone phosphate (as sodium phosphate)	In 5 mL.[1]
Decadron Phosphate, Rx (Merck)	**Solution:** 0.01% dexa- methasone phosphate (as sodium phosphate)	In 5 mL Ocumeters.[2]
Maxidex, Rx (Alcon)	**Suspension:** 0.1% dexamethasone	In 5 mL and 15 mL Drop- Tainers.[3]

Corticosteroids

Generic Name Trade Name	Doseform/ Strength	How Supplied
Dexamethasone Sodium Phosphate, Rx (Bausch & Lomb)	**Ointment:** 0.05% dexamethasone phosphate (as sodium phosphate)	In 3.5 g.
AK-Dex, Rx (Akorn)	**Ointment:** 0.05% dexamethasone phosphate (as sodium phosphate)	In 3.5 g.[4]
Fluorometholone		
Fluorometholone, Rx, (Various, eg, Bausch & Lomb, Falcon)	**Solution:** 1%	In 5, 10, and 15 mL.
Fluor-Op, Rx (Novartis)	**Suspension:** 0.1%	In 5, 10, and 15 mL.[5]
FML, Rx (Allergan)	**Suspension:** 0.1%	In 1, 5, 10, and 15 mL.[5]
Flarex, Rx (Alcon)	**Suspension:** 0.1% fluorometholone acetate	In 2.5, 5, and 10 mL DropTainers.[6]
eFLone, Rx (Novartis)	**Suspension:** 0.1% fluorometholone acetate	In 5 and 10 mL.[6]
FML Forte, Rx (Allergan)	**Suspension:** 0.25% fluorometholone acetate	In 2, 5, 10, and 15 mL.[7]
FML S.O.P., Rx (Allergan)	**Ointment:** 0.1%	In 3.5 g.[8]
Loteprednol Etabonate		
Alrex, Rx (Bausch & Lomb)	**Suspension:** 0.2%	In 5 and 10 mL.[9]
Lotemax, Rx (Bausch & Lomb)	**Suspension:** 0.5%	In 2.5, 5, and 10 mL.[9]
Medrysone		
HMS, Rx (Bausch & Lomb)	**Suspension:** 0.1%	In 15 mL.[10]
Prednisolone		
Pred Mild, Rx (Allergan)	**Suspension:** 0.12% prednisolone acetate	In 5 and 10 mL.[11]
Econopred, Rx (Alcon)	**Suspension:** 0.125% prednisolone acetate	In 5 and 10 mL DropTainers.[12]
AK-Pred, Rx (Akorn)	**Solution:** 0.125% prednisolone sodium phosphate	In 5 mL.[13]
Inflamase Mild, Rx (Novartis)	**Solution:** 0.125% prednisolone sodium phosphate	In 3, 5, and 10 mL.[14]

CHAPTER SUMMARIES

Corticosteroids

Generic Name Trade Name	Doseform/ Strength	How Supplied
Econopred Plus, Rx (Alcon)	**Suspension**: 0.1% prednisolone acetate	In 5 and 10 mL Drop-Tainers.[12]
Pred Forte, Rx (Allergan)	**Suspension**: 1% prednisolone acetate	In 1, 5, 10, and 15 mL.[11]
Prednisolone Acetate Ophthalmic, Rx (Falcon)	**Suspension**: 1% prednisolone acetate	In 5 and 10 mL.[12]
Prednisolone Sodium Phosphate, Rx (Various, eg, Bausch & Lomb)	**Solution**: 1% prednisolone sodium phosphate	In 5, 10, and 15 mL.
AK-Pred, Rx (Akorn)	**Solution**: 1% prednisolone sodium phosphate	In 5 and 15 mL.[13]
Inflamase Forte, Rx (Novartis)	**Solution**: 1% prednisolone sodium phosphate	In 3, 5, 10, and 15 mL.[14]
Rimexolone *Vexol, Rx* (Alcon)	**Suspension**: 1%	In 5 and 10 mL Drop-Tainers.

[1] With 0.01% benzalkonium chloride, EDTA, and hydroxyethylcellulose.
[2] With polysorbate 80, EDTA, 0.1% sodium bisulfite, 0.25% phenylethanol, and 0.02% benzalkonium chloride.
[3] With 0.01% benzalkonium chloride, EDTA, 0.5% hydroxypropyl methylcellulose, and polysorbate 80.
[4] With lanolin anhydrous, parabens, PEG-400, white petrolatum, and mineral oil.
[5] With 0.004% benzalkonium chloride, EDTA, polysorbate 80, and 1.4% polyvinyl alcohol.
[6] With 0.01% benzalkonium chloride, EDTA, hydroxyethylcellulose, and tyloxapol.
[7] With 0.005% benzalkonium chloride, EDTA, polysorbate 80, and 1.4% polyvinyl alcohol.
[8] With 0.0008% phenylmercuric acetate, white petrolatum, mineral oil, petrolatum, and lanolin alcohol.
[9] With 0.01% benzalkonium chloride, EDTA, glycerin, povidone, and tyloxapol.
[10] With 0.004% benzalkonium chloride, EDTA, 1.4% polyvinyl alcohol, and hydroxypropyl methylcellulose.
[11] With 0.01% benzalkonium chloride, EDTA, polysorbate 80, hydroxypropyl methylcellulose, and glycerin.
[12] With 0.01% benzalkonium chloride, EDTA, hydroxypropyl methylcellulose, and sodium bisulfite.
[13] With 0.01% benzalkonium chloride and EDTA.
[14] With 0.01% benzalkonium chloride, polysorbate 80, and EDTA in carbapol gel.

Decongestants and Antihistamines

Trade Name	Decongestant	Antihistamine	How Supplied
Naphcon-A Solution, otc (Alcon)	naphazoline HCl 0.025%	pheniramine maleate 0.3%	In 15 mL Drop-Tainers.[1]
Opcon-A Solution, otc (Bausch & Lomb)	naphazoline HCl 0.027%	pheniramine maleate 0.315%	In 15 mL. [2]
Vasocon-A Solution, otc (Ciba Vision)	naphazoline HCl 0.05%	antazoline phosphate 0.5%	In 15 mL.[3]

[1] With 0.01% benzalkonium chloride, and EDTA.
[2] With 0.5% hydroxypropyl methylcellulose, 0.01% benzalkonium chloride, 0.1% EDTA, and boric acid.
[3] With 0.01% benzalkonium chloride, PEG 8000, polyvinyl alcohol, and EDTA.

Mast Cell Inhibitors

Generic Name Trade Name	Doseform/ Strength	How Supplied
Cromolyn Sodium		
Cromolyn Sodium, Rx (Various, eg, Akorn, Falcon, Teva)	**Solution**: 4%	In 10 mL opaque polyethylene bottle with controlled dropper tip.[1]
Crolom, Rx (Bausch & Lomb)	**Solution**: 4%	In 2.5 and 10 mL bottles with controlled drop tip.
Opticrom, Rx (Allergan)	**Solution**: 4%	In 10 mL opaque polyethylene eye drop bottles.[1]
Lodoxamide Tromethamine		
Alomide, Rx (Alcon)	**Solution**: 0.1%	10 mL Drop-Tainers.
Nedocromil Sodium		
Alocril, Rx (Allergan)	**Solution**: 2%	In 5 mL bottle with a controlled dropper tip.[2]
Pemirolast Potassium		
Alamast, Rx (Santen)	**Solution**: 0.1%	In 10 mL bottles with a controlled dropper tip.[3]

[1] With 0.01% benzalkonium chloride and 0.1% EDTA.
[2] With 0.01% benzalkonium chloride, 0.5% sodium chloride, and 0.05% EDTA.
[3] With 0.005% lauralkonium chloride, glycerin, dibasic sodium phosphate, monobasic sodium phosphate, phosphoric acid, and sodium hydroxide.

Nonsteroidal Anti-Inflammatory Agents (NSAIDs)

Generic Name Trade Name)	Doseform/ Strength	How Supplied
Diclofenac Sodium		
Diclofenac Sodium Ophthalmic, Rx (Various, eg, Falcon, Geneva)	**Solution**: 0.1%	In 15 mL.
Voltaren, Rx (Novartis)	**Solution**: 0.1%	In 2.5 and 5 mL dropper bottles.[2]
Flurbiprofen Sodium		
Ocufen, Rx (Allergan)	**Solution**: 0.03%	In 2.5, 5, and 10 mL dropper bottles.[3]
Flurbiprofen Sodium Ophthalmic, Rx (Various, eg, Bausch & Lomb)	**Solution**: 0.03%	In 2.5 mL.[3]

CHAPTER SUMMARIES

Nonsteroidal Anti-Inflammatory Agents (NSAIDs)

Generic Name Trade Name)	Doseform/ Strength	How Supplied
Ketorolac Tromethamine		
Acular, Rx (Allergan)	**Solution**: 0.5%	In 5 mL dropper bottles.[4]
Acular PF, Rx (Allergan)	**Solution**: 0.5%	In 12 single-use 0.4 mL vials.[5]
Suprofen		
Profenal, Rx (Alcon)	**Solution**: 1%	In 2.5 mL Drop-Tainers.[6]

[1] With 1 mg/mL EDTA, boric acid, polyoxyl 35 castor oil, 2 mg/mL sorbic acid, and tromethamine.
[2] With 1.4% polyvinyl alcohol, 0.005% thimerosal, and EDTA.
[3] With 0.01% benzalkonium chloride, 0.1% EDTA, and octoxynol 40.
[4] With 0.5% ketorolac tromethamine.
[5] With 0.005% thimerosol, 2% caffeine, EDTA.

Artificial Tear Solutions

Trade Name	Doseform/Strength	How Supplied
20/20 Tears, otc (S.S.S.)	**Solution**: 1.4% PVA, 0.01% benzalkonium Cl, 0.05% EDTA, KCl, NaCl	Thimerosal free. In 15 mL.
Akwa Tears, otc (Akorn)	**Solution**: 1.4% PVA, 0.005% benzalkonium Cl, EDTA, NaCl, sodium phosphate	In 15 mL.
AquaSite, otc (Novartis)	**Solution**: 0.2% PEG-400, 0.1% dextran 70, polycarbophil, NaCl, EDTA, sodium hydroxide	Preservative free. In 6 mL (single-use 24s).
Artificial Tears, otc (Various, eg, Rugby, United)	**Solution**: 1.4% PVA, 0.01% benzalkonium Cl, EDTA, NaCl, KCl	In 15 mL.
Bion Tears, otc (Alcon)	**Solution**: 0.1% dextran 70, 0.3% hydroxypropyl methylcellulose 2910, sodium hydroxide, carbon dioxide, hydrochloric acid	Preservative free. In 0.45 mL (UD 28s).
Celluvisc, otc (Allergan)	**Solution**: 1% carboxymethylcellulose, calcium chloride, NaCl, KCl, sodium lactate	Preservative free. In 0.1 mL (UD 30s and 50s).
Dry Eye Therapy, otc (Bausch & Lomb)	**Solution**: 0.3% glycerin, NaCl, KCl, sodium citrate, sodium phosphate	Preservative free. In 3 mL.
GenTeal, otc (Novartis)	**Solution**: 0.3% hydroxypropyl methylcellulose, boric acid, NaCl, KCl, phosphoric acid, sodium perborate	In 15 and 25 mL.
HypoTears, otc (Novartis)	**Solution**: 1% PVA, 1% PEG-400, 0.01% benzalkonium Cl, dextrose, EDTA	In 15 and 30 mL.
HypoTears PF, otc (Novartis)	**Solution**: 1% PVA, 1% PEG-400, dextrose, EDTA	Preservative free. In 0.5 mL (UD 30s).

Artificial Tear Solutions

Trade Name	Doseform/Strength	How Supplied
Isopto Plain, otc (Alcon)	**Solution**: 0.5% hydroxypropyl methyl-cellulose 2910, 0.01% benzalkonium Cl, NaCl, sodium phosphate, sodium citrate	In 15 mL Drop-Tainers.
Isopto Tears, otc (Alcon)	**Solution**: 0.5% hydroxypropyl methyl-cellulose 2910, 0.01% benzalkonium Cl, NaCl, sodium phosphate, sodium citrate	In 15 mL.
Just Tears, otc (Blairex)	**Solution**: Benzalkonium Cl, 1.4% PVA, EDTA, NaCl, KCl	In 15 mL.
Liquifilm Tears, otc (Allergan)	**Solution**: 1.4% PVA, 0.5% chlorobuta-nol, NaCl	In 15 and 30 mL.
Moisture Eyes, otc (Bausch & Lomb)	**Solution**: 1% propylene glycol, 0.3% glycerin, 0.01% benzalkonium Cl	In 15 and 30 mL.
Moisture Eyes Preservative Free, otc (Bausch & Lomb)	**Solution**: 0.95% propylene glycol, boric acid, EDTA, KCl, NaCl, sodium borate	In 0.6 mL (UD 32s).
Murine Tears, otc (Ross)	**Solution**: 0.5% PVA, 0.6% PVP, benzal-konium Cl, dextrose, EDTA, NaCl, sodium bicarbonate, sodium phosphate, KCl, sodium citrate	In 15 and 30 mL.
Murocel, otc (Bausch & Lomb)	**Solution**: 1% methylcellulose, propyl-ene glycol, NaCl, 0.028% methylpara-ben, 0.012% propylparaben, boric acid, sodium borate	In 15 mL.
Nu-Tears II, otc (Optopics)	**Solution**: 1% PVA, 1% PEG-400, EDTA, benzalkonium Cl	In 15 mL.
OcuCoat, otc (Bausch & Lomb)	**Solution**: 0.1% dextran 70, 0.8% hydroxypropyl methylcellulose, sodium phosphate, KCl, NaCl, 0.01% benzal-konium Cl, dextrose	In 15 mL.
OcuCoat PF, otc (Bausch & Lomb)	**Solution**: 0.1% dextran 70, 0.8% hydroxypropyl methylcellulose, sodium phosphate, KCl, NaCl, dextrose	Preservative free. In 0.5 mL (UD 28s).
Puralube Tears, otc (Fougera)	**Solution**: 1% PVA, 1% PEG-400, EDTA, benzalkonium Cl	In 15 mL.
Refresh, otc (Allergan)	**Solution**: 1.4% PVA, 0.6% PVP, NaCl	Preservative free. In 0.3 mL (UD 30s and 50s).
Refresh Plus, otc (Allergan)	**Solution**: 0.5% carboxymethylcellulose sodium, KCl, NaCl, calcium chloride, magnesium chloride, sodium lactate	Preservative free. In 0.3 mL (UD 30s and 50s).
Refresh Tears, otc (Allergan)	**Solution**: 0.5% carboxymethylcellulose sodium, boric acid, calcium chloride, magnesium chloride, KCl, NaCl, stabi-lized oxychloro complex	In 15 mL.

Artificial Tear Solutions

Trade Name	Doseform/Strength	How Supplied
Teargen, otc (Zenith-Goldline)	**Solution**: 0.01% benzalkonium Cl, EDTA, NaCl, 1.4% sodium phosphate	In 15 mL.
Teargen II, otc (Zenith-Goldline)	**Solution**: 0.4% hydroxypropyl methylcellulose 2910, sodium phosphate, 0.01% benzalkonium Cl, EDTA, KCl, NaCl	In 15 mL.
Tearisol, otc (Novartis)	**Solution**: 0.5% hydroxypropyl methylcellulose, 0.01% benzalkonium Cl, EDTA, boric acid, sodium carbonate	In 15 mL.
Tears Naturale, otc (Alcon)	**Solution**: 0.1% dextran 70, 0.01% benzalkonium Cl, 0.3% hydroxypropyl methylcellulose, NaCl, EDTA, hydrochloric acid, sodium hydroxide, KCl	In 15 and 30 mL.
Tears Naturale II, otc (Alcon)	**Solution**: 0.1% dextran 70, 0.3% hydroxypropyl methylcellulose 2910, 0.001% polyquarternium-1, NaCl, KCl, sodium borate	In 15 and 30 mL Drop-Tainers.
Tears Naturale Free, otc (Alcon)	**Solution**: 0.3% hydroxypropyl methylcellulose 2910, 0.1% dextran 70	Preservative free. In 0.6 mL (UD 32s).
Tears Plus, otc (Allergan)	**Solution**: 1.4% PVA, 0.6% PVP, 0.5% chlorobutanol, NaCl	In 15 and 30 mL.
Tears Renewed, otc (Akorn)	**Solution**: 0.01% benzalkonium Cl, EDTA, 0.1% dextran 70, NaCl, 0.3% hydroxypropyl methylcellulose 2906, hydrochloric acid, KCl, NaCl, sodium hydroxide	In 15 mL.
Thera Tears, otc (Advanced Vision)	**Solution**: 0.25% sodium carboxymethylcellulose, NaCl, KCl, sodium phosphate, borate buffers, calcium chloride, magnesium chloride, sodium bicarbonate	Preservative free. In 0.6 mL (UD 32s).
Ultra Tears, otc (Alcon)	**Solution**: 1% hydroxypropyl methylcellulose 2910, 0.01% benzalkonium Cl, NaCl, sodium citrate, sodium phosphate	In 15 mL.
Visine Tears, otc (Pfizer)	**Solution**: 1% PEG-400, 0.2% hydroxypropyl methylcellulose, 0.2% glycerin, ascorbic acid, benzalkonium Cl, boric acid, dextrose, disodium phosphate, glycine, KCl, magnesium chloride, NaCl, sodium borate, sodium citrate, sodium lactate	In 15 mL.
Viva-Drops, otc (Vision Pharm)	**Solution**: Polysorbate 80, citric acid, NaCl, EDTA, retinyl palmitate, mannitol, sodium citrate, pyruvate	Preservative free. In 10 and 15 mL.

Ocular Lubricants, Ointments and Gels

Trade Name	Doseform/Strength	How Supplied
Akwa Tears, otc (Akorn)	**Ointment**: White petrolatum, mineral oil, lanolin	Preservative free. In 3.5 g.
Artificial Tears, otc (Rugby)	**Ointment**: 83% white petrolatum, 15% mineral oil, lanolin oil	In 3.5 g.
Dry Eyes, otc (Bausch & Lomb)	**Ointment**: White petrolatum, mineral oil, lanolin	Preservative free. In 3.5 g.
Duratears Naturale, otc (Alcon)	**Ointment**: White petrolatum, anhydrous liquid lanolin, mineral oil	Preservative free. In 3.5 g.
HypoTears, otc (Novatis)	**Ointment**: White petrolatum, light mineral oil	Preservative and lanolin free. In 3.5 g.
Lacri-Lube NP, otc (Allergan)	**Ointment**: 57.3% white petrolatum, 42.5% mineral oil	Preservative free. In 0.7 g.
Lacri-Lube S.O.P., otc (Allergan)	**Ointment**: 56.8% white petrolatum, 42.5% mineral oil, chlorobutanol, lanolin alcohols	In 0.7, 3.5, and 7 g.
Moisture Eyes PM, otc (Bausch & Lomb)	**Ointment**: 80% white petrolatum, 20% mineral oil	Preservative free. In 3.5 g.
Puralube, otc (Fougera)	**Ointment**: White petrolatum, light mineral oil	In 3.5 g.
Refresh PM, otc (Alllergan)	**Ointment**: 56.8% white petrolatum, 41.5% mineral oil, lanolin alcohols, NaCl	Preservative free. In 3.5 g.
Stye, otc (Del Pharm)	**Ointment**: 57.7% white petrolatum, 31.9% mineral oil, stearic acid, wheat germ oil, microcrystalline wax	In 3.5 g.
Tears Naturale P.M., otc (Alcon)	**Ointment**: White petrolatum, anhydrous liquid lanolin, mineral oil	Preservative free. In 3.5 g.
Tears Renewed, otc (Akorn)	**Ointment**: White petrolatum, light mineral oil	Preservative free. In 3.5 g.
GenTeal Gel, otc (Novartis)	**Gel**: 0.3% hydroxypropyl methylcellulose, 0.028% sodium perborate, carbopol 980, phosphoric acid, sorbitol	In 10 mL.

Artificial Tear Insert

Trade Name	Doseform/Strength	How Supplied
Lacrisert, Rx (Merck & Co.)	**Insert**: 5 mg hydroxypropyl cellulose	Preservative free. In 60s with applicator.

Punctal Plugs

Trade Name	Doseform/Strength	How Supplied
Eagle FlexPlug, Rx (Eagle Vision)	**Plug**: Silicone plug.	In 0.4, 0.5, 0.6, 0.7, 0.8 and 0.9 mm sizes (single packs).
EaglePlug, Rx (Eagle Vision)	**Plug**: Silicone plug	In 0.4, 0.5, 0.6, 0.7, and 0.8 mm sizes (packs of 2 plugs).
Herrick Lacrimal Plug, Rx (Lacrimedics)	**Plug**: Silicone plug	In 0.3, 0.5, and 0.7 mm sizes (packs of 2 plugs).
Ready-Set Punctum Plugs, Rx (FCI Ophthalmics)	**Plug**: Silicone plug	In 0.4, 0.5, 0.7, 0.8, and 1 mm sizes (packs of 2 plugs).
Tears Naturale, Rx (Alcon)	**Plug**: Silicone plug	In 0.4, 0.5, 0.6, 0.7, and 0.8 mm sizes.
TearSaver, Rx (Ciba Vision)	**Plug**: Silicone plug	In 0.4, 0.5, 0.6, 0.7, and 0.8 mm sizes (packs of 2 plugs).

Collagen Implants

Trade Name	Doseform/Strength	How Supplied
Collagen Implant, Rx (Lacrimedics)	**Implant**: Collagen implant	In 0.2, 0.3, 0.4, 0.5, and 0.6 mm sizes (72s).
Soft Plug, Rx (Oasis)	**Implant**: Collagen implant	In 0.3 and 0.4 mm sizes (60s).
Tears Naturale, Rx (Alcon)	**Implant**: Collagen implant	In 0.2, 0.3, and 0.4 mm sizes (60s).
TearSaver, Rx (Ciba Vision)	**Implant**: Collagen implant	In 0.2, 0.3, 0.4, 0.5, and 0.6 mm sizes.
Temporary Punctal/Canalicular Collagen Implant, Rx (Eagle Vision)	**Implant**: Collagen implant	In 0.2, 0.3, 0.4, 0.5, and 0.6 mm sizes (72s).

Cleaning/Lubricant for Artificial Eyes

Generic Name Trade Name	Doseform/Strength	How Supplied
Tyloxapol		
Enuclene, otc (Alcon)	**Solution**: 0.25%[1]	In 15 mL Drop-Tainers.

[1] 0.02% benzalkonium Cl.

Antibiotics

Generic Name Trade Name	Doseform/ Strength	How Supplied
Bacitracin		
Bacitracin, Rx (Various)	**Ointment**: 500 units/g	In 3.5 and 3.75 g.
AK-Tracin, Rx (Akorn)	**Ointment**: 500 units/g	Preservative free. In 3.5 g.[1]
Polymyxin B Sulfate		
Polymyxin B Sulfate Sterile, Rx (Bedford)	**Powder for Solution**: 500,000 units	In 20 mL vials.
Chloramphenicol		
Chloramphenicol, Rx (Ivax)	**Solution**:[2] 5 mg/mL	In 7.5 and 15 mL.[3]
AK-Chlor, Rx (Akorn)	**Solution**: 5 mg/mL	In 7.5 and 15 mL.[3]
Chloromycetin, Rx (Monarch)	**Solution**: 5 mg/mL	In 15 mL.[3]
Chloroptic, Rx (Allergan)	**Solution**: 5 mg/mL	In 2.5 and 7.5 mL.[4]
AK-Chlor, Rx (Akorn)	**Ointment**: 10 mg/g	In 3.5 g.[5]
Chloroptic S.O.P., Rx (Allergan)	**Ointment**: 10 mg/g	In 3.5 g.
Chloromycetin, Rx (Monarch)	**Powder for Solution**: 25 mg/vial	Preservative free. In 15 mL with diluent.
Erythromycin		
Erythromycin, Rx (Various)	**Ointment**: 5 mg/g	In 3.5 g.
Ilotycin, Rx (Dista)	**Ointment**: 5 mg/g	In 3.5 g.[6]
Gentamicin Sulfate		
Gentamicin Ophthalmic, Rx (Various)	**Solution**: 3 mg/mL	In 5 and 15 mL.
Garamycin, Rx (Schering)	**Solution**: 3 mg/mL	In 5 mL dropper bottles.[7]
Genoptic, Rx (Allergan)	**Solution**: 3 mg/mL	In 1 and 5 mL dropper bottles.[8]
Gentacidin, Rx (Novartis)	**Solution**: 3 mg/mL	In 3 and 5 mL dropper bottles.[7]
Gentak, Rx (Akorn)	**Solution**: 3 mg/mL	In 5 and 15 mL dropper bottles.[7]
Gentamicin Ophthalmic, Rx (Various)	**Ointment**: 3 mg/g	In 3.5 g.

CHAPTER SUMMARIES

395

Antibiotics

Generic Name Trade Name	Doseform/ Strength	How Supplied
Garamycin, Rx (Schering)	**Ointment**: 3 mg/g	In 3.5 g.[9]
Genoptic S.O.P., Rx (Allergan)	**Ointment**: 3 mg/g	In 3.5 g.[9]
Gentacidin, Rx (Novartis)	**Ointment**: 3 mg/g	In 3.5 g.[1]
Gentak, Rx (Akorn)	**Ointment**: 3 mg/g	In 3.5 g.[9]
Tobramycin		
Tobramycin, Rx (Various)	**Solution**: 0.3%	In 5 mL bottle.
AKTob, Rx (Akorn)	**Solution**: 0.3%	In 5 mL.[10]
Tobrex, Rx (Alcon)	**Solution**: 0.3%	In 5 mL Drop-Tainers.[11]
Tobrex, Rx (Alcon)	**Ointment**: 3 mg/g	In 3.5 g.[12]
Ciprofloxacin		
Ciloxan, Rx (Alcon)	**Solution**: 0.3% (equivalent to 3 mg base)	In 2.5, 5, and 10 mL Drop-Tainers.[13]
Ciloxan, Rx (Alcon)	**Ointment**: 0.3% (equivalent to 3 mg base)	in 3.5 g tube.[1]
Norfloxacin		
Chibroxin, Rx (Merck)	**Solution**: 3 mg/mL	In 5 mL Ocumeters.[14]
Ofloxacin		
Ocuflox, Rx (Allergan)	**Solution**: 0.3%	In 1, 5, and 10 mL.[15]

[1] With white petrolatum and mineral oil.
[2] Refrigerate until dispensed.
[3] With 0.5% chlorobutanol, boric acid, sodium borate, hydroxypropyl methylcellulose, sodium hydroxide, and hydrochloric acid.
[4] With 0.5% chlorobutanol, PEG-300, polyoxyl 40 stearate, and sodium hydroxide or hydrochloric acid.
[5] With white petrolatum, mineral oil, and polysorbate 80.
[6] With white petrolatum and mineral oil.
[7] With 0.1 mg/mL benzalkonium chloride, 1.4% sodium phosphate, and NaCl.
[8] With benzalkonium chloride, 1.4% polyvinyl alcohol, EDTA, sodium phosphate dibasic, NaCl, and hydrochloric acid or sodium hydroxide
[9] With white petrolatum and parabens.
[10] With 0.01% benzalkonium chloride, boric acid, and sodium sulfate.
[11] With benzalkonium chloride, tyloxapol, boric acid, and NaCl.
[12] With white petrolatum, mineral oil, and 0.5% chlorobutanol.
[13] With 0.006% benzalkonium chloride, 4.6% mannitol, and 0.05% EDTA.
[14] With 0.0025% benzalkonium chloride, EDTA, and NaCl.
[15] With 0.005% benzalkonium chloride and NaCl.

Combination Antibiotics

Trade Name	Antibiotics	How Supplied
Triple Antibiotic Ophthalmic Ointment, Rx (Various, eg, Fougera)	Polymyxin B Sulfate (units/g or mL): 10,000 Neomycin Sulfate (mg/g or mL): 3.5 Bacitracin Zinc (units/g): 400)	In 3.5 g.
Bacitracin Neomycin Polymyxin B Ointment, Rx (Various, eg, Fougera)		In 3.5 g.
AK-Spore Ointment, Rx (Akorn)		Preservative free. White petrolatum, mineral oil. In 3.5 g.
Neosporin Ophthalmic Ointment, Rx (GlaxoSmithKline)		White petrolatum. In 3.5 g.
Neomycin Sulfate-Polymyxin B Sulfate-Gramicidin Solution, Rx (Various, eg, Rugby, Steris)	Polymyxin B Sulfate (units/g or mL): 10,000 Neomycin Sulfate (mg/g or mL): 1.75 Gramicidin: 0.025 mg/mL)	In 2 and 10 mL.
AK-Spore Solution, Rx (Akorn)		In 2 and 10 mL.[1]
Neosporin Ophthalmic Solution, Rx (GlaxoSmithKline)		In 10 mL Drop Dose.[1]
Bacitracin Zinc and Polymyxin B Ointment, Rx (Bausch & Lomb)	Polymyxin B Sulfate (units/g or mL): 10,000 Bacitracin Zinc (units/g): 500)	White petrolatum and mineral oil. In 3.5 g.
AK-Poly-Bac Ointment, Rx (Akorn)		Preservative free. White petrolatum, mineral oil. In 3.5 g.
Polysporin Ophthalmic Ointment, Rx (Monarch)		White petrolatum, mineral oil. In 3.5 g.
Terramycin w/Polymyxin B Ointment, Rx (Roerig)	Polymyxin B Sulfate (units/g or mL): 10,000 Oxytetracycline HCl: 5 mg/g	White and liquid petrolatum. In 3.5 g.
Terak Ointment, Rx (Akorn)		White and liquid petrolatum. In 3.5 g.

Combination Antibiotics

Trade Name	Antibiotics	How Supplied
Trimethoprim Sulfate and Polymyxin B Sulfate Ophthalmic Solution, Rx (Bausch & Lomb)	Polymyxin B Sulfate (units/g or mL): 10,000 Trimethoprim: 1 mg/mL	In 10 mL.[2]
Polytrim Ophthalmic Solution, Rx (Allergan)		In 10 mL.[2]

[1] With 0.001% thimerosal, 0.5% alcohol, propylene glycol, and polyoxyethylene polyoxypropylene.
[2] With 0.004% benzalkonium chloride and NaCl.

Sulfonamides

Generic Name Trade Name	Doseform/ Strength	How Supplied
Sulfisoxazole Diolamine		
Gantrisin, Rx (Roche)	**Solution**: 4%	With 1:100,000 phenylmercuric nitrate. In 15 mL with dropper.
Sulfacetamide Sodium		
Sulster, Rx (Akorn)	**Solution**: 1%	In 5 and 10 mL.
Sulfacetamide Sodium, Rx (Various, eg, Bausch & Lomb, Fougera)	**Solution**: 10%	In 15 mL.
AK-Sulf, Rx (Akorn)	**Solution**: 10%	In 2, 5, and 15 mL.[1]
Bleph-10, Rx (Allergan)	**Solution**: 10%	In 2.5, 5, and 15 mL.[2]
Ocusulf-10, Rx (Optopics)	**Solution**: 10%	In 2, 5, and 15 mL.[3]
Sodium Sulamyd, Rx (Schering)	**Solution**: 10%	In 5 and 15 mL.[1]
Sulf-10, Rx (Novartis)	**Solution**: 10%	In 1 mL Dropperettes.[4]
Sulfacetamide Sodium, Rx (Various, eg, Schein, Steris)	**Solution**: 30%	In 15 mL.
Sodium Sulamyd, Rx (Schering)	**Solution**: 30%	In 15 mL.[5]
Sulfacetamide Sodium, Rx (Various, eg, Fougera, Moore)	**Ointment**: 10%	In 3.5 g.
AK-Sulf, Rx (Akorn)	**Ointment**: 10%	In 3.5 g.[6]
Bleph-10, Rx (Allergan)	**Ointment**: 10%	In 3.5 g.[7]
IsoptoCetamide, Rx (Alcon)	**Ointment**: 10%	In 3.5 g.[8]

OPHTHALMIC DRUG FACTS

Sulfonamides

Generic Name Trade Name	Doseform/ Strength	How Supplied
Sodium Sulamyd, Rx (Schering)	**Ointment**: 10%	In 3.5 g.[9]
Sulfonamide/Decongestant Combination		
Vasosulf, Rx (Ciba Vision)	**Solution**: 15% sodium sulfacetamide and 0.125% phenylephrine	With sodium thiosulfate, pol- xamer 188, and parabens. In 5 and 15 mL.

[1] With 3.1 mg sodium thiosulfate pentahydrate, 5 mg methylcellulose, 0.5 mg methylparaben, and 0.1 mg propylparaben per mL.

[2] With 1.4% polyvinyl alcohol, 0.005% benzalkonium chloride, polysorbate 80, sodium thiosulfate, and EDTA.

[3] With parabens, 1.4% polyvinyl alcohol, and sodium thiosulfate.

[4] With sodium thiosulfate, 0.005% thimerosal, and boric acid.

[5] With 1.5 mg sodium thiosulfate pentahydrate, 0.5 mg methylparaben, and 0.1 mg propylparaben per mL.

[6] With 0.5 mg methylparaben, 0.1 mg propylparaben, 0.25 mg benzalkonium chloride, and petrolatum base per g.

[7] With 0.0008% phenylmercuric acetate, white petrolatum, mineral oil, petrolatum, and lanolin alcohol.

[8] With 0.05% methylparaben, 0.01% propylparaben, white petrolatum, anhydrous liquid lanolin, and mineral oil.

[9] With 0.5 mg methylparaben, 0.1 mg propylparaben, 0.25 mg benzalkonium chloride, and petrolatum base per g.

CHAPTER SUMMARIES

Steroid and Sulfonamide Combinations, Suspensions and Solutions

Trade Name	Steroid	Sulfonamide	How Supplied
FML-S Suspension, Rx (Allergan)	0.1% fluorometholone	10% sodium sulfacetamide	In 5 and 10 mL.[1]
Blephamide Suspension, Rx (Allergan)	0.2% prednisolone acetate	10% sodium sulfacetamide	In 5 and 10 mL.[2]
Isopto Cetapred Suspension, Rx (Alcon)	0.25% prednisolone acetate	10% sodium sulfacetamide	In 5 and 15 mL Drop-Tainers.[3]
AK-Cide Suspension, Rx (Akorn)	0.5% prednisolone acetate	10% sodium sulfacetamide	In 5 mL dropper bottle.[4]
Metimyd Suspension, Rx (Schering)			In 5 mL.[5]
Sulfacetamide Sodium and Prednisolone, Rx (Schein)	0.25% prednisolone acetate	10% sodium sulfacetamide	In 5 and 10 mL.[6]
Sulster Solution, Rx (Akorn)			In 5 and 10 mL.[7]

[1] EDTA, 1.4% polyvinyl alcohol, 0.006% benzalkonium chloride, polysorbate 80, povidone, sodium thiosulfate, and sodium chloride.
[2] EDTA, 1.4% polyvinyl alcohol, polysorbate 80, sodium thiosulfate, and benzalkonium chloride.
[3] 0.5% hydroxypropyl methylcellulose 2910, EDTA, polysorbate 80, sodium thiosulfate, 0.025% benzalkonium chloride, 0.05% methylparaben, and 0.01% propylparaben.
[4] 5 mg phenethyl alcohol, tyloxapol, sodium thiosulfate, 0.25 mg benzalkonium chloride, and EDTA per mL.
[5] 0.5% phenylethyl alcohol, 0.025% benzalkonium chloride, sodium thiosulfate, EDTA, and tyloxapol.
[6] 0.01% mg thimerosal, EDTA, and boric acid.
[7] 0.01% mg thimerosal and EDTA.

Steroid and Sulfonamide Combinations, Ointments

Trade Name	Steroid	Sulfonamide	How Supplied
Blephamide S.O.P., Rx (Allergan)	0.2% prednisolone acetate	10% sodium sulfacetamide	In 3.5 g.[1]
Cetapred, Rx (Alcon)	0.25% prednisolone acetate	10% sodium sulfacetamide	In 3.5 g.[2]
AK-Cide, Rx (Akorn)	0.5% prednisolone acetate	10% sodium sulfacetamide	In 3.5 g applicator tube.[3]
Metimyd, Rx (Schering)			In 3.5 g.[4]
Vasodine, Rx (Novartis)			In 3.5 g.[5]

[1] 0.0008% phenylmercuric acetate, mineral oil, white petrolatum, and lanolin alcohol.
[2] Mineral oil, white petrolatum, lanolin oil, 0.05% methylparaben, and 0.01% propylparaben.
[3] 0.5 mg methylparaben, 0.1 mg propylparaben per g, mineral oil, and white petrolatum.
[4] Mineral oil, white petrolatum, 0.05% methylparaben, and 0.01% propylparaben.
[5] Mineral oil and white petrolatum.

Steroid and Antibiotic Ointments

Trade Name	Steroid (per g)	Antibiotic (per g)	How Supplied
Bacitracin Zinc/Neomycin Sulfate/Polymyxin B Sulfate/ Hydrocortisone, Rx (Various, eg, Fougera)	1% hydrocortisone	Neomycin sulfate equivalent to 0.35% neomycin base, 400 units bacitracin zinc, 10,000 units polymyxin B sulfate	In 3.5 g.
AK-Spore H.C., Rx (Akorn)			Preservative free. In 3.5 g.[1]
Cortisporin, Rx (Monarch)			In 3.5 g.[2]
Pred-G S.O.P., Rx (Allergan)	0.6% prednisolone acetate	Gentamicin sulfate equivalent to 0.3% gentamicin base	In 3.5 g.[3]
Neomycin/Polymyxin B Sulfate/Dexamethasone, Rx (Various)	0.1% dexamethasone	Neomycin sulfate equivelent to 0.35% neomycin base, 10,000 units polymyxin B sulfate.	In 3.5 g.
AK-Trol, Rx (Akorn)			In 3.5 g.[4]
Dexacidin, Rx (Novartis)			In 3.5 g.[1]

[1] White petrolatum and mineral oil.
[2] White petrolatum.
[3] 0.5% chlorobutanol, white petrolatum, mineral oil, petrolatum, and lanolin alcohol.
[4] White petrolatum, lanolin oil, mineral oil, and parabens.
[5] White petrolatum, anhydrous liquid lanolin, and parabens.

Steroid and Antibiotic Solutions and Suspensions

Trade Name	Steroid (per mL)	Antibiotic (per mL)	How Supplied
Neomycin/Polymyxin B Sulfate/Hydrocortisone, Rx (Various)	1% hydrocortisone	Neomycin sulfate equivalent to 0.35% neomycin base, 10,000 units polymyxin B sulfate	In 7.5 and 10 mL.
AK-Spore H.C. Ophthalmic Suspension, Rx (Akorn)			In 7.5 mL.[3]
Cortisporin Suspension, Rx (Monarch)			In 7.5 mL Drop Dose.[1]

Steroid and Antibiotic Solutions and Suspensions

Trade Name	Steroid (per mL)	Antibiotic (per mL)	How Supplied
Poly-Pred Suspension, Rx (Allergan)	0.5% prednisolone acetate	Neomycin sulfate equivalent to 0.35% neomycin base, 10,000 units poly-myxin B sulfate	In 5 and 10 mL.[2]
Pred-G Suspension, Rx (Allergan)	1% prednisolone acetate	Gentamicin sulfate equivalent to 0.3% gentramicin base	In 2, 5, and 10 mL.[3]
Neomycin Sulfate/ Dexamethasone Sodium Phosphate Solution, Rx (Various)	0.1% dexametha-sone phosphate (as sodium phosphate)	Neomycin sulfate equivalent to 0.35% neomycin base	In 5 mL.
NeoDecadron Solution, Rx (Merck)			In 5 mL Ocu-meters.[4]
Neo-Dexameth, Rx (Major)			In 5 mL.[5]
TobraDex Suspension, Rx (Alcon)	0.1% dexametha-sone	0.3% tobramycin	In 2.5, 5, and 10 mL Drop-Tainers.[6]
Neomycin/Polymyxin B Sulfate/Dexametha-sone Suspension, Rx (Various)	0.1% dexametha-sone	Neomycin sulfate equivalent to 0.35% neomycin base, 10,000 units poly-myxin B sulfate	In 5 mL.
AK-Trol Suspension, Rx (Akorn)			In 5 mL.[7]
Maxitrol Suspension, Rx (Alcon)			In 5 mL Drop-Tainers.[8]

[1] 0.001% thimerosal, cetyl alcohol, glyceryl monostearate, polyoxyl 40 stearate, propylene glycol, mineral oil, and NaCl.
[2] 1.4% polyvinyl alcohol, 0.001% thimerosal, polysorbate 80, and propylene glycol.
[3] 1.4% polyvinyl alcohol, 0.005% benzalkonium chloride, EDTA, hydroxypropyl methylcellulose, polysorbate 80, and NaCl.
[4] Polysorbate 80, EDTA, 0.2% benzalkonium chloride, 0.1% sodium bisulfite.
[5] 0.01% benzalkonium chloride, EDTA, polysorbate 80, and sodium bisulfite.
[6] 0.01% benzalkonium chloride, tyloxapol, EDTA, hydroxyethylcellulose, sodium sulfate, and NaCl.
[7] 0.004% benzalkonium chloride, polysorbate 20, 0.5% hydroxypropyl methylcellulose, and NaCl.
[8] 0.5% hydroxypropyl methylcellulose, polysorbate 20, 0.004% benzalkonium chloride.

OPHTHALMIC DRUG FACTS

Anti-infective Agents

Generic Name Trade Name	Doseform/ Strength	How Supplied
Zinc Sulfate Solution		
20/20 Eye Drops, otc (S. S. S.)	**Solution:** 0.25%	In 15 mL.[1]
Clear Eyes ACR Eye Drops, otc (Ross)	**Solution:** 0.25%	In 15 and 30 mL.[2]
Vasoclear A Eye Drops, otc (Novartis)	**Solution:** 0.25%	In 15 mL.[3]
Visine AC, otc (Pfizer)	**Solution:** 0.25%	In 15 mL.[4]
Zincfrin, otc (Alcon)	**Solution:** 0.25%	In 15 mL.[5]

[1] With 0.4% glycerin, 0.12% naphazoline HCl, EDTA, KCl, and camphor.
[2] With 0.2% glycerin, 0.12% naphazoline HCl, benzalkonium chloride, boric acid, EDTA, NaCl, and sodium citrate.
[3] With 0.02% naphazoline HCl, 1% polyethylene glycol 40, 0.0025% PVA, NaCl, and EDTA.
[4] With 0.05% tetrahydrozoline HCl, EDTA, boric acid, and NaCl.
[5] With 0.12% phenylephrine HCl, 0.01% benzalkonium chloride, polysorbate 80, sodium citrate, and sodium hydroxide.

Epinephrines

Generic Name Trade Name	Doseform/ Strength	How Supplied
Epinephrine HCl		
Epifrin, Rx (Allergan)	**Solution:** 0.5% (as base)	In 15 mL dropper bottles.[1]
Epifrin, Rx (Allergan)	**Solution:** 1% (as base)	In 15 mL dropper bottles.[1]
Glaucon, Rx (Alcon)	**Solution:** 1%	In 10 mL Drop-Tainers.[2]
Epifrin, Rx (Allergan)	**Solution:** 2% (as base)	In 15 mL dropper bottles.[1]
Glaucon, Rx (Alcon)	**Solution:** 2%	In 10 mL Drop-Tainers.[2]
Epinephryl Borate		
Epinal, Rx (Alcon)	**Solution:** 0.5%	In 7.5 mL.[3]
Epinal, Rx (Alcon)	**Solution:** 1%	In 7.5 mL.[3]

CHAPTER SUMMARIES

Epinephrines

Generic Name Trade Name	Doseform/ Strength	How Supplied
Dipivefrin HCl **(Dipivalyl epinephrine))**		
Dipivefrin HCl, Rx (Falcon)	**Solution:** 0.1%	In 5, 10, and 15 mL.
Propine, Rx (Allergan)	**Solution:** 0.1%	In 5, 10, and 15 mL C Cap Compliance Cap B.I.D.[4]

[1] With benzalkonium chloride, sodium metabisulfite, EDTA, and hydrochloric acid.
[2] With 0.01% benzalkonium chloride, sodium metabisulfite, EDTA, sodium chloride, hydrochloric acid, and sodium hydroxide.
[3] With 0.01% benzalkonium chloride, ascorbic acid, acetylcysteine, boric acid, and sodium carbonate.
[4] With 0.005% benzalkonium chloride, sodium chloride, EDTA, and hydrochloric acid.

Alpha$_2$ Adrenergic Agonists

Generic Name Trade Name	Doseform/ Strength	How Supplied
Apraclonidine HCl		
Iopidine, Rx (Alcon)	**Solution:** 0.5%	With 0.01% benzalkonium chloride. In 5 and 10 mL Drop-Tainers.
Iopidine, Rx (Alcon)	**Solution:** 1%	With 0.01% benzalkonium chloride. In 0.1 mL (2s).
Brimonidine Tartrate		
Alphagan, Rx (Allergan)	**Solution:** 0.2%	With polyvinyl alcohol, NaCl, 0.05 mg benzalkonium chloride per mL. In 5, 10, and 15 mL dropper bottles.
Alphagan, Rx (Allergan)	**Solution:** 0.15%	With sodium borate, boric acid, NaCl, KCl. In 5, 10, and 15 mL dropper bottles.

Beta-Adrenergic Blocking Agents

Generic Name Trade Name	Doseform/ Strength	How Supplied
Betaxolol HCl		
Betopic, Rx (Alcon)	**Solution:** 5.6 mg (equivalent to 5 mg base) per mL (0.5%)	In 10 mL Drop-Tainers.[1]
Betopic S, Rx (Alcon)	**Suspension:** 2.8 mg (equivalent to 2.5 mg base) per mL (0.25%)	In 5, 10, and 15 mL Drop-Tainers.[2]
Carteolol HCl		
Ocupress, Rx (Novartis)	**Solution:** 1%	In 5, 10 and 15 mL dropper bottles.[3]
Levobetaxolol HCl		
Betaxon, Rx (Alcon)	**Suspension, ophthalmic:** 0.5% as base (5.6 mg/mL)	In 5, 10, and 15 mL Drop-Tainers.[4]
Levobunolol HCl		
Levobunolol, Rx (Various, eg, Bausch & Lomb)	**Solution:** 0.25%	In 5 and 10 mL.
Betagen Liquifilm, Rx (Allergan)	**Solution:** 0.25%	In 5 and 10 mL dropper bottles with B.I.D. C Cap.[5]
Levobunolol, Rx (Various, eg, Bausch & Lomb)	**Solution:** 0.5%	In 5, 10, and 15 mL.
Betagen Liquifilm, Rx (Allergan)	**Solution:** 0.5%	In 2, 5, 10, and 15 mL bottles with B.I.D. and Q.D. C Cap.[5]
Metipranolol HCl		
OptiPranolol, Rx (Bausch & Lomb)	**Solution:** 0.3%	In 5 or 10 mL dropper bottles.[6]
Timolol Hemihydrate		
Betimol, Rx (Novartis)	**Solution:** 0.25%	In 2.5, 5, 10, and 15 mL.[7]
Betimol, Rx (Novartis)	**Solution:** 0.5%	In 2.5, 5, 10, and 15 mL.[7]
Timolol Maleate		
Timolol Maleate, Rx (Various)	**Solution:** 0.25%	In 2.5, 5, 10, and 15 mL.
Timoptic, Rx (Merck)	**Solution:** 0.25%	Preservative free. In UD 60s Ocudose.[8]

Beta-Adrenergic Blocking Agents

Generic Name Trade Name	Doseform/ Strength	How Supplied
Timpotic, Rx (Merck)	**Solution**: 0.25%	In 2.5, 5, 10, and 15 mL Ocumeters[9]
Timolol Maleate, Rx (Various)	**Solution**: 0.5%	In 2.5, 5, 10, and 15 mL.
Timpotic, Rx (Merck)	**Solution**: 0.5%	Preservative free. In UD 60s Ocudose.[8]
Timpotic, Rx (Merck)	**Solution**: 0.5%	In 2.5, 5, 10, and 15 mL Ocumeters[9]
Timolol Maleate Ophthalmic, Rx (Falcon)	**Solution, gel-forming**: 0.25%	In 2.5 and 5 mL.[9]
Timoptic-XE, Rx (Merck)	**Solution, gel-forming**: 0.25%	In 2.5 and 5 mL Ocumeters.[10]
Timolol Maleate Ophthalmic, Rx (Falcon)	**Solution, gel-forming**: 0.5%	In 2.5 and 5 mL.[9]
Timoptic-XE, Rx (Merck)	**Solution, gel-forming**: 0.5%	In 2.5 and 5 mL Ocumeters.[10]

[1] With 0.01% benzalkonium chloride, NaCl, hydrochloric acid or sodium hydroxide, and EDTA.
[2] With 0.01% benzalkonium chloride, mannitol, poly sulfonic acid, carbomer 934P, hydrochloric acid or sodium hydroxide, and EDTA.
[3] With 0.005% benzalkonium chloride, NaCl, and sodium phosphate.
[4] With 0.01% benzalkonium chloride, EDTA, hydrochloric acid, and boric acid.
[5] With 1.4% polyvinyl alcohol, 0.004% benzalkonium chloride, sodium metabisulfite, and EDTA.
[6] With 0.004% benzalkonium chloride and EDTA.
[7] With 0.01% benzalkonium chloride, and monosodium and disodium phosphate dihydrate.
[8] Use immediately after opening; discard remaining contents. With monobasic and dibasic sodium phosphate and sodium hydroxide
[9] With 0.01% benzalkonium chloride, sodium hydroxide, and monobasic and dibasic sodium phosphate.
[10] With 0.012% benzododecinium bromide.

Miotics, Direct-Acting

Generic Name Trade Name	Doseform/ Strength	How Supplied
Acetylcholine Chloride, Intraocular		
Miochol-E, Rx (Novartis)	**Solution**: 1:100 acetyl- choline chloride when reconstituted	In 2 mL dual chamber univial (lower chamber 20 mg lyophi- lized acetylcholine chloride and 56 mg mannitol; upper chamber 2 mL electrolyte dilu- ent[1] and sterile water for injec- tion).
Carbachol, Intraocular		
Carbastat, Rx (Novartis)	**Solution**: 0.01%	In 1.5 mL vials.[2]
Miostat, Rx (Alcon)	**Solution**: 0.01%	In 1.5 mL vials.[2]
Carbachol, Topical		
Isopto Carbachol, Rx (Alcon)	**Solution**: 0.75%	In 15 and 30 mL Drop- Tainers.[3]
Isopto Carbachol, Rx (Alcon)	**Solution**: 1.5%	In 15 and 30 mL Drop- Tainers.[3]
Isopto Carbachol, Rx (Alcon)	**Solution**: 2.25%	In 15 mL Drop-Tainers.[3]
Isopto Carbachol, Rx (Alcon)	**Solution**: 3%	In 15 and 30 mL Drop- Tainers.[3]
Carboptic, Rx (Optopics)	**Solution**: 3%	In 15 mL.[4]
Pilocarpine HCl		
Isopto Carpine, Rx (PolyMedica)	**Solution**: 0.25%	In 15 mL.[5]
Pilocarpine HCl, Rx (Various, eg, Martec)	**Solution**: 0.5%	In 15 mL.
Isopto Carpine, Rx (PolyMedica)	**Solution**: 0.5%	In 15 and 30 mL.[5]
Pilocar, Rx (Novartis)	**Solution**: 0.5%	In 15 mL and twin-pack (2 × 15 mL).[6]
Pilocarpine HCl, Rx (Various, eg, Alcon)	**Solution**: 1%	In 2, 5, and 15 mL and twin- pack (2 × 15 mL).
Akarpine, Rx (Akorn)	**Solution**: 1%	In 15 mL.
Isopto Carpine, Rx (Alcon)	**Solution**: 1%	In 15 and 30 mL.[5]

Miotics, Direct-Acting

Generic Name Trade Name	Doseform/ Strength	How Supplied
Pilocar, Rx (Novartis)	**Solution**: 1%	In 15 mL, twin-pack (2 × 15 mL) and 1 mL Dropperettes.[6]
Pilocarpine HCl, Rx (Various, eg, Alcon)	**Solution**: 2%	In 2 and 15 mL and twin-pack (2 × 15 mL).
Akarpine, Rx (Akorn)	**Solution**: 2%	In 15 mL dropper bottles.
Isopto Carpine, Rx (Alcon)	**Solution**: 2%	In 15 and 30 mL.[5]
Pilocar, Rx (Novartis)	**Solution**: 2%	In 15 mL, twin-pack (2 × 15 mL) and 1 mL Dropperettes.[6]
Pilostat, Rx (Bausch & Lomb)	**Solution**: 2%	In 15 mL and twin-pack (2 × 15 mL).[7]
Isopto Carpine, Rx (Alcon)	**Solution**: 3%	In 15 mL.[5]
Pilocar, Rx (Novartis)	**Solution**: 3%	In 15 mL, twin-pack (2 × 15 mL).[6]
Pilocarpine HCl, Rx (Various, eg, Alcon)	**Solution**: 4%	In 2 and 15 mL.
Akarpine, Rx (Akorn)	**Solution**: 4%	In 15 mL dropper bottles.
Isopto Carpine, Rx (Alcon)	**Solution**: 4%	In 15 and 30 mL.[5]
Pilocar, Rx (Novartis)	**Solution**: 4%	In 15 mL, twin-pack (2 × 15 mL), and 1 mL Dropperettes.[6]
Pilopto-Carpine, Rx (Lebeh Pharmacal)	**Solution**: 4%	In 15 mL.
Isopto Carpine, Rx (Alcon)	**Solution**: 5%	In 15 and 30 mL.[5]
Pilocarpine HCl, Rx (Various, eg, Alcon)	**Solution**: 6%	In 15 mL.
Isopto Carpine, Rx (Alcon)	**Solution**: 6%	In 15 mL.[5]
Pilocar, Rx (Ciba Vision)	**Solution**: 6%	In 15 mL and twin-pack (2 × 15 mL).[7]
Pilocarpine HCl, Rx (Alcon)	**Solution**: 8%	In 2 mL.
Isopto Carpine, Rx (Alcon)	**Solution**: 8%	In 15 mL.[5]
Isopto Carpine, Rx (PolyMedica)	**Solution**: 10%	In 15 mL.[5]
Pilopine HS, Rx (Alcon)	**Gel**: 4%	In 3.5 g.[10]

OPHTHALMIC DRUG FACTS

Miotics, Direct-Acting

Generic Name Trade Name	Doseform/ Strength	How Supplied
Pilocarpine Nitrate		
Pilagan, Rx (Allergan)	**Solution**: 1%	In 15 mL.[8]
Pilagan, Rx (Allergan)	**Solution**: 2%	In 15 mL.[8]
Pilagan, Rx (Allergan)	**Solution**: 4%	In 15 mL.[8]
Pilocarpine Ocular Therapeutic System		
Ocusert Pilo-20, Rx (Akorn)	**Ocular Therapeutic System**: Releases 20 mcg pilocarpine per hour for 1 week	In packs of 8 individ. sterile systems.
Ocusert Pilo-40, Rx (Akorn)	**Ocular Therapeutic System**: Releases 40 mcg pilocarpine per hour for 1 week	In packs of 8 individ. sterile systems.

[1] With sodium chloride, potassium chloride, magnesium chloride hexahydrate, and calcium chloride dihydrate.
[2] With 0.64% sodium chloride, 0.075% potassium chloride, 0.048% calcium chloride dihydrate, 0.03% magnesium chloride hexahydrate, 0.39% sodium acetate trihydrate, 0.17% sodium citrate dihydrate, sodium hydroxide, and hydrochloric acid.
[3] With 0.005% benzalkonium chloride, 1% hydroxypropyl methylcellulose, sodium chloride, boric acid, and sodium borate.
[4] With benzalkonium chloride, polyvinyl alcohol, and sodium phosphate dibasic and monobasic.
[5] With 0.5% hydroxypropyl methylcellulose and 0.01% benzalkonium chloride.
[6] With hydroxypropyl methylcellulose, benzalkonium chloride, and EDTA.
[7] With 0.008% benzalkonium chloride, carbopol 940, and EDTA.
[8] With 1.4% polyvinyl alcohol, 0.5% chlorobutanol, menthol, camphor, phenol, and eucalyptol.

Cholinesterase Inhibitors

Generic Name Trade Name	Doseform/ Strength	How Supplied
Physostigmine		
Eserine Sulfate, Rx (Fougera)	**Ointment**: 0.25% (as sulfate)	In 3.5 g.[1]
Demecarium Bromide		
Humorsol, Rx (Merck)	**Solution**: 0.125%	In 5 mL Ocumeters.[2]
Humorsol, Rx (Merck)	**Solution**: 0.25%	In 5 mL Ocumeters.[2]
Echothiophate Iodide		
Phospholine Iodide, Rx (Wyeth)	**Powder for reconstitution**: 1.5 mg to make 0.03%	With 5 mL diluent.[3]

CHAPTER SUMMARIES

Cholinesterase Inhibitors

Generic Name Trade Name	Doseform/ Strength	How Supplied
Phospholine Iodide, Rx (Wyeth)	**Powder for reconstitution**: 3 mg to make 0.06%	With 5 mL diluent.[3]
Pilocarpine and Epinephrine		
E-Pilo-1, Rx (Ciba Vision)	**Solution**: 1% pilocarpine HCl, 1% epinephrine bitartrate	In 10 mL dropper bottles.[4]
P₁E₁, Rx (Alcon)	**Solution**: 1% pilocarpine HCl, 1% epinephrine bitartrate	In 15 mL Drop-Tainers.[5]
E-Pilo-2, Rx (Ciba Vision)	**Solution**: 2% pilocarpine HCl, 1% epinephrine bitartrate	In 10 mL dropper bottles.[4]
P₂E₁, Rx (Alcon)	**Solution**: 2% pilocarpine HCl, 1% epinephrine bitartrate	In 15 mL Drop-Tainers.[5]
E-Pilo-4, Rx (Ciba Vision)	**Solution**: 4% pilocarpine HCl, 1% epinephrine bitartrate	In 10 mL dropper bottles.[4]
P₄E₁, Rx (Alcon)	**Solution**: 4% pilocarpine HCl, 1% epinephrine bitartrate	In 15 mL Drop-Tainers.[5]
E-Pilo-6, Rx (Ciba Vision)	**Solution**: 6% pilocarpine HCl, 1% epinephrine bitartrate	In 10 mL dropper bottles.[4]
P₆E₁, Rx (Alcon)	**Solution**: 6% pilocarpine HCl, 1% epinephrine bitartrate	In 15 mL Drop-Tainers.[5]

[1] With lanolin, white petrolatum, and mineral oil.
[2] With 1:5000 benzalkonium chloride and sodium chloride.
[3] With potassium acetate, 0.55% chlorobutanol, and 1.2% mannitol.
[4] With benzalkonium chloride, EDTA, mannitol, and sodium bisulfite.
[5] With 0.01% benzalkonium chloride, methylcellulose, EDTA, chlorobutanol, polyethylene glycol, and sodium bisulfite.

Carbonic Anhydrase Inhibitors

Generic Name Trade Name	Doseform/ Strength	How Supplied
Acetazolamide		
Acetazolamide, Rx (Various, eg, Mutual, URL)	**Tablets**: 125 mg	In 50s, 100s, 250s, 500s, and 1000s.
Diamox, Rx (Wyeth)	**Tablets**: 125 mg	In 100s.

OPHTHALMIC DRUG FACTS

Carbonic Anhydrase Inhibitors

Generic Name Trade Name	Doseform/ Strength	How Supplied
Acetazolamide, Rx (Various, eg, Qualitest, Schein)	**Tablets**: 250 mg	In 50s, 100s, 250s, 500s, and 1000s.
Dazamide, Rx (Major)	**Tablets**: 250 mg	In 100s, 250s, 1000s, and UD 100s.
Diamox Sequels, Rx (Wyeth)	**Capsules, sustained-release**: 500 mg	In 30s and 100s.
Acetazolamide, Rx (Various, eg, Bedford)	**Powder for injection, lyophilized**: 500 mg (as sodium)	In vials.
Diamox, Rx (Wyeth)	**Powder for injection, lyophilized**: 500 mg (as sodium)	In vials.
Dichlorphenamide		
Daranide, Rx (Merck)	**Tablets**: 50 mg	Lactose. In 100s
Methazolamide		
Methazolamide, Rx (Various, eg, Teva)	**Tablets**: 25 mg	In 100s and 1000s.
GlaucTabs, Rx (Akorn)	**Tablets**: 25 mg	In 100s.
Neptazane, Rx (Wyeth)	**Tablets**: 25 mg	In 100s.
Methazolamide, Rx (Various, eg, Teva)	**Tablets**: 50 mg	In 100s and 1000s.
GlaucTabs, Rx (Akorn)	**Tablets**: 50 mg	In 100s.
Neptazane, Rx (Wyeth)	**Tablets**: 50 mg	In 100s.
Dorzolamide HCl		
Trusopt, Rx (Merck)	**Solution**: 2%	In 5 and 10 mL.[1]
Brinzolamide		
Azopt, Rx (Alcon)	**Suspension**: 1%	In 5, 10, and 15 mL Drop-Tainers.

[1] 0.0075% benzalkonium chloride.

CHAPTER SUMMARIES

Carbonic Anhydrase Inhibitor/Beta-Adrenergic Blocking Agent

Generic Name Trade Name	Doseform/ Strength	How Supplied
Dorzolamide/Timolol Maleate *Cosopt, Rx* (Merck)	**Solution**: 20 mg dorzol-amide, 5 mg timolol maleate	In 5 and 10 ml dispenser with controlled tip.[1]

[1] With sodium citrate, hydroxyethyl cellulose, sodium hydroxide, and mannitol. Benzalkonium chloride 0.0075% is added as a preservative.

Prostaglandins

Generic Name Trade Name	Doseform/ Strength	How Supplied
Latanoprost *Xalatan, Rx* (Pharmacia)	**Solution**: 0.005%	In 2.5 mL plastic ophthalmic dispenser bottle with dropper tip.[1]
Travoprost *Travatan, Rx* (Alcon)	**Solution**: 0.004%	In 2.5 mL Drop-Tainers.[2]
Bimatoprost *Lumigan, Rx* (Allergan)	**Solution**: 0.03%	In 2.5 and 5 mL.[3]
Unoprostone Isopropyl *Rescula, Rx* (Novartis)	**Solution**: 0.15%	In 5 mL.[4]

[1] With 0.2% benzalkonium chloride, sodium chloride, sodium dihydrogen phosphate monohydrate, and disodium hydrogen phosphate anhydrous.
[2] 0.015% benzalkonium chloride, EDTA.
[3] 0.05 mg benzalkonium chloride/mL.
[4] 0.015% benzalkonium chloride, EDTA, sodium hydroxide, hydrochloric acid.

Hyperosmotic Agents

Generic Name Trade Name	Doseform/ Strength	How Supplied
Glucose, Topical *Glucose-40, Rx* (Ciba Vision)	**Ointment**: 40%	White petrolatum, anhydrous lanolin, parabens. In 3.5 g.
Glycerin, Topical *Ophthalagan, Rx* (Wyeth)	**Solution**: Glycerin	0.55% chlorobutanol. In 7.5 mL.

Hyperosmotic Agents

Generic Name Trade Name	Doseform/ Strength	How Supplied
Sodium Chloride, Hypertonic		
Adsorbonac, Rx (Alcon)	**Solution**: 2%	In 15 mL.[1]
Muro 128, Rx (Bausch & Lomb)	**Solution**: 2%	In 15 mL.[2]
Adsorbonac, Rx (Alcon)	**Solution**: 5%	In 15 mL.[1]
AK-NaCl, Rx (Akorn)	**Solution**: 5%	In 15 mL.[3]
Muro 128, Rx (Bausch & Lomb)	**Solution**: 5%	In 15 and 30 mL.[4]
AK-NaCl, Rx (Akorn)	**Ointment**: 5%	Preservative free. In 3.5 g.[5]
Muro 128, Rx (Bausch & Lomb)	**Ointment**: 5%	In 3.5 g single and twin packs.[6]
Glycerin (Glycerol)		
Osmōglyn, Rx (Alcon)	**Solution**: 50% (0.6 g glycerin/mL)	Lime flavor. In 180 and 220 mL.
Isosorbide		
Ismotic, Rx (Alcon)	**Solution**: 45% (100 g per 220 mL)	With 4.6 mEq sodium and 0.9 mEq potassium per 220 mL. Alcohol, saccharin, sorbitol. Vanilla-mint flavor. In 220 mL.
Mannitol		
Osmitrol, Rx (Clintec)	**Injection**: 5%	In 1000 mL.
Mannitol, Rx (Various, eg, Astra)	**Injection**: 10%	In 1000 mL.
Osmitrol, Rx (Clintec)	**Injection**: 10%	In 500 and 1000 mL.
Osmitrol, Rx (Clintec)	**Injection**: 15%	In 500 mL.
Mannitol, Rx (Various, eg, Astra)	**Injection**: 20%	In 250 and 500 mL.
Osmitrol, Rx (Clintec)	**Injection**: 20%	In 250 and 500 mL.
Mannitol, Rx (Various, eg, Astra)	**Injection**: 25%	In 50 mL.

[1] With povidone, hydroxyethylcellulose 2910, PEG-90M, poloxamer 188, 0.004% thimerosal, and EDTA.
[2] With hydroxypropyl methylcellulose 2910, 0.028% methylparaben, 0.01% propylparaben, propylene glycol, and boric acid.
[3] With hydroxypropyl methylcellulose 2906, propylene glycol, 0.023% methylparaben, 0.01% propylparaben, and boric acid.
[4] With boric acid, hydroxypropyl methylcellulose 2910, propylene glycol, 0.023% methylparaben, and 0.01% propylparaben.
[5] With mineral oil, white petrolatum, and lanolin oil.
[6] With mineral oil, white petrolatum, and lanolin.

CHAPTER SUMMARIES 413

Surgical Adjuncts		
Generic Name Trade Name	**Doseform/ Strength**	**How Supplied**
Intraocular Irrigating Solutions		
Balanced Salt Solution, Rx (B. Braun)	**Solution**: 0.64% NaCl, 0.075% KCl, 0.03% magnesium chloride, 0.048% calcium chloride, 0.39% sodium acetate, 0.17% sodium citrate and sodium hydroxide acid or hydrochloric acid	In 500 mL.
BSS, Rx (Alcon)	**Solution**: 0.64% NaCl, 0.075% KCl, 0.03% magnesium chloride, 0.048% calcium chloride, 0.39% sodium acetate, 0.17% sodium citrate and sodium hydroxide or hydrochloric acid	Preservative free. In 15, 30, 250, and 500 mL.
Iocare Balanced Salt, Rx (Ciba Vision)	**Solution**: 0.64% NaCl, 0.075% KCl, 0.03% magnesium chloride, 0.048% calcium chloride, 0.39% sodium acetate, 0.17% sodium citrate and sodium hydroxide or hydrochloric acid	Preservative free. In 15 mL.
BSS Plus, Rx (Alcon)	**Solution**: Part 1: 7.44 mg NaCl, 0.395 mg KCl, 0.433 mg dibasic sodium phosphate, 2.19 mg sodium bicarbonate, hydrochloric acid or sodium hydroxide/mL *Mix aseptically just prior to use.*	Preservative free. In 240 mL.
	Solution: Part 2: 3.85 mg calcium chloride dihydrate, 5 mg magnesium chloride hexahydrate, 23 mg dextrose, 4.6 mg glutathione disulfide/mL *Mix aseptically just prior to use.*	Preservative free. In 10 mL.
B-Salt Forte, Rx (Akorn)	**Solution**: Part 1: 7.14 mg NaCl, 0.38 mg KCl, 0.154 mg calcium chloride dihydrate, 0.2 mg magnesium chloride hexahydrate, 0.92 mg dextrose, hydrochloric acid or sodium hydroxide/mL	Preservative free. In 515 mL.
	Solution: Part 2: 1081 mg sodium bicarbonate, 216 mg dibasic sodium phosphate (anhydrous), 95 mg glutathione disulfide (oxidized glutathione)/vial	Preservative free. In 60 mL.
Povidone Iodine		
Betadine 5% Sterile Ophthalmic Prep Solution, Rx (Alcon)	**Solution**: 5%	In 50 mL.[1]
Sodium Hyaluronate		
Biolon, Rx (Akorn)	**Injection**: 10 mg/mL[2]	In 0.5 and 1 mL disp. syringes.

Surgical Adjuncts

Generic Name Trade Name	Doseform/ Strength	How Supplied
Healon, Rx (Pharmacia)	**Injection**: 10 mg/mL[2]	In 0.4, 0.55, 0.85, and 2 mL disp. syringes.
ProVisc, Rx (Alcon)	**Injection**: 10 mg/mL[2]	In 0.4, 0.55, and 0.85 mL disp. glass syringes.
Amvisc, Rx (Chiron)	**Injection**: 12 mg/mL[3]	In 0.5 or 0.8 mL disp. syringes.
Healon GV, Rx (Pharmacia)	**Injection**: 14 mg/mL[2]	In 0.85 mL disp. syringes.
Amvisc Plus, Rx (Chiron)	**Injection**: 16 mg/mL[3]	In 0.5 or 8 mL disp. syringes.
AMO Vitrax, Rx (Allergan)	**Injection**: 30 mg/mL[4]	In 0.65 mL disp. syringes.
Sodium Hyaluronate and Chondroitin Sulfate		
Viscoat, Rx (Alcon)	**Solution**: ≤ 40 mg sodium chondroitin sulfate, 30 mg sodium hyaluronate per mL	0.45 mg sodium dihydrogen phosphate hydrate, 2 mg disodium hydrogen phosphate, 4.3 mg sodium chloride per mL. In 0.5 mL disp. syringes.
Hydroxyethylcellulose		
Gonioscopic, Rx (Alcon)	**Solution**: Hydroxyethylcellulose	0.004% thimerosal, 0.1% EDTA. In 15 mL Drop-Tainers.
Hydroxypropyl Methylcellulose		
Gonak, Rx (Akorn)	**Solution**: 2.5%	In 15 mL.[5]
Goniosol, Rx (Novartis)	**Solution**: 2.5%	In 15 mL.[6]
Absorbable Gelatin Film, Sterile		
Gelfilm, Rx (Pharmacia)	**Film**: 100 mm × 125 mm	In 1s.
Gelfilm Ophthalmic, Rx (Pharmacia)	**Film**: 25 mm × 50 mm	In 6s.

CHAPTER SUMMARIES

Surgical Adjuncts

Generic Name Trade Name	Doseform/ Strength	How Supplied
Miotics, Direct-Acting Acetylcholine Chloride, Intraocular		
Miochol-E, Rx (Novartis)	**Solution**: 1:100 acetylcholine chloride when reconstituted	In 2 mL dual chamber univial (lower chamber 20 mg lyophilized acetylcholine chloride and 56 mg mannitol; upper chamber 2 mL electrolyte diluent[7] and sterile water for injection).
Miotics, Direct-Acting Carbachol, Intraocular		
Carbastat, Rx (Novartis)	**Solution**: 0.01%	In 1.5 mL vials.[8]
Miostat, Rx (Alcon)	**Solution**: 0.01%	In 1.5 mL vials.[8]
Polydimethylsiloxane (Silicone Oil)		
AdatoSil 5000, Rx (Escalon Ophthalmics)	**Injection**: Polydimethysiloxane oil	In single-use 10 and 15 mL vials.
Botulinum Toxin Type A		
Botox, Rx (Allergan)	**Powder for injection, lyophilized**: 100 units of lyophilized *Clostridium botulinum* toxin type A.[9]	Preservative free. 0.05 mg albumin (human), 0.9 mg sodium chloride. In vials.
Verteporfin		
Visudyne, Rx (Novartis)	**Lyophilized cake**: 15 mg (reconstituted to 2 mg/mL)[10]	In single-use vials.

[1] With glycerin, sodium chloride, sodium hydroxide, and sodium phosphate.
[2] With 8.5 mg NaCl per mL.
[3] With 9 mg NaCl per mL.
[4] With 3.2 mg NaCl, 0.75 mg KCl, 0.48 mg calcium chloride, 0.3 mg magnesium chloride, 3.9 mg sodium acetate, and 1.7 mg sodium citrate per mL.
[5] With 0.01% benzalkonium chloride, EDTA, boric acid, KCl, sodium borate, hydrochloric acid or sodium hydroxide.
[6] With 0.01% benzalkonium chloride, boric acid, KCl, and EDTA.
[7] With sodium chloride, potassium chloride, magnesium chloride hexahydrate, and calcium chloride dihydrate.
[8] With 0.64% sodium chloride, 0.075% potassium chloride, 0.048% calcium chloride dihydrate, 0.03% magnesium chloride hexahydrate, 0.39% sodium acetate trihydrate, 0.17% sodium citrate dihydrate, sodium hydroxide, and hydrochloric acid.
[9] One unit corresponds to the calculated median lethal intraperitoneal dose (LD_{50}) in mice of the reconstituted drug injected.
[10] Egg phosphatidylglycerol.

OPHTHALMIC DRUG FACTS

416

Nonsurgical Adjuncts

Generic Name Trade Name	Doseform/ Strength	How Supplied
Dapiprazole HCl		
Rēv-Eyes, otc (Lederle)	**Powder, lyophilized**: 25 mg (0.5% solution when reconstituted)	In vial with 5 mL diluent and dropper.[1]
Extraocular Irrigating Solutions		
AK-Rinse, otc (Akorn)	**Solution**: Sodium carbonate, KCl, boric acid, EDTA, 0.01% benzalkonium chloride	In 30 and 118 mL.
Collyrium for Fresh Eyes Wash, otc (Wyeth Ayerst)	**Solution**: Boric acid, sodium borate, benzalkonium chloride	In 120 mL.
Dacriose, otc (Novartis)	**Solution**: NaCl, KCl, sodium phosphate, sodium hydroxide, 0.01% benzalkonium chloride, EDTA	In 15 and 120 mL.
Eye Stream, otc (Alcon)	**Solution**: 0.64% NaCl, 0.075% KCl, 0.03% magnesium chloride hexahydrate, 0.048% calcium chloride dihydrate, 0.39% sodium acetate trihydrate, 0.17% sodium citrate dihydrate, 0.013% benzalkonium chloride	In 30 and 118 mL.
Eye Wash, otc (Bausch & Lomb)	**Solution**: Boric acid, KCl, EDTA, sodium carbonate, 0.01% benzalkonium chloride	In 118 mL.
Eye Wash, otc (Zenith-Goldline)	**Solution**: Boric acid, KCl, EDTA, anhydrous sodium carbonate, 0.01% benzalkonium chloride	In 118 mL.
Eye Wash, otc (Lavoptik)	**Solution**: 0.49% NaCl, 0.4% sodium biphosphate, 0.45% sodium phosphate, 0.0005% benzalkonium chloride	In 180 mL with eye cup.
Eye Irrigating Solution, otc (Rugby)	**Solution**: Sodium borate, NaCl, boric acid, sorbic acid, EDTA	In 180 mL with eyecup.
Optigene, otc (Pfeiffer)	**Solution**: NaCl, mono- and dibasic sodium phosphate, benzalkonium Cl, EDTA	In 118 mL.
Lid Scrubs		
Eye-Scrub, otc (Ciba Vision)	**Solution**: PEG-200 glyceryl tallowate, disodium laureth sulfosuccinate, cocoamidopropylamine oxide, PEG-78 glyceryl cocoate, benzyl alcohol, EDTA	In UD 30s (pads) and kit (120 mL and 60 pads).

CHAPTER SUMMARIES

417

Nonsurgical Adjuncts

Generic Name Trade Name	Doseform/ Strength	How Supplied
Lid Wipes-SPF, otc (Akorn)	**Solution**: PEG-200 glyceryl tallowate, PEG-80 glyceryl cocoate, laureth-23, cocoamidopropylamine oxide, NaCl, glycerin, sodium phosphate, sodium hydroxide	Preservative free. In UD 30s (pads).
OCuSOFT, otc (OCuSOFT)	**Solution**: PEG-80 sorbitan laurate, sodium trideceth sulfate, PEG-150 distearate, cocoamidopropyl hydroxysultaine, lauroamphacarboxyglycinate, sodium laureth-13 carboxylate, PEG-15 tallow polyamine, quarternium-15	Alcohol and dye free. In UD 30s (pads), 30, 120, and 240 mL and compliance kit (120 mL and 100 pads).
Tear Test Strips		
Sno-Strips, otc (Akorn)	**Strips**: Sterile tear flow test strips	In 100s.
Schirmer Tear Test, otc (Alcon)	**Strips**: Sterile test strips	In 250s.
Zone-Quick, otc (Menicon USA)	**Threads**: Phenol red threads (PRT)	In 50 Aluminum package sets (100 threads).
Zinc Sulfate Solution		
Eye-Sed, otc (Scherer)	**Solution**: 0.25%	In 15 mL.[2]
Vitamins and Minerals		
Vitamin A Palmitate, otc (Freeda)	**Tablets**: 10,000 IU	In 100s and 250s.
Vitamin A Palmitate, otc (Freeda)	**Tablets**: 15,000 IU	In 100s and 250s.
Vitamin A Palmitate, otc (Freeda)	**Tablets**: 25,000 IU	In 100s.
Beta Carotene, otc (Freeda)	**Tablets**: 10,000 IU	In 100s, 250s, and 500s.
Palmitate-A, otc (Akorn)	**Tablets**: 15,000 IU vitamin A palmitate	In 100s.
Palmitate-A 5000, otc (Akorn)	**Tablets**: 5000 IU vitamin A	In 100s.
Icaps Plus, otc (Alcon)	**Tablets**: 6000 IU vitamin A,[3] 200 mg C, 20 mg B_2, 60 IU E, 40 mg Zn,[4] 2 mg Cu, 5 mg Mn, 20 mcg Se	In 60s, 120s, and 180s.
Icaps Time Release, otc (Alcon)	**Tablets**: 7000 IU vitamin A,[3] 200 mg C, 20 mg B_2, 100 IU E, 40 mg Zn,[4] 2 mg Cu, 20 mcg Se	In 60s.

Nonsurgical Adjuncts

Generic Name Trade Name	Doseform/ Strength	How Supplied
AntiOxidants, otc (Akorn)	**Caplets**: 5000 IU vitamin A,[3] 400 mg C,[5] 200 IU E,[6] 40 mg Zn,[7] 5 mg L-glutathione, 3 mg sodium pyruvate, 2 mg Cu,[8] 40 mcg Se[9]	In 60s.
Oxi-Freeda, otc (Freeda)	**Tablets**: 5000 IU beta carotene, 150 IU E, 20 mg B_1, 20 mg B_2, 20 mg B_6, 10 mcg B_{12}, 15 mg elemental Zn, 50 mcg Se, 20 mg calcium pantothenate, 40 mg glutathione, 40 mg B_3, 100 mg C, 75 mg L-cysteine	In 100s and 250s.
One-A-Day Extras Antioxidant, otc (Bayer)	**Capsules, softgel**: 5000 IU vitamin A,[3] 200 IU E, 250 mg C, 7.5 mg Zn, 1 mg Cu, 15 mcg Se, 1.5 mg Mn	(One-A-Day) Tartrazine. In 50s.
OCuSOFT VMS, otc (OCuSOFT)	**Tablets**: 5000 IU vitamin A, 30 IU E, 60 mg C, 40 mg Zn, 2 mg Cu, 40 mcg Se	Film coated. In 60s.
Ocuvite, otc (Bausch & Lomb)	**Tablets**: 40 mg elemental Zn,[10] 2 mg elemental Cu,[11] 40 mcg elemental Se,[12] 5000 IU vitamin A,[3] 30 IU E,[5] 60 mg C[6]	In 75s.
Ocuvite Extra, otc (Bausch & Lomb)	**Tablets**: 40 mg elemental Zn,[10] 2 mg elemental Cu,[11] 200 mg C, 50 IU E, 6000 IU vitamin A,[3] 40 mcg elemental Se, 3 mg B_2, 40 mg B_3, 5 mg elemental Mn, 5 mg L-glutathione	In 50s.

[1] With 2% mannitol, 0.4% hydroxypropyl methycellulose, 0.01% EDTA, 0.01% benzalkonium chloride, and sodium chloride.
[2] With 0.05% tetrahydrozoline HCl, EDTA, benzalkonium chloride, and sodium chloride.
[3] As beta carotene.
[4] As zinc acetate.
[5] As ascorbic acid.
[6] As dl-alpha tocopheryl acetate.
[7] As zinc ascorbate.
[8] As copper ascorbate.
[9] As L-selenomethionine.
[10] As zinc oxide.
[11] As cupric oxide.
[12] As sodium selenate.

CHAPTER SUMMARIES

419

Antiviral and Antifungal Agents

Generic Name Trade Name	Doseform/ Strength	How Supplied
Natamycin		
Natacyn, Rx (Alcon)	**Suspension**: 5%	With 0.02% benzalkonium. In 15 mL.
Vidarabine (Adenine Arabino- side; Ara-A)		
Vira-A, Rx (Monarch)	**Ointment**: 3% vidara- bine monohydrate (equivalent to 2.8% vidarabine)	In a liquid petrolatum base. In 3.5 g.
Trifluridine (Trifluorothymidine)		
Viroptic, Rx (Monarch)	**Solution**: 1%	In aqueous solution with NaCl and 0.001% thimerosal. In 7.5 mL Drop-Dose.
Ganciclovir (DHPG)		
Cytovene, Rx (Roche)	**Capsules**: 250 mg	In 180s.
Cytovene, Rx (Roche)	**Capsules**: 500 mg	In 180s.
Cytovene, Rx (Roche)	**Powder for injection, lyophilized**: 500 mg/vial ganciclovir (as sodium)	In 10 mL vials.
Ganciclovir Intravitreal Implant		
Vitrasert, Rx (Bausch & Lomb Surgical)	**Implant**: Minimum 4.5 mg	In individal unit boxes in a ster- ile Tyvek package.
Foscarnet Sodium (Phosphono- formic Acid))		
Foscavir, Rx (Astra)	**Injection**: 24 mg/mL	In 250 and 500 mL bottles.
Fomivirsen Sodium		
Vitravene, Rx (Novartis)	**Injection**: 6.6 mg/mL	In 0.25 mL single-use vials.[1]
Cidofovir		
Vistide, Rx (Gilead Sciences)	**Injection**: 75 mg/mL	5 mL amps.

[1] With sodium bicarbonate, NaCl, and sodium carbonate.

INDEX

This **Index** lists all generic names, brand names *(italics)*, and group names included in *Ophthalmic Drug Facts*. Additionally, many drug tables, synonyms, pharmacological actions, and therapeutic uses for the agents listed are included.

Index entries may refer to more than one form of a product (eg, tablets, solutions, suspensions, ointments) when all forms are included on the single page. Separate index entries are included when multiple forms of a product appear on different pages or when products are listed in more than one therapeutic group.

9-Cis-Retinoic Acid, 354
20/20 Eye Drops, 64, 135, 296
20/20 Tears, 102

Absorbable Gelatin Film, 264, 273
Acanthamoeba keratitis, 304
Accutane, 332
Acetaminophen, 342
Acetaminophen with Codeine, 342
Acetaminophen with Hydrocodone, 342
Acetazolamide, 226, 227, 332, 345
Acetylcholine Chloride, Intraocular, 208, 264, 275
Acetylcysteine, 311, 348
Acular, 98, 348
Acular PF, 98
Acute Anterior Uveitis: Treatment and Follow-up, 365
Acyclovir, 341, 348
Adaprolol Maleate, 356
AdatoSil 5000, 278
Adenine Arabinoside, 137
Adenosine Regulating Agents, 356
ADL 2-1294, 356
Adsorbonac, 256
Agents for Glaucoma, see Glaucoma
AGN-190342, 356
AGN-192151 (AGN-191151), 356
AI-RSA, 354
AK-Chlor, 119, 120
AK-Cide, 134
AK-Cide Suspension, 133
AK-Con, 65
AK-Dex, 91
AK-Dilate, 47
AK-Fluor, 18
AK-Homatropine, 52
AK-NaCl, 256
AK-Nefrin, 64
AK-Pentolate, 53

AK-Poly-Bac Ointment, 124
AK-Pred, 92, 93
AK-Rinse, 293
AK-Spore, 124
AK-Spore H.C., 127
AK-Spore H.C. Ophthalmic Suspensions, 125
AK-Sulf, 130, 131
AK-T-Caine PF, 37
AK-TAINE, 37
AK-Tob, 122
AK-Tracin, 118
AK-Trol, 127
AK-Trol Suspension, 126
Akarpine, 210, 211
Akwa Tears, 102, 105
Alamast, 80
Albalon, 65
Alcaine, 37
Alcohol, 332
Alcon Saline Especially for Sensitive Eyes, 317
Allegra, 343
Allergan Enzymatic, 319
Allergic Conditions, 57
Allergy Drops, 64
Allergy Drops Maximum Strength, 65
Alocril, 78
Alomide, 76, 348
Alond, 361
Alpha-1 Antichymotrypsin, 356
Alpha$_2$-Adrenergic Agonists, 180, 187
Alphagan, 193, 354
Alphagan P, 193
Alrex, 91
Alteplase, 330
American Optometric Association Clinical Practice Guidelines, 363
Amicar, 345, 348
Amikacin, 330

Aminocaproic Acid, 345, 348, 354
Aminoglycosides, 341
Amiodarone, 331, 333, 337
Amitriptyline, 332
AMO Vitrax, 271
Amoxicillin, 340
Amoxicillin/Clavulanate, 340
Amphetamines, 332
Amphotericin B, 342
Amvisc, 271, 348, 349
Amvisc Plus, 271
Analgesics, 342
Ancobon, 342
Anecortave Acetate, 356
Anesthetics, Local, 25, 329
Anti-Glaucoma Agent, 356
Anti-Infective Agents, 112
Anti-Inflammatory Agents, 85, 343
Antiallergy and Decongestant Agents, 57
Antianxiety Agents, 331
Antibacterials (Table), 340
Antibiotic Agents, 112
Antibiotic and Steroid Ointments, 127
Antibiotic and Steroid Solutions/Suspensions, 125
Antibiotic Treatment for Common Ocular Conditions (Table), 114
Antibiotics, 114, 340
Anticholinergics, 332, 334, 335
Antidepressants, 332
Antifungal Agent, 113 (Table), 342
Antihistamines, 332, 334, 343
Antiallergy and Decongestants, 66
Antihistamines, Mast Cell Stabilizers, and NSAIDs, 59
Antihistamine/Ophthalmic Decongestant Combinations, 83
Antimalarial Drugs, 331

422 OPHTHALMIC DRUG FACTS

Antimetabolites, 329
Antimicrobial Agents, 339
AntiOxidants, 297
Antistaphylococcal Penicillins, 341
Antiviral Agents, 113
    (Table), 341
Antiviral Agents for Ophthalmic
    Conditions, 113
AOSept, 316, 317
Apraclonidine HCl, 187
    Drug Interactions (Table), 189
AquaSite, 102
Aqueous Tear Secretion, Drugs
    that Decrease, 334
Ara-A, 137
Aralen Phosphate, 332
Artificial Tear Insert, 106
Artificial Tear Solutions, 99, 102
Artificial Tear Solutions and Ocu-
    lar Lubricants, 99
Artificial Tears, 102, 105
Aspirin, 332, 344, 348, 349
Atabrine HCl, 332
Atenolol, 332
Atopic Keratoconjunctivitis, 58
Atropine, 332
Atropine Care, 51
Atropine Sulfate, 51
Atropisol, 51
Augmentin, 340
Auranofin, 332
Aurolate, 332
Axokine, 356
Azathioprine, 344, 345
Azelastine HCl, 81
Azithromycin, 340
Azopt, 233

B-*Salte Forte,* 268
Bacitracin, 118
Bacitracin Neomycin, Polymyxin
    B Ointment, 124
Bacitracin Zinc and Polymyxin B
    Ointment, 124
Bacitracin Zinc/Neomycin Sulfate/
    Polymyxin B Sulfate Hydrocorti-
    sone, 127
Bactericidal/Permeability-increas-
    ing Protein, 356
BAK, 307
Balanced Salt Solution, 268
Barbiturates, 332
Batimastat, 356
Bayer, 332, 336, 348
BB-94/ISV-120, 356
BCX-34, 356
Benadryl, 332
Benzalkonium Chloride (BAK), 307
Benzyl Alcohol, 307
Beta-Adrenergic Blocking Agents,
    181, 193
    Pharmacokinetics of (Table), 194
β-Blockers, 332
Beta Blockers, 335
    Drug Interactions (Table), 197
Beta Carotene, 296
*Betadine 5% Sterile Ophthalmic
    Prep Solution,* 269
Betagan Liquifilm, 202
BetaSite, 359
Betaxolol, 201
Betaxon, 202
Betimol, 203, 204
Betoptic, 201

Betoptic S, 201
Bicarbonate, 308
Biguanide, 350
Bimatoprost, 237
Biolon, 271
Bion Tears, 102
Blairex Sterile Saline, 317
Bleph-10, 130, 131
Blephamide S.O.P., 134
Blephamide Suspension, 133
Boric Acid, 308
Boston Advance Cleaner, 312
*Boston Advance Comfort Formula
    Conditioning,* 310
*Boston One-Step Liquid Enzymatic
    Cleaner,* 313
Boston Original Formula Cleaner,
    312
*Boston Original Formula Condi-
    tioning,* 310
Boston Rewetting Drops, 314
Boston Simplicity Multi-Action,
    310, 311
Botox, 284, 354
Botulinum Toxin Type A, 265, 279,
    354
    Dilution of (Table), 283
Botulinum Toxin Type F, 354
BPI-21, 356
Brimonidine, 354, 356
Brimonidine Tartrate, 191
Brinzolamide, 231
Bromocriptine, 344
BSS, 268
BSS Plus, 268
Buffers, 2, 308
Bupivacaine HCl, 34
Bupivacaine HCl and Bupivacaine
    Combinations, 34

Cal*Optic,* 361
Caprogel, 356
Carbachol, Intraocular, 208, 264,
    275
Carbastat, 209, 276
Carbonic Anhydrase Inhibitors,
    181, 221, 332
    Drug Interactions (Table), 223
    Pharmacokinetics of (Table), 221
    (Table), 345
Carbonic Anhydrase Inhibitor/
    Beta-Adrenergic Blocking Agent,
    246
Carboptic, 209
Cardio-Green, 21
Carteolol HCl, 201
Cefazolin, 329, 341
Cefixime, 340
Ceftazidime, 330
Ceftriaxone, 340, 341
Cell Adhesion Molecule (CAM)
    Inhibitors, 356
Celluvisc, 102
Central Nervous System Stimu-
    lants, 332, 335
Cephalexin, 340
Cereport, 360
Cetapred, 134
Cetirazine, 343
Chapter Summaries, 377
Chibroxin, 123
Chlor-Trimeton, 332
Chlorambucil, 345
Chloramphenicol, 119, 332, 338

Chlordiazepoxide, 331
Chlorhexidine, 307, 338
Chloromycetin, 119, 120, 332
Chloroptic, 119
Chloroptic S.O.P., 120
Chloroquine, 332, 336
Chlorpheniramine, 332, 343
Chlorpromazine, 332, 334
Cholinesterase-Inhibiting Miotics,
    185, 214
Cholinesterase Inhibitors, 213
    Drug Interactions (Table), 216
Chondroitin Sulfate, 271, 348
Chondroitinase, 356
Cidofovir, 171, 341, 356
    Pharmacokinetic Parameters
    (Table), 172
    *Dosing of, with Renal Function
    Impairment* (Table), 177
Ciliary Neurotrophic Factor, 356
Ciloxan, 122
Ciprofloxacin, 122
Citrate, 308
Claris Cleaning and Soaking, 311,
    312
Claris Rewetting Drops, 314
Claritin, 343
Cleaner/Lubricant for Artificial
    Eyes, 109
Clear Conscience Multi-Purpose,
    315
Clear Conscience Saline, 317
Clear Eyes, 64
Clear Eyes ACR, 64, 135, 296
*Clerz 2 Lubricating & Rewetting
    Drops* 320
Clindamycin, 341
*Clostridium Botulinum Toxin Type
    A,* 356, 357
*Clostridium Botulinum Toxin Type
    F,* 357
CNS-1237, 357
CNS-5065, 357
Cocaine, 332
Codeine, 332, 335
Colchicine, 345
Collagen Implants, 108, 109
Collagenase, 357
Collyrium for Fresh Eyes Wash,
    293
Collyrium Fresh, 66
Combination Antibiotic Products,
    124
Combination Products,
    Antihistamines, Mast Cell Stabi-
    lizers, and NSAIDs, 59
*ComfortCare GP Wetting & Soak-
    ing,* 310
*Complete Lubricating and Rewet-
    ting Drops,* 320
*Complete Weekly Enzymatic
    Cleaner,* 319
Concentrated Cleaner, 312
Conjunctiva and Lids, Drugs
    Affecting, 334
Consept, 317
ContaClair, 311, 315
Contact Lens Care, 299
Contact Lens Care Compliance,
    301

INDEX

Contact Lens Care Products, 309
  Buffers, 308
  Components of, 307
  Preservatives, 307
Contact Lens, Disinfection, In-Office, 305
Contact Lens Guidelines, 302
Contact Lens Material and Composition, 299
Contact Lens Non-Compliance and Management (Table), 303
Contact Lens Use, Precautions, 304
Cordarone, 331
Cornea and Lens, Drugs Affecting, 331
Corneaplasty, 357
Corticosteroids, 332, 333
  Anti-inflammatory Agents, 85 (Table), 343
  Topical, 88
Cortisol, 332
Cortisporin, 125, 127
Cosopt, 250
Crack Cocaine, 332
Crolom, 74
Cromolyn Sodium, 73, 74, 354
Cronassial, 354
Curdlan Sulfate, 357
Cyclogyl, 53
Cyclomydril, 55
Cyclopentolate HCl, 53
Cyclophosphamide, 345
Cycloplegia, Drugs Causing, 336
Cycloplegics and Mydriatics, Introduction, 39, 40
  Group monograph, 47
  Pharmacology (Table), 47
Cyclosporine, 357
Cyclosporine A, 344
Cymeval, 361
Cysteamine HCl, 357
Cytoxan, 345
Cytovene, 155

Daclizumab *Monoclonal Antibody,* 357
Dacriose, 293
Daily Cleaner for Sensitive Eyes, 318
Dapiprazole HCl, 289, 291
Dapsone, 345
Daranide, 227
Daraprim, 341
Dazamide, 226
Decadron Phosphate, 91
Decongestants, 58, 61
Decongestants and Anti-Allergy Agents, 57
Decongestant, Ophthalmic, and Antihistamine Combination, 83
Dehydrex, 354, 357
Demecarium Bromide, 218
Devices, 7
Dexacidin, 127
Dexamethasone, 91, 329, 354
Dexamethasone Sodium Phosphate, 91
Dexanabinol, 357
Dexedrine, 332
Dextran 70, 332, 354
Diamox, 226, 227, 332
Diamox Sequels, 227

Dichlorphenamide, 227
Diclofenac, 357
Diclofenac Sodium, 97, 348, 349
Dicloxacillin, 340
Diflucan, 342
Digitalis Glycosides, 332, 337
Digoxin, 332
Dilantin, 332
Diphenhydramine, 332, 343
Dipivefrin HCl, 185, 187
Disinfection, Chemical Non-Hydrogen Peroxide, Soft Lenses, 314
Disinfection, Hydrogen Peroxide (Oxidative), Soft Lenses, 315
Disinfection, Thermal (Heat), Soft Lenses, 316
Disinfecting/Cleaning Solutions, RGP Lenses, 311
Disinfecting/Wetting/Soaking Solutions, RGP Lenses, 310
Disinfecting/Wetting/Soaking Solutions, Soft Lenses, 320
Disodium EDTA, 307
Diuretics, 332
Dorzolamide HCl, 227
Dorzolamide HCl/Timolol Maleate, 246
  Drug Interactions (Table), 248
Dosage Forms and Routes of Administration, 1
Doxycycline, 340
Dronabinol, 357
Drug Interactions,
  Injectable Local Anesthetics (Table), 31
  Sympathomimetics, Ophthalmic (Table), 62
Drug Packaging Standards (Table), 2
Dry Eye Therapy, 103
Dry Eyes, 105
Duranest, 34
Duratears Naturale, 105
Dynacin, 332
Dysport, 354, 356

E*-Pilo-1,* 221
E-Pilo-2, 221
E-Pilo-4, 221
E-Pilo-6, 221
Eagle FlexPlug, 108
EaglePlug, 108
Echothiophate Iodide, 218
Econopred, 92
Econopred Plus, 92
EDTA, 307
eFlone, 92
Elavil, 332
Elevated Serum Creatine with IV Ganciclovir (Table), 150
Eliprodil, 357
Emadine, 73
Emedastine Difumarate, 72
Engineered Cells, 357
Enuclene, 110
Enzymatic Cleaners, RGP Lenses, 313
Enzymatic Cleaners, Soft Lenses, 319
Enzyme-Based Iodine Technology, 357
Enzymes, Surgical, 265
Epifrin, 185
Epinal, 185

Epinastine, 357
Epinephrine HCl, 185
Epinephrines, 179, 183
Epinephryl Borate, 185
Erythromycin, 120, 340
Esotropia, Cycloplegic and Mydriatics Use in, 40
Ethambutol, 332, 338
Ethylenediamine Tetra Acetate, see EDTA
Etidocaine HCl, 34
Excipient Glossary, 367
Extemporaneous Preparations, 323
  Isotinicity of, 325
  Stability of, 324
  Sterility of, 324
  Vehicles of, 325
Extraocular Muscles, Drugs Affecting, 335
Extraocular Irrigating Solutions, 289, 292
Eye Irrigating Solution, 293
Eye•Scrub, 294
Eye Stream, 293
Eye Wash, 293
Eyesine, 66

Famciclovir, 341
Famvir, 341
Fetal Liver Kinase-1 Receptor/Tyrosin Kinase Antagonist, 358
Fexofenadine, 343
Fibroblast Growth Factor, 358
FIK-1 RTK Antagonist, 358
FK-366, 361
Flarex, 92
Flex-Care Rinising, Disinfectina dn Storage Especially for Sensitive Eyes, 310, 315
Floxin, 340
Flucinolone, 354
Fluconazole, 342
Flucytosine, 342
Fluimucil, 359
Fluor-Op, 92
Fluoracaine, 39
Fluorescein Sodium, 13, 16, 348, 349
Fluorescite, 18, 348, 349
Fluoresoft, 19
Fluorets, 18
Fluorexon, 14, 18
Fluorometholone, 91
Fluorosilicone/Acrylate F-S/A, 282
Flurbiprofen Sodium, 97
Fluress, 38
FML, 92
FML Forte, 92
FML S.O.P., 92
FML-S Suspension, 133
Focus Lens Drops, 320
Fomivirsen, 358
Fomivirsen Sodium, 158
Foscarnet, 330, 341
Foscarnet Sodium/ddl, 358
Foscarnet Sodium (Phosphonoformic Acid), 162
  Plasma Concentrations (Table), 163
  Dosing Guide Based on CCr (Table), 171
Foscavir, 171, 341, 358

424 OPHTHALMIC DRUG FACTS

Freedox IV Solution, 360
Frequency and Composition of Visits for Conjunctivitis, 363
Frequency and Composition of Visits for Open Angle Glaucoma, 364
Ful-Glo, 18

Galardin MMPI, 358
Ganciclovir, 330, 341
  Adverse Reactions (Table), 149
  Elevated Serum Creatine with IV (Table), 150
  (DHPG) Capsules and Powder for Injection, 142
  Drug Interactions (Table), 148
  Intravitreal Implant, 155
  IV Dosing in Renal Impairment (Table), 153
  IV Pharmacokinetics in Patients with Renal Impairment (Table), 143
  Oral Dosing in Renal Impairment (Table), 153
  Oral Pharmacokinetics in Patients with Renal Impairment (Table), 143
  Patients with Positive CMV Cultures Following IV (Table), 144
  Patients with Positive CMV Cultures Following Oral (Table), 144
Gangliosides as Sodium Salts, 354
Gantrisin, 130, 332
Garamycin, 121
Gelatin Film, Adsorbable, 264, 273
Gelfilm, 274
Gelfilm Ophthalmic, 121, 274
GEM-132, 358
Gene Therapy, Retinal Detachment, 358
Geneye, 66
Genoptic, 121
Genoptic S.O.P., 121
Gentak, 121
Gentamicin, 329, 340
Gentamicin Ophthalmic, 121
Gentamicin Sulfate, 121
GenTeal, 103, 105
Giant Papillary Conjunctivitis, 58
Glaucoma,
  Agents for, 179
  Agents for (Table), 180
Glaucon, 185
GlaucTabs, 227
Glucose-40, 254
Glucose, Topical, 254, 256
Glutamate Ion Channel Blockers, Glaucoma, 358
Glycerin 50%-75%, 346
Glycerin Topical, 254, 256
Glycerol, 256
GM6001, 358
Gold Salts, 332, 333
Gold Sodium Thiomalate, 332
Gonak, 273
Gonioscopic, 273
Goniosol, 273
Granulocytopenia/Thrombocytopenia with IV Ganciclovir (Table), 150

Hard Contact Lenses, 299
Healon, 271
Healon GV, 271
Heroine, 332
Herrick Lacrimal Plug, 108
HMS, 92
Homatropine HBr, 52
Hormone Growth Hormone (hGH) Receptor Antagonist, 358
HsS, 358
HU-211, 357
Human Immunodeficiency Virus (HIV), 305
Humorsol, 218
Hyaluronidase, 358
Hydrochlorothiazide, 332
HydroDIURIL, 332
Hydrogel (Soft) Contact Lenses, 300, 314
Hydrogel Lens Classification (Table), 300
Hydroxychloroquine, 332, 336
Hydroxyethylcellulose, 273
Hydroxypropyl Methylcellulose, 272
Hylan A, 358
Hylashield, 358
Hylasol, 358
Hyoscine HBr, 52
Hypericin (Aromatic Polycyclic Dione), 358
Hyperosmotic Agents, 181, 251, (Table), 346
Hypertonic solutions, 325
HypoTears, 103, 105
HypoTears PF, 103
Hypotonic Solutions, 325

I-PREX, 356
Ibuprofen, 342, 344
Icaps Plus, 297, 346
Icaps Time Release, 297
Ilotycin, 120
Imidazole Derivatives, 59
Immunosuppressive Agents (Table), 344
Imuran, 345
Inactive Ingredients, 1
Indocyanine Green, 14, 20
Indocin, 332
Indomethacin, 332, 333, 337, 344
Inflamase Forte, 93
Inflamase Mild, 92
Injectable Local Anesthetic Drug Interactions (Table), 31
Injectable Local Anesthetic Pharmacokinetics (Table), 28
INS 358, 365
Insulin-Like Growth Factor (IGF)/BP3 Complex, 359
Intracameral Administration, 9
Intraocular Administration, 326
Intraocular Agents, 330
Intraocular Irrigating Solutions, 263, 267
Intraocular Pressure, Drugs Affecting, 328
Intravitreal Administration, 10
Investigational New Drugs, 355, 356
Iocare Balanced Salt, 268
Ioperamide/Peripheral Mu Agonist Opioid, 359

Iopidine, 191
Irrigating Solutions,
  Extraocular, 292
  Intraocular, 263, 267
ISIS-2922, 358
ISIS-13312, 359
Ismotic, 258, 346
Isopropyl Unoprostone, 359
Isopto Atropine, 51
Isopto Carbachol, 209
Isopto Carpine, 210, 211
Isopto Cetapred Suspension, 133
Isopto Homatropine, 52
Isopto Hyoscine, 53
Isopto Plain, 103
Isopto Tears, 103
Isosorbide 45%, 257, 346
Isotretinoin, 332, 334, 335, 337
ISV-205, 357
ISV-900, 359
Itraconazole, 342

Just Tears, 103
Just Tears Lubricant Drops, 320

Keratase, 358
Keratitis, 304
Keratitis,
  Steps to Minimize Risks Associated with Contact Lens Wear (Table), 304
Ketoconazole, 342
Ketorolac, 342
Ketorolac Tromethamine, 97, 343
Ketotifen Fumarate, 69

Lacri-Lube NP, 105
Lacri-Lube S.O.P., 105
Lacrisert, 107
Lanoxin, 332
Latanoprost, 242
LC-65 Daily Contact Lens Cleaner, 312, 318
Lens and Cornea, Drugs Affecting, 331
Lens Drops, 314, 320
Lens Plus Daily Cleaner, 318
Lens Plus Rewetting Drops, 320
Lens Plus Sterile Solution, 317
Leukeran, 345
Levobetaxolol, 202
Levobunolol HCl, 202, 359
Levocabastine, 70, 354
Levofloxacin, 123
LEX001, 356
Lexipafant (BB-882), 359
LGD-1550, 359
Librium, 331
Lid Scrub-Cotton Tipped Applicator, 6
Lid Scrub-Gauze, 6
Lid Scrubs, 289
Lid Wipes-SPF, 294
Lidocaine HCl and Lidocaine Combinations, 33
Lidocaine, w/Epinephrine, 28
Lids and Conjunctiva, Drugs Affecting, 334
Liquid Perfluorocarbons, 349
Liquifilm Tears, 103
Lisinopril, 359
Lissamine Green, 15, 22
Livostin, 71

INDEX

Local Anesthetic Combinations, Miscellaneous, 38
Local Anesthetics, 25, 329
Classification (Table), 25
Injectable, 28
Injectable, Drug Interactions (Table), 31
Injectable, Pharmacokinetics (Table), 28
Ophthalmic Uses (Table), 27, 28, 35
Topical, 34
Lodoxamide, 348
Anti-Allergy and Deconges-tants, 75
Lotemax, 91, 359
Loteprednol Etabonate, 91
Loteprednol Etabonate/Tobra-mycin, 359
Lubricant/Cleaning for Artifical Eyes, 109
Lumigan, 239

Mannitol, 259, 261, 346
Manufacturer's Index, 371
Marinol, 357
Mast Cell Stabilizers, Antihista-mines, and NSAIDs, 59
Maxidex, 91
Maxitrol, 126
Medications, 2
Medrysone, 92
Mellaril, 332
Memantine, 359
Mepivacaine HCl, 33
Methazolamide, 227, 345
Methotrexate, 344
Methoxsalen, 332
Methylcellulose, 2, 309, 325
Methylphenidate, 332
Methylprednisone, 344
Metimyd, 134
Metimyd Suspension, 133
Metipranolol HCl, 202
Minerals and Vitamins, 290, 296
Minocin, 332
Minocycline, 332, 334
Miochol-E, 208, 275
Miosis, Drugs Causing, 335
Miostat, 212, 276
Miotics, Direct-Acting, 181, 204, 274
Miosis Induction of (Table), 204
MiraFlow Extra-Strength Daily Cleaner, 318
MiraSept, 317
Miscellaneous Local Anesthetic Combinations, 38
Mitomycin, 329
Moisture Eyes, 103
Moisture Eyes PM, 105
Moisture Eyes Preservative Free, 103
Monoclonal Antibody (MAb), Anti-VEGF, 359
Morphine, 332
Motexafin Lutetium, 359
Mucomyst, 348
Murine Tears, 103
Murine Tears Plus, 66
Muro 128, 256
Murocel, 103
Murocoll-2, 55

Myambutol, 332
Mydfrin 2.5, 47
Mydriacyl, 54
Mydriasis, Drugs Causing, 335
Mydriatic Combinations, 54
Mydriatics, 39
Mydriatics and Cycloplegics, 39
Myopia, Drugs Causing, 335

N-acetylcysteine (NAC), 359
Nafazair, 65
Nafcillin, 341
Naphazoline HCl, 64
Naphcon, 64
Naphcon-A Solution, 84
Naphcon Forte, 65
Naproxen, 344
Narcotic Analgesics (Table), 342
Nasolacrimal Occlusion, 4
Natacyn, 135
Natamycin, 135
Nedocromil Sodium, 76, 359
Neo-Dexameth, 126
Neo-Synephrine, 47
Neo-Synephrine Viscous, 47
NeoDecadron Solution, 126
Neomycin/Polymyxin B Sulfate/Dexamethasone, 127
Neomycin/Polymyxin B Sulfate/Dexamethasone Suspension, 126
Neomycin/Polymyxin B Sulfate/Hydrocortisone, 125
Neomycin Sulfate Dexametha-sone Sodium Phosphate Solu-tion, 126
Neomysin Sulfate-Polymyxin B Sulfate Gramicidin Solution, 124
Neoral, 344
Neosporin Ophthalmic, 124
Neptazane, 227
Neurotrophic Factors, 359
New Drug Development, 355
Nolvadex, 332
Non-Narcotic Analgesics (Table), 342
Non-Sedating Antihistamines (Table), 343
Nonsteroidal Anti-Inflammatory Agents (NSAIDS),
Anti-Inflammatory Agents, 86, 93
(Table), 341
Nonsteroidal Anti-Inflammatory Ophthalmic Agents (Table), 93
Nonsurgical Adjuncts, 289
Norfloxacin, 122
NRT Technology, Degenerative Retinal Disease, 359
NSAIDs, Mast Cell Stabilizers, and Antihistamines, 59
Nu-Tears II, 103

OcuClear, 66
OcuCoat, 103
OcuCoat PF, 103
Ocufen, 97
Ocuflox, 123
Ocular Hypotensive Agents, 345
Ocular Lubricants (Ointments and Gels), 99, 104
Ocular Lubricants and Artificial Tear Solutions, 99
OcuNex, 359
Ocupress, 201

Ocusert Pilo-20, 213
Ocusert Pilo-40, 213
OCuSOFT, 294
OCuSOFT VMS, 297
Ocusulf-10, 130
Ocuvite, 297, 346
Ocuvite Extra, 297
Off-Labeled Drugs with Ophthal-mic Uses, 347
Ofloxacin, 340
Anti-Infective Agents, 123
Ointments, 5,
Ointments and Gels, 104
Ocular Lubricants, 99
Ointments, Recommended Proce-dures for Administration (Table), 4
Oligonucleotide Antisense Com-pounds, 359
Olopatadine HCl, 80
One-A-Day Extras Antioxident, 297
Opcon-A Solution, 84
Ophthalgan, 255
Ophthalmic Decongestant/Antihis-tamine Combinations, 83
Ophthalmic Drug Therapy, Topi-cal, General Considerations (Table), 8
Ophthalmic Dyes, 13
Ophthalmic Sympathomimetic Drug Interactions (Table), 62
Ophthalmic Uses of Local Anes-thetics (Table), 26, 27, 28, 35
Ophthalmic Vasoconstrictors (Table), 61
Ophthetic, 37
Opiates, 332
Opti-Clean II Daily Cleaner Espe-cially for Sensitive Eyes, 312, 318
Opti-Free Daily Cleaner, 318
Opti-Free Express MultiPurpose Disinfecting, 315
Opti-Free Rewetting Drops, 320
Opti-Free Rinsing, Disinfecting and Storage, 315
Opti-Free Supra Clens Daily Pro-tein Removal, 313, 318, 319
Opti-One Multi-Purpose, 315
Opti-One Rewetting Drops, 320
Opti-Soak Daily Cleaner Especially for Sensitive Eyes, 311, 312
Opti-Tears Soothing Drops, 314, 320
Opti-Zyme Enzymatic Cleaner Especially for Sensitive Eyes, 313, 319
Optic Nerve, Drugs Affecting, 337
Opticrom, 74, 354
Optigene, 294
Optigene 3, 66
Optimum C/D/S, 311, 314
Optimum Extra Strength Cleaner, 311
OptiPranolol, 203
Optivar, 83
Optrin, 359
Oral Administration, 8, 238
Orphan and Investigational Drugs, 353
Orphan Drug Development, Gov-ernment Incentives (Table), 353

OPHTHALMIC DRUG FACTS

Orphan Drug Information Sources (Table), 355
Orphan Drugs (Table), 354
Osmitrol, 261, 346
Osmoglyn, 257, 346
Osmotic Diuretic Pharmacokinetics (Table), 252
Oxi-Freeda, 297
Oxsoralen, 332
Oxymetazoline HCl, 66

P₁E₁, 221P₂E₁, 221P₄E₁, 221P₆E₁, 221
Packaging Standards, 2
Palmitate-A, 296
Palmitate-A 5000, 296
PAPB, 307
Parenteral Administration, 8
Patanol, 81
Pegvisomant, 360
Pemirolast Potassium, 78
Penicillin G, 341
Periocular Administration, 326
Periocular Agents, 329
Periocular/Peribulbar Administration, 9
pH/Buffering, of Extemporaneous Preparations, 324
Pharmacologic Management of Antihistamines, Mast Cell Stabilizers, and NSAIDs, 59
Phenobarbital, 332
Phenylephrine HCl,
 Cycloplegics and Mydriatics, 39
 Decongestants and Anti-Allergy Agents, 58, 64
 Monograph, 43
 Pharmacology Table, 43
 Product Table, 47
Phenytoin, 332
PHMB, 329
Phospholipids, 360
Phospholine Iodide, 220
Phosphonoformic Acid, see Foscarnet Sodium
Photopoint, 360
Photosensitizing Drugs, 333
Physostigmine, 218
Physostigmine Sulfate, 218
Pilagel, 318
PilaSite, 360
Piligan, 211
Pilocar, 210, 211
Pilocarpine, 360
Pilocarpine and Epinephrine, 220
Pilocarpine HCl, 209, 210, 211
Pilocarpine Nitrate, 211
Pilocarpine Ocular Therapeutic System, 212
Pilopto-Carpine, 211
Pilostat, 211
Piroxicam, 360
Plaquenil Sulfate, 332
Pliagel, 327
PMMA, 299
Polocaine, 33
Polocaine MPF, 33
Poloxamer 407, 309
Poly-Pred Suspension, 125
Polyaminopropyl Biguanide, 307
Polydimethylsiloxane (Silicone Oil), 264, 276
Polyhexamethylene Biguanide, 348

Polymyxin B Sulfate, 118
Polymyxin B Sulfate Sterile, 118
Polyquad, 308
Polysporin Ointment, 124
Polytrim Solution, 124
Polyvinyl Alcohol (PVA), 309
Povidone Iodine, 263, 268, 360
Pred-G S.O.P., 127
Pred-G Suspension, 126
Pred Forte, 92
Pred Mild, 92
Prefrin Liquifilm, 64
Prednisolone, 92
Prednisolone Acetate, 92
Prednisolone Sodium Phosphate, 93
Prednisone, 332, 344
Preservative Free Saline Solutions, Soft Lenses, 317
Preservatives, 307
Preserved Saline Solutions, Soft Lenses, 317
Prinomastat Matrix Metalloproteinase Inhibitor, 360
Procaterol, 360
Processed Pericardium, 264
Profenal, 98, 348, 349
ProFree/GP Weekly Enzymatic Cleaner, 313
Proparacaine HCl, 37, 329, 360
Propine, 187
ProSite, 360
Prostaglandins, 181, 234
Protovir, 360
ProVisc, 271
Psoralens, 332
Punctal Plugs, 100, 107
Puralube, 105
Puralube Tears, 103
Pure Eyes, 316, 317
Purilens UV Disinfection System, 315
Purlytin, 360
Pyridoxine (B₆), 346
Pyrimethamine, 341

Quick CARE, 315
Quinacrine, 332
Quinamm, 332
Quinine, 332, 336
Quixin, 123

Rare Diseases and Orphan Treatment, Information Sources, 355
Ready-Set Punctum Plugs, 108
Recommended Procedures for Administration of Ointments (Table), 4
Recommended Procedures for Administration of Solutions and Suspensions (Table), 3
Refresh, 103
Refresh Plus, 103
Refresh PM, 105
Refresh Tears, 103
Relief, 64
ReNu 1 Step Enzymatic Cleaner, 319
ReNu Effervescent Enzymatic Cleaner, 319
ReNu Lubricating & Rewetting Drops, 320
ReNu MultiPlus Lubricating & Rewetting Drops, 321

ReNu MultiPlus Multi-Purpose, 320
Renu Multi-Purpose, 315
ReNu Saline, 317
Rescula, 242, 359
Resolve/GP Daily Cleaner, 312
Restasis, 357
Retina, Drugs Affecting, 336
Retinal Pigment Epithelial Cells, 360
Retinamide, 360
Rēv-Eyes, 292
Rewetting Solutions,
 RGP Lenses, 313
 Soft Lenses, 320
Ridaura, 332
Rigid Gas Permeable Lenses (RGP), 299, 310
Rimexolone, 93
Ritalin, 332
RMP-7, 360
Rose Bengal, 14, 22
Rosets, 22
Rostaporfin (SnET2) Tin Ethyl Etiopurpurin, 360

Sabril, 332
Salicylates, 332
Saline, 317
Schirmer Tear Test, 295
Scopolamine HBr, 332
 Cycloplegic Mydriatics, 52
Seasonal Allergic Conjunctivitis, 57
Sedating Antihistamines (Table), 343
Sensitive Eyes Daily Cleaner, 318
Sensitive Eyes Drops, 321
Sensitive Eyes Enzymatic Cleaner, 319
Sensitive Eyes Plus, 317
Sensitive Eyes Preservative Free Sterile Saline, 317
Sensitive Eyes Saline, 317
Sensitive Eyes Saline/Cleaning, 318
Sensorcaine MPF, 34
Sevirumab, 360
Sildenafil, 332, 337
Silicone Oil, see Polydimethylsiloxane
Sno-Strips, 295
Sodium Borate, 308
Sodium Chloride, Hypertonic, 255
Sodium Fluorescein 16
Sodium Hyaluronate, 269, 271, 348
Sodium Sulamyd, 130, 131, 360
Soft Lenses, 300, 314
Softplug, 109
SofWwear Saline for Sensitive Eyes, 317
Solid Devices,
 Artifical Tear Solutions and Ocular Lubricants, 100
SOLO-Care Multi-Purpose, 315
Solution Preparation (Table), 119
Solutions and Suspensions – Drops, 3
Solutions and Suspensions, Recommended Procedures for Administration (Table), 3
Solutions, Artificial Tear 2, 99, 102
SomatoKine, 359

INDEX

Sorbic Acid, 308
Sporanox, 342
Sterile Daily Cleaner, 318
Sterile Preserved Saline, 317
Sterile Sereine Wetting Solution, 314
Steroid and Antibiotic Ointments, 127
Steroid and Antibiotic Solutions and Suspensions, 125
Steroid and Sulfonamide Combinations, Ointments, 134
Steroid and Sulfonamide Combinations, Suspensions and Solutions, 131
Stye, 105
Sulf-10, 130
Sulfacetamide, 360
Sulfacetamide Sodium, 130, 131
Sulfacetamide Sodium & Prednisolone Sodium Phosphate, 133
Sulfadiazine, 341
Sulfisoxazole, 332
Sulfisoxazole Diolamine, 130
Sulfonamide and Steroid Combinations, Ointments, 134
Sulfonamide and Steroid Combinations, Suspensions and Solutions, 131
Sulfonamide/Decongestant Combination, 131
Sulfonamides, 332
    Anti-Infective Agents, 128
Sulster, 130
Sumycin, 332
Suprax, 340
Suprofen, 98, 348
Surfactant Cleaning Solutions, RGP Lenses, 312
    Soft Lenses, 318
Surgical Adjuncts, 263
Surgical Enzymes, 265
Suspensions and Solutions, Recommended Procedures for Administration (Table), 3
Systemic Agents, 251
Systemic Drugs Affecting the Eye (Table), 331
Systemic Medications Used for Ocular Conditions, 339

Talc, 336
Tamoxifen, 332, 337
Tazarotene, 360
Tazorac, 360
Tear Test Strips, 294
Teargen, 103
Teargen II, 104
Tearisol, 104
Tears Naturale, 104, 108, 109
Tears Naturale II, 104
Tears Naturale Free, 104
Tears Naturale P.M., 105
Tears Plus, 104
Tears Renewed, 104, 105
TearSaver, 108, 109
Tear Secretion, Aqueous, Drugs that Decrease, 334
Temporary Punctual/Canalicular Collagen Implant, 108, 109
Tenormin, 332

Terak Ointment, 124
Terramycin w/Polymyxin B Ointment, 124
Tetracaine HCl, 37
Tetracycline, 332, 340
Tetracyclines, 334
Tetrahydrozoline HCl, 65, 66
Tetrasine, 66
Tetrasine Extra, 66
Thalidomide, 360
Thera Tears, 104
Thimerosal, 307
Thioridazine, 332, 336
Tilavist, 359
Timolol Maleate, 203, 204
Timolol Maleate/Dorzolamide HCl, 246
    Drug Interactions (Table), 248
Timoptic, 203, 204
Timoptic XE, 204
Tin Ethyl Etiopurpurin, 360
Tirilazad Mesylate, 360
Tissue Plasminogen Activator (tPA), 261, 330
TobraDex Suspension, 126
Tobramycin, 121, 126, 329
Tobrex, 122
Topical Administration, 1
Topical Agents, 251, 329
Topical Corticosteroids, 88
Topical Local Anesthetics, 34
Topical Ophthalmic Antibiotic Preparations (Table), 112
Topical Ophthalmic Drug Packaging Standards (Table), 2
Topical Ophthalmic Drug Therapy, General Considerations (Table), 8
Topical Preparations, 325
Toradol, 342
Tramadol, 342
Transforming Growth Factor-Beta 2, 354
Trentinoin, 354
Tavoprost, 234
Travatan, 237
Triamcinolone Acetonide, 329
Trifluorothymidine, 139
Trifluridine, 139
Trimethoprim Sulfate and Polymyxin B Sulfate Ophthalmic Solution, 124
Triple Antibiotic Ophthalmic Ointment, 124
Tropicacyl, 54
Tropicamide, 54
Trovert, 358
Trusopt, 231
Tryptase Inhibitor, 361
Tyloxapol, 109

Ultra Tears, 104
UltraCare, 316
Ultram, 342
Ultrazyme Enzymatic Cleaner, 319
Unisol 4, 317
Unisol Plus, 317
Unizyme Enzymatic Cleaner, 319
Unlabeled Uses, Ophthalmics (Table), 348
Unoprostone Isopropyl, 240
Uveitis, Cycloplegics and Mydriatics Use in, 41

Valacyclovir, 341
Valganciclovir, 361
Valtrex, 341
Vancomycin, 329, 330
Vascular Endothelial Growth Factor, 361
Vasocine, 134
VasoClear, 65, 296
VasoClear A, 65, 135
Vasocon-A Solution, 84
Vasocon Regular, 65
Vasoconstrictors, Ophthalmic (Table), 61
Vasosulf, 131
Verapamil HCl, 361
Vernal Conjuctivitis, 57
Verteporfin, 265, 284
Vexol, 93
Viagra, 332
Vidarabine, 137
Vigabatrin, 332, 337
VIMRxyn, 358
Vira-A, 139
Virologic Response to IV Ganciclovir Treatment (Table), 144
Viroptic, 141
Viscoat, 272, 348
Viscoelastic Agents, 263, 351
Visine, 66
Visine A.C., 66, 135, 296
Visine Advanced Relief, 66
Visine L.R., 66
Visine Tears, 104
Vistide, 177, 356
Visudyne, 287
Vitamin A, 346
Vitamin A Palmitate, 296
Vitamin B_{12}, 271, 346
Vitamins and Minerals, 290, 296, 346
Vitrase, 358, 361
Vitrasert, 158
Vitravene, 162
Viva-Drops, 104
Vizoral, 342
Voltaren, 97, 348, 349

Wet-N-Soak, 311
Wet-N-Soak Plus, 311
Wetting Agents, 309
Wetting & Soaking Solution, 311

Xalatan, 246
XMP-200, 361
Xylocaine, 33
Xylocaine MPF, 33

Zaditor, 70
Zenapax, 357
Zenarestat, 361
Zestril Diabetes, 359
Zinc Sulfate Solution, 295
    Anti-Infective Agents, 135
Zincfrin Solution, 64, 135, 296
Zithromax, 340
Zone-Quick, 295
Zopolrestat, 361
Zovirax, 348
Zyrtec, 343